NEUROSCIENCE RESEARCH PROGRESS

# EPIDEMIOLOGY OF SPINAL CORD INJURIES

# NEUROSCIENCE RESEARCH PROGRESS

Additional books in this series can be found on Nova's website
under the Series tab.

Additional e-books in this series can be found on Nova's website
under the e-book tab.

# NEUROLOGY – LABORATORY AND CLINICAL RESEARCH DEVELOPMENTS

Additional books in this series can be found on Nova's website
under the Series tab.

Additional e-books in this series can be found on Nova's website
under the e-book tab.

NEUROSCIENCE RESEARCH PROGRESS

# EPIDEMIOLOGY OF SPINAL CORD INJURIES

## VAFA RAHIMI-MOVAGHAR
## SEYED BEHZAD JAZAYERI
### AND
## ALEXANDER R. VACCARO
### EDITORS

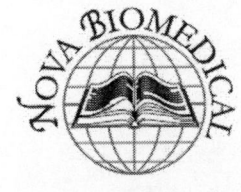

Nova Science Publishers, Inc.

New York

**Library of Congress Cataloging-in-Publication Data**

Library of Congress Control Number: 2011946295
ISBN: 978-1-61942-894-2

*Published by Nova Science Publishers, Inc.† New York*

# CONTENTS

# PREFACE

Spinal cord injury (SCI) is a devastating condition with enormous financial, social and personal costs. SCI is the most expensive traumatic condition in the United States. Overall, most frequent etiologies of injury are motor vehicle crashes and falls, followed by violence, sports-related injuries, and work-related accidents. Research on SCI prevention, regeneration and long term care has progressed steadily over the past decade making an introductory foray into the epidemiology of SCI and important undertaking. This book is designed as a general reference book reviewing the epidemiology of SCI throughout the world with potential insight to cause and effect as well as the difficulties and boundaries to minimize this unfortunate occurrence.

Chapter 1 - The estimated incidence of spinal cord injury (SCI) in the United States is about 40 cases per million population, or approximately 12,000 new cases per year (excluding those patients who die at the scene of the accident).

Chapter 2 - The pathogenesis of adult nontraumatic (NT) spinal cord injury (SCI) includes such etiologies as vertebral spondylosis (spinal stenosis), neoplastic and infectious-related injury, vascular ischemia, and multiple sclerosis. Other etiologies include inflammatory disease, transverse myelitis, motor neuron disease, radiation myelopathy, syringomyelia, paraneoplastic syndrome, and vitamin B12 deficiency. The clinical presentation and SCI-related medical complications in individuals with nontraumatic SCI warrant an interdisciplinary approach to maximize their medical, functional and psychosocial outcomes. The demographic and clinical comparisons between nontraumatic and traumatic SCI reveal several differences that may be of importance when considering these outcomes. Though they make up a significant percentage of patients with SCI admitted for rehabilitation, their outcomes have not been as thoroughly studied as in those with traumatic etiology. A better understanding of these issues will assist in the medical management, rehabilitation and long-term follow up for individuals with nontraumatic SCI.

Chapter 3 - This chapter provides an overview of the epidemiology of spinal cord injuries (SCIs) in the general United States (U.S.) population, followed by an in-depth discussion of the prevalence, causes, and complications of SCIs in children and adolescents. The annual incidence of SCIs in the U.S. is approximately 40 cases per million population or approximately 12,000 new cases each year. Approximately 20% of traumatic SCIs occur in individuals younger than 21 years of age, with 3% to 5% of injuries occurring in those younger than 15.Compared to adult-onset SCI, individuals with pediatric-onset SCI are unique in several ways. Because of their younger age at injury and longer lifespan, they will be more susceptible to long-term complications such as cardiovascular disease, and overuse syndromes. The pediatric-onset SCI population also has developmental needs and experiences relatively unique complications, such as scoliosis and hip dysplasia, which will impact them throughout their life-span. Moreover, demographic and injury related factors vary as a function of age at injury, including pediatric-specific etiologies and presentations, such as lap-belt injuries, neonatal SCI, transverse myelitis, and SCI associated with Down syndrome, juvenile idiopathic arthritis and skeletal dysplasias as well as SCI without radiographic abnormality.

Chapter 4 - An understanding of region specific spinal cord injury(SCI) epidemiology is important for the targeting of primary preventive efforts and to understand deficiencies in current clinical care practices. The epidemiology of traumatic SCI in Canada appears similar to data published from other developed countries throughout the world such as the United States and the United Kingdom. Current estimates of SCI incidence in Canada range from approximately 23 to 52 per million per year with prevalence estimated at 1290 per million. As the Canadian population continues to age, we anticipate a greater number of elderly patients presenting to acute care centers predominately with cervical SCI. Throughout this chapter we will explore in detail the available Canadian epidemiologic data for traumatic SCI while making comparisons to data from countries around the world.

Chapter 5 - Spinal cord injury (SCI) occurrence is more common in recent years due to increasing urban violence. The sequelae of spinal cord injury leads to a health problem as many cases are irreparable.

Chapter 6 - In 2010, Brazil had almost 200 million inhabitants. It is a large country that has a population with a varied economic and development distribution. The population´s age has changed in recent years with a smaller proportion of people younger than 25 years-old and a greater proportion of older people then 65 years old (7,4%).

Chapter 7 - Although fall-induced injuries among older adults are said to be a major public health concern in modern societies with aging populations, reliable epidemiologic information on their secular trends is limited.

We assessed the secular trend in the number and incidence (per 100 000 persons) of fall-induced severe cervical spine injuries (fracture, cord injury, or both) of older adults in Finland, an EU-country with a well-defined white population of 5.3 million, by taking into account all persons 60 years of age or older who were admitted to Finnish hospitals for primary treatment of such injuries in 1970-2009. Similar patients aged 20 through 49 years served as a reference group.

The number and raw incidence of fall-induced cervical spine injury among Finns 60 years of age or older rose considerably between the years 1970 and 2009, from 37 (number) and 5.7 (incidence) in 1970 to 280 and 21.7 in 2009. The relative increases were 657% and 280%, respectively. Throughout the study period, the age-adjusted incidence of injury was higher in men than women and showed a clear increase in both sexes in 1970-2009: from 9.7 to 30.0 in men, and from 3.0 to 13.2 in women. A similar finding was observed in the age-specific incidences of the study group. In the reference group, the annual number and incidence of injury decreased somewhat over time. Assuming that the observed increase in the age-adjusted or age-specific injury incidence continues in the 60-year-old or older Finns and the size of this population increases as predicted, the annual number of fall-induced cervical spine injuries in this population will be almost two-times higher in the year 2030 than it was in 2009.

In Finnish persons aged 60 years or older, the number of fall-induced severe cervical spine injuries seems to show an alarming rise with a rate that cannot be explained merely by demographic changes. The finding underscores an increasing influence of falls and subsequent injuries on health and well-being of our older adults, and therefore, wide-scale fall-prevention measures should be urgently adopted to control this development.

Chapter 8 - The mean annual incidence of traumatic spinal cord injuries (TSCI) increased from 5.9 per million inhabitants in the period 1952–1961 to 21.2 per million inhabitants in the period 1992–2001 based on hospital data from two counties in western Norway. On January 1st, 2002, the total prevalence of TSCI was 365 per million inhabitants.

The mean age at time of injury was 42.9 years, and the male: female ratio was 4.7:1. The most frequent cause of injury was falls (45.5 %), followed by traffic accidents (34.2 %). The frequency of TSCI due to traffic accidents has increased especially among men less than 30 years of age. The frequency of TSCI due to falls and the frequency of incomplete cervical lesions have increased especially among men over the age of 60 at the time of injury.

In our study the level of injury was cervical in 52.4%, thoracic in 29.5% and lumbar/sacral in 18.2 %. The lesion was clinically incomplete in 58.6 % and complete in 41.4%.

Among patients with TSCI, 3.9 % were age 0–14 years at the time of injury, and 13.1 % were 15–19 years at time of injury. The average age-adjusted incidence was 2.4 per million children, and 25.1 per million adolescences. The age-adjusted incidence of TSCI among adolescents has increased, while the age-adjusted incidence among children has remained low. TSCI was highly associated with car and pedestrian accidents among children. Among adolescents, TSCI was most often associated with car and motorcycle accidents.

Among patients with TSCI, 46.7 % had a clinical concomitant traumatic brain injury (TBI). Clinical TBI was classified as mild in 30.1 %, moderate in 11.0 % and severe in 5.7 %. Alcohol was the strongest risk factor for clinical TBI (OR = 3.69) followed by completeness of TSCI (OR = 2.18).

There is an increasing number of elderly patients sustaining TSCI in Norway. In a study of TSCI in patients older than 60, fall from height was the most common mode of injury (77%). The cervical spine was the most common region of the spine injured (71%). Cervical spinal stenosis increases the risk of TSCI caused by minor trauma. Patients older than 60 years of age at the time of injury benefitted significantly from rehabilitation.

TSCI patients have a 1.85 increase in mortality rate relative to the Norwegian population, with the first ten years after injury being associated with the highest. Complete injury is associated with reduced survival regardless of the level of injury (4.23 versus 1.25). Women have reduced survival compared to men (2.88 versus 1.72). Median survival time was 7.4 years. The cause specific standardized mortality ratio for respiratory disease was 1.96, and for suicide including 3.70 for men and 37.59 for women.

Chapter 9 - The country of Sweden has an unusually long tradition of population registration, dating back to 1749 when a specific governmental institution, *"Tabellverket"* was founded for this specific purpose. Since then, several nationwide population-based disease or effect registers have been developed. The drop-out rates are typically very low, usually under 5%. The registers are frequently utilized for research, evaluation, planning and other purposes by a variety of users.

Furthermore, there is a unique system of individual so-called personal registration numbers (PRN) for the identification of every Swedish resident.

This, together with availability of modern computer-based techniques, provides facilities for easy linkage of exposure and outcome data down to the level of individual patients.

Population-based administrative registers are practical and cost-effective when utilized for epidemiological purposes. However, there are caveats when using such databases for scientific research. Since the primary purpose of many such registers is administrative rather than scientific, this may reflect negatively on data quality.

Chapter 10 - Traumatic spinal cord injury (SCI) often results in profound and long-term disability, which is life changing for the injured individual and his or her family. These injuries also have tremendous social costs associated with expensive health care treatment, rehabilitation, and lost productivity. The estimated annual incidence of traumatic SCI is 12.7 per million inhabitants in Turkey. The mortality rate of SCI is estimated to be 12%-15% in Turkey. SCI patients became either tetraplegic (32.18%) and paraplegic (67.82%) after injury. The most common level of injury was C5 among tetraplegics, T12 and L1 for paraplegics. The most prevalent associated injury was head trauma followed by extremity fractures. Regarding the etiology, traffic accident is the most common cause of spinal cord injury, the second most-common cause is falls from height and the third is gunshot injury. The incidences of gunshot wounds and injuries from falls are higher in Turkey than other countries, which can be explained by special socio-economic and cultural differences. The high incidence of gunshot wounds is the result of the violence experienced mainly in south-eastern of Turkey. Moreover, the higher frequency of falls from height can be associated with the fact that most falls occurred in the summer when it is very hot in this region and people are forced to sleep on the top of their houses, which do not have barriers along the roof perimeter. Traumatic SCI is more frequent among males than females and among those between the ages of 15 and 39 years. Considering that traffic accidents, falls from height and gunshot wounds are the leading cause of traumatic SCI, it can be concluded that the prevention measures should be focused mainly on these types of traumas in order to reduce the frequency of SCI in Turkey.

Chapter 11 - The incidence of SCI is widely variable, from 9 to 53 cases per million population inhabitants per year in the international literature. The life expectancy of patients with spinal cord injury (SCI) has been improved over the years through enhancements in emergency care, acute medical and surgical stabilization and rehabilitation. In the past, the main focus of researchers has been the prevention and treatment of complications such as urinary tract infection and skin break down. However recently, the focus of research has been expanded to include methods of mobility restoration and optimization of an affected individual's quality of life. This report will attempt to summarize the available data on SCI care in certain large medical systems in Europe.

Chapter 12 - In India, approximately 1.5 million people live with deficits caused by spinal cord injury. Every year, 10,000 new cases are added to this group. The majority of SCIs occur in males in the 16-30 age group. However, this is only an estimate since there is no reliable national database. There is a decline in the male to female SCI ratio which reflects the changing social norms as females in India become more active and outgoing. There is a gradual trend towards an increased incidence of road traffic accidents indicating a gradual urbanization of society and an increase in the number of vehicles on the roads in India. In earlier studies, pressure sores and urinary tract infections were the most prevalent morbidities in individuals with spinal cord injury. In more recent studies, on the other hand, pain and spasticity were found to be more prevalent. Psychiatric morbidity in individuals with spinal cord injury is given more attention than in the past. There is scant literature on quality of life, re-integration into the community and employment of patients with spinal cord injury in India. Major barriers for community reintegration are architectural and environmental obstacles, poor socio-economic status and associated co-morbidities. Most studies from India are hospital based and there is still no existing national database. Thus, there is a need to have a multi-centric effort in India to establish a reliable national database.

Chapter 13 - The abrupt onset of spinal cord injury (SCI) is tragic and has a profound impact on the individuals and their families. Knowledge of epidemiology of spinal cord injuries in a given country is important not only for planning of resources, but also for adequate treatment and rehabilitation. In the Indian setup, as in most developing countries, very little is known about the exact incidence of SCI as there is no national database. In India, approximately 1.5 million people live with SCI. Approximate 20,000 new cases of SCI are added every year and 60-70% of them are illiterate, poor villagers. Majority of them are males in the age group of 16-30 years, signifying higher incidence in young, active and productive population of the society. There has been substantial decrease in male female ratio from the past which reflects changing face of social norms where females are becoming more active and outgoing in the modern era. In India fall from height rates highest among the etiological factors. There is a gradual trend towards increasing incidence of road traffic accidents indicating gradual urbanization of society and increase in number of vehicles on roads in India. Seasonal distribution of SCI shows a marked increase during summer, signifying increased movement of people in this season. Head injury is the most common associated trauma. The incidence of secondary medical problems in SCI population is high compared to the western world. There is tremendous lack of basic infrastructure and trained medical personnel, especially in rural areas, involved in initial management of patient. Vast majority of people lack basic knowledge about the initial immobilization and transportation of these patients to higher centers and by the time patient reaches a general or institutional hospital; there may be an extensive damage to neurological status, which could have been prevented.

To conclude, in India, management and rehabilitation of patients with SCI lags far behind. Rescue and retrieval systems for these patients are inadequate. There are few specialized centers for the management of such patents. The frequency of decubitus ulcers and UTI is unacceptably high. There is a strong need to identify the risk factors and to take steps to control them by disseminating information to masses, to train paramedical staff in rural areas about initial handling and transportation of patients having spinal cord injuries. A comprehensive multidisciplinary management and rehabilitation approach is the need of the hour to reintegrate patients with SCI to the community.

Chapter 14 - Iran is a Middle Eastern country with a surface area of 1,745,150 square kilometers and a population of 74,169,000; 69% living in urban areas. In 2009, the gross national income per capita of Iran was $10,850 USD. Total expenditure on health per capita was $685 USD and total expenditure on health as percentage of GDP was 5.5%. Life expectancy for male and female was 70 and 75 years.

Trauma is one of the highest burdens of disease in the world and traumatic spinal cord injury (SCI) is a major permanent sequel of trauma. The burden of SCI in Tehran (the capital of Iran) in the year 2008 was 0.7 per 1000 population. By applying this proportion to the country population, the national burden of SCI is estimated as 51,918 DALYs.

Chapter 15 - Epidemiological research on Spinal Cord Injuries (SCI) in Pakistan is limited to hospital based surveys. Further limitations are the absence of a national trauma registry, a small sample size in reported studies, under-representation of certain regions and a lack of focus on non-traumatic spinal cord injuries (NTSCI). The demographics of SCI in Pakistan described in this chapter are based on a diverse research methodology. It comprises of a electronic and manual literature search, interviews with professional colleagues throughout the country who manage SCI patients and the personal experience of the authors working at the largest spinal rehabilitation unit in Pakistan.

Fall from height is the most common etiology for Traumatic SCI (TSCI) followed by road traffic accidents (RTA) and acts of violence. The majority of the patients are young males in their second and third decade. Pre-hospital care and evacuation from the site of trauma is inadequate most of the time due to the lack of widespread implementation of cervical spine precautions following injury. This is likely because of a deficiency of trained emergency personnel throughout the region. Paraplegia is the most frequent presentation and most of the patients have a complete neurological injury at admission. Surgical interventions are carried out in most of the cases of TSCI but rehabilitation referrals are often delayed and multidisciplinary SCI rehabilitation is not widely available. Spinal Tuberculosis is the most common cause of NTSCI followed by transverse myelitis and degenerative spinal disorders. NTSCI is more common in males in their fifth and sixth decades. The complication profile of SCI patients in Pakistan is similar to the reported complications in developed countries with a notably increased incidence. Social support systems and community re-integration programs for SCI patients are not well established and patients face social, financial and mobility barriers while attempting community re-integration.

There is a need to establish a national trauma registry, improve pre-hospital care for SCI, improve the existing neurosurgical services, and develop multidisciplinary SCI rehabilitation and social services for SCI patients in Pakistan.

Chapter 16 - Spinal cord injuries also afflict inhabitants of Oceania islands countries and territories. Selected data from the region is presented. Fiji has a well developed healthcare sector with post-acute rehabilitation of all spinal cord injury (SCI) being provided at the rehabilitation hospital. The incidence of new SCI admitted to the rehabilitation hospital was 18.7 per million population per year comprising 53.6% traumatic and 46.4% non-traumatic causes. The incidence varied according to gender and ethnicity with Fijian males being at the highest (41.85) risk. Among traumatic SCI, 38.7% were due to falls, 25.3% motor vehicle accidents, 20% sports, 8% shallow water dive and 4% each deep sea diving and others, whereas among non-traumatic SCI, 52.3% were due to unknown causes, 32.3% infections, 9.2% neoplasms and 6.2% others. The male/female ratio was 4:1. The 16-30 year age group accounted for 35% of SCI. 31% had tetraplegia and 52.1% had complete lesions. The subset of the sample that experienced traumatic SCI were more likely to be employed, aged between 16-30 years at the time of injury and to sustain complete tetraplegia. Those who experienced incomplete paraplegia were more likely to be unemployed, aged 46-60 years and educated to primary level at the time of injury. There was a high proportion of complete spinal lesion when compared with other studies. The incidence of secondary complications such as pressure sores and UTI were also found to be high when compared with other studies. The data support the view that young Fijian males are most prone to sustaining traumatic spinal cord injury, and that there is a high incidence of secondary preventable complications.

Chapter 17 - In this chapter, the available literature is reviewed on epidemiology of spinal cord injuries (SCI) from countries that have not been covered in other chapters. The epidemiology of SCI in pediatrics based on available evidence is also appraised.

# SECTION I: EPIDEMIOLOGY OF SPINAL CORD INJURIES IN AMERICA

In: Epidemiology of Spinal Cord Injuries
Editors: V. Rahimi-Movaghar, S. B. Jazayeri et al.

ISBN: 978-1-61942-894-2
©2012 Nova Science Publishers, Inc.

*Chapter 1*

# EPIDEMIOLOGY OF SPINAL CORD INJURY IN THE UNITED STATES

### *Todd B. Francis and Edward C. Benzel\**

Neurological Institute, Center for Spine Health, Cleveland Clinic, Ohio, US

## INTRODUCTION

The estimated incidence of spinal cord injury (SCI) in the United States is about 40 cases per million population, or approximately 12,000 new cases per year (excluding those patients who die at the scene of the accident). [SCI facts and figures at a glance, The National SCI Statistical Center].

As of 2010, there are approximately 265,000 people living with SCI in the United States. Regarding the incidence of SCI, there is currently a trend towards older patients. In the 1970s the average age at injury was 28.7 years, whereas since 2005, the average age has increased to 40.7 years.

A possible explanation for this, among others, is the increased median age of the population of the United States. SCI is more common among males (roughly 80% to 20% male:female ratio) and is trending upward in the African-American and Hispanic races (which most likely reflects the evolving population distribution in the United States).

Interestingly, motor vehicle accidents account for nearly half of all SCIs, and another one quarter is attributable to falls. Of the remaining 25%, violence (primarily gunshot wounds) accounts for 15% and sports-related injuries account for 8%. Both of the latter have been on the decline in recent years. Over half of patients with SCI reported being employed at the time of their injury, and roughly half also are not married at the time of injury. The relatively younger age of incidence explains the latter.

Most patients with SCI are discharged from the hospital to a private setting (most commonly their home); only about 5% are sent to nursing homes. The estimated lifetime cost of SCI for a 25 year old at the time of injury ranges from $3 million to $4.5 million for a tetraplegic and $2 million for a paraplegic.[1]

---

\*E-mail: benzele@ccf.org, Telephone: (216) 444-7381, Fax: (216) 445-9999.

## DATA COLLECTION

Most of the epidemiological data regarding SCI in the United States is collected in the National SCI Database. This database was created in 1973 and encompasses data from only about 13% of new SCI cases. Since its creation, the NSCI database has collected data from 26 federally funded SCI model systems around the country, of which only 14 remain. Between 1973 and 1981 the National SCI Data Research Center oversaw data collection into the NSCI database until the University of Alabama at Birmingham's Department of Rehabilitation Medicine took over data collection, creating the federally funded National Spinal Cord Injury Statistical Center (NSCISC). This organization oversees SCI data collection from all 14 SCI model systems throughout the country as well as 7 Form II centers that are subcontracted to gather and submit follow-up data (all are former SCI model systems). The current SCI model systems are located in Alabama, Colorado, Georgia, Illinois, Massachusetts, Michigan, New Jersey, New York, Ohio, Pennsylvania (two are located in this state), Texas, Washington state, and Washington, DC. For each patient with SCI evaluated in the model systems, two forms are submitted (Form I and Form II). Form I is completed for SCI patients who are admitted to any of the 14 model systems.

It records data from time of patient admission to discharge, including patient demographics, neurologic exam on presentation and discharge, and hospital course. Form II is concerned with follow up data and can be filled out by any of the 14 model systems or one of the 7 subcontracted Form II centers. Form II records the patient's course in inpatient and outpatient rehabilitation. The survival analyses calculated by the NSCISC, uses the Collaborative SCI Survival Study database, which contains many more patients than the NSCI database. This database draws from patients outside of the Form I and II patients from the national SCI centers.

## THE 2010 ANNUAL STATISTICAL REPORT FOR THE SPINAL CORD INJURY MODEL SYSTEMS: FACTS, FIGURES, AND TRENDS [2]

### Cause of Death

As of October, 2010 there are 10,409 deceased patients in the Collaborative SCI survival Study database. These include patients with SCI treated at model systems since 1973 within 1 year of their injury. Of these patients, there are 1,413 patients who died of unknown causes; these patients were excluded from the survival analyses. The leading cause of death in the remaining patients was respiratory (67.4% of these were cases of pneumonia). The second leading cause of death was infection, usually septicemia brought on by chronic infections or decubitus ulcers.

The third leading cause is hypertensive and ischemic heart disease, followed by neoplasms (predominantly lung cancer). Of interest, suicide was the tenth leading cause of death. Of note, there were an additional 28 unintentional suicides included in another category (subsequent trauma of uncertain nature). If these unintentional suicides are counted in the suicide category, then suicide becomes the eighth leading cause of death.[2]

## Long Term Survival and Life Expectancy

The cumulative 20-year survival rate for patients with SCI is 68.6%, while the 30-year survival rate is 52.9%. These rates need to be cautiously interpreted, as there are many patients lost to follow up (many of whom may have died) and there is notorious underreporting of patients that suffer SCI and die at the accident scene.

Life expectancy for patients with SCI was assessed for several age groups (10 years to 80 years old) surviving at least 24 hours and at least 1 year post injury. Intuitively, the results varied based on age and level of SCI, with decreasing life expectancy for older patients and higher neurological levels. Life expectancy drops off significantly for any patient who is ventilator dependent, regardless of neurologic level. For example, a 25 year old patient who survives at least 24 hours post injury will, on average, survive 40.8 years if paraplegic and 31.8 years if a C1-C4 tetraplegic. If this patient is ventilator dependent, the life expectancy drops to 14.9 years. On the contrary, a 60 year old patient with SCI who survives at least 24 hours post injury has an average life expectancy of 12.8 years if paraplegic, 7.7 years if C1-C4 tetraplegic, and 1.5 years if ventilator dependent.[2]


## Age, Gender, Race, and Etiology

The age range of patients in the database is less than one year to 98 years of age. The mean age of all patients is 33.9 years. The most common age at time of injury is 19, reaffirming the trend that SCI is a disease of young people. 25% of all patients with SCI in the database were between 17 and 22 years of age, and 50% of all injuries occurred between 16 and 30 years of age. Only roughly 10% of all SCI occurred at age 60 or greater.

80.7% of all patients with SCI in the database are male. This did not vary greatly between individual trauma systems, as the majority of patients suffering SCI at all of the national centers were invariably male. There was, however, significant variability between the SCI centers in race. The proportion of Caucasian patients varied between 37.7% and 90.6%, while the ratio of African Americans ranged from 3.1% to 57.4% at some centers. More interestingly, there has been, on average, a growing number of African Americans enrolled in the database since 1979. Concurrently, there has been a decrease in the percentage of Caucasians in the database. The number of Caucasians enrolled in the database dropped from 76.8% in 1979 to 66.5% after 2005, while the number of African Americans jumped from 14.2% to 26.8% in the same time period. This trend is thought to result from underlying race-specific SCI incidence rates, since the change is too large to be explained solely by changes in the United States general population and model system enrollment fluctuations. The percentage of Hispanic patients has increased slightly since the inception of the database, but has been trending down as of late. There is also a slight increase in the percent of Asian/Pacific Islanders in the study.

For both males and females, the most common causes of SCI are auto accidents, falls, and gunshot wounds (GSW). Among males, diving accidents and motorcycle accidents ranked fourth and fifth. In females, medical/surgical complications was fourth while diving accidents were fifth. Proportionally, auto accidents and medical/surgical complications were significantly more common in women, while motorcycle accidents, diving accidents, and falling objects were significantly more common in males. When etiologies are grouped according to gender, females are more likely to sustain an SCI in auto accidents while males are more likely to sustain SCI in sports injuries and violence. When grouped according to race, auto accidents were the leading cause of SCI among all of the races except for African Americans. In this latter population, violence is the leading cause. In the Hispanic population, both vehicular accidents and violence were the leading cause of SCI (auto accidents were only slightly more common than violence).[2]

## Work Injuries, Marital Status, and Level of Education

Roughly 10% of spinal cord injuries in the database that were sustained since 2001 were work-related. On average, 57.3% of participants were employed at the time of injury. This trend has actually increased since the database was created, from roughly 11% to 35% of respondents reporting that they were employed at the time of injury. Furthermore, the amount of unemployed participants is trending down since inception of the database, from 55.6% to 23.9%.

Given the preponderance of young patients with SCI, greater than ½ of patients in the database were never married at the time of injury. Interestingly, only 59.5% of participants were at least high school graduates at the time on injury. One would expect a much higher number given the fact that 85.6% of participants were at least 19 years of age at the time on injury. 9.2% of patients had an eighth grade education or less, despite the fact that only 2% of participants were 15 years old or less at the time of injury.[2]

## Hospital Course and Neurologic Status

Most of the patients in the database had sustained a cervical SCI (53.4%), followed by thoracic (35.5), and lumbar (10.7%). Only 0.4% of patients had sacral lesions. 46% of patients in the database had an injury to C4-7, the majority (30%) were at C4 or C5. The next two most common sites of injury were T12 and L1. At the time of discharge, most patients were incomplete tetraplegics (30.6%). The other patients were either complete paraplegics (25.3%), complete tetraplegics (20%), or incomplete paraplegics (18.6%). When grouped by etiology, violence most commonly resulted in complete paraplegia, while all of the other etiologies most commonly resulted in incomplete tetraplegia. Of note, almost all sports injuries resulted in tetraplegia and nearly 70% of all violence caused paraplegia. When the data is stratified to examine ASIA impairment scores, complete injuries (A) are the largest category (45.3%) at discharge, followed by functional motor incomplete (D). Between the time of admission and discharge from rehabilitation (for those patients admitted to the hospital within 24 hours of their injury), there was a decline in the 3 most severe ASIA grades: complete (A) patients dropped from 46.8% to 43.1%, sensory incomplete (B) patients dropped from 12.5% to 9.8%, and non-functional motor incomplete (C) participants dropped from 14.4% to 11.45%. Conversely, the number of functional motor incomplete patients (D) rose from 17.8% to 30.5, suggesting a positive effect of rehabilitation on improvement in ASIA grades for those patients admitted within 1 day of their injury.

The Functional Independence measure (FIM) is an instrument used to assess the functional status of SCI patients throughout their hospital stay and at discharge. It consists of

18 items, but only the motor scores are recorded in the national SCI database. Both Form I and Form II require FIM data, and it is only collected for patients greater than 6 years old. The motor scores include categories such as activities of daily living, locomotion, bowel and bladder control, and the like. The FIM total motor score ranges from 13 to 91, with 91 being the best possible score. Intuitively, mean FIM total motor scores were considerably higher for those patients admitted to rehabilitation with incomplete paraplegia-minimal deficit (41.4) than those patients with complete tetraplegia (15). Importantly, mean FIM scores nearly doubled in both the latter and the former categories (78.9 and 29, respectively).

Median days hospitalized were, not surprisingly, greater for patients with complete tetraplegia than for those patients with incomplete tetraplegia. For both categories, however, median hospital days fell, on average, from the 1980s to the year 2010. For patients with neurologically complete tetraplegia, the median days hospitalized were 23 (down from 30 from 1980-1984), and for incomplete tetraplegics, 10 (down from 22 in 1980-1984). In fact, median hospital days decreased or remained the same in nearly all of the neurological categories since the 1980s. A very similar pattern is noticed in the median days hospitalized in rehabilitation units.[2]

## INTERPRETATION OF THE SCI DATABASE TRENDS

The mean age of patients with SCI has been slowly increasing since the 1970s. The proportion of patients who are over 60 years of age is also slightly increasing. This is explainable by the gradual increase in age of the United States population. It is, however, possible that age-specific incidence rates may have contributed to this trend.[3] For example, injuries in females has slightly increased over time, and SCI at older ages is more common in females. Also, falls have become more common causes of SCI as of late. Since falls are the leading cause of SCI in patients greater than 45, this may also serve to explain the increase in age of patients with SCI.[3] For nearly every year that the database has been in existence, the top five etiologies have been automobile accidents, falls, GSW, diving, and motorcycle accidents (in that order). Nobunaga and colleagues noticed an alarming trend in violence as the cause of injury in 1999. At this time, persons sustaining an SCI tended to be young, non-white males. The 1990s showed a significant trend toward violence as a leading cause of SCI, especially among non-white ethnic groups.[4] This trend has significantly decreased from the year 2000 to the present, and is now less common a cause of SCI than it was in the 1970s and 1980s. The average education level of patients with SCI has also increased as of late, as has the percentage of patients discharged to a nursing home after their hospital stay. The latter is likely explained by the increase in age of patients with SCI.[3]

This increase in age of patients sustaining SCI also may have significant implications in average location and severity of SCI. The database shows an increase in the amount of patients with high cervical injuries, ventilator dependency, and incomplete neurologic injury.[3] When older patients fall they tend to suffer incomplete cervical injuries. These trends may also be explained by increasing survival of patients with high cervical injuries.

The trends in SCI life expectancy, survivability, and mortality are somewhat disappointing. Strauss and colleagues demonstrate that, although there was a significant increase in survival in the first 2 post-injury years after SCI, there is no evidence for increased survival after that period of time.[5] This is contrary to popular belief in the medical community in the United States, which previously relied on older data on SCI to draw conclusions. Strauss cites many plausible explanations, such as critical care improvements postponing the death of SCI patients, for this finding, however none have been proven through specific studies.

To complicate matters, interpretation of the SCI database is difficult due to many inherent limitations of the data within. The database only records 13% of patients with SCI in the United States, and only those treated at model systems. Furthermore it excludes several important comorbidities that may have a significant impact on survival, and it often contains incomplete or missing information.

# CONCLUSION

The national SCI database provides a snapshot of the epidemiology of SCI in the United States. SCI continues to be predominantly a disease of young males, with the average age of patients enrolled in the database at 34 years old and 80.7% of the patients in the database male. The average age of patients with SCI, however, is increasing and this may be due to any number of factors. The increasing age of the American population, the increased survivability of patients in the short term, and better post-injury care are all potential explanations. The most common cause of SCI in the United States is motor vehicle accidents. Women are much more likely to sustain a SCI in a motor vehicle crash than males, and young non-Caucasian males most commonly sustain SCI through acts of violence, although this etiology is decreasing in frequency. Average hospital and rehabilitation stays are steadily decreasing and ASIA and neurologic scores are improving, suggesting better critical care and rehab therapy. While the database provides an excellent cross section of the epidemiology of SCI in the United States, more data still needs to be collected from more SCI centers and further stratification of the data will be helpful.

# REFERENCES

[1]    Spinal cord injury facts and figures at a glance. *The journal of spinal cord medicine* 33:439-440, 2010.

[2]    The National Spinal Cord Injury Statistical Center University of Alabama at Birmingham.. *The 2010 Annual Statistical Report for the Spinal Cord Injury Model Systems.* 2011.

[3]    DeVivo MJ, Chen Y: Trends in new injuries, prevalent cases, and aging with spinal cord injury. *Archives of physical medicine and rehabilitation* 92:332-338, 2011.

[4]    Nobunaga AI, Go BK, Karunas RB: Recent demographic and injury trends in people served by the Model Spinal Cord Injury Care Systems. *Archives of physical medicine and rehabilitation* 80:1372-1382, 1999.

[5]    Strauss DJ, Devivo MJ, Paculdo DR, Shavelle RM: Trends in life expectancy after spinal cord injury. *Archives of physical medicine and rehabilitation* 87:1079-1085, 2006.

In: Epidemiology of Spinal Cord Injuries
Editors: V. Rahimi-Movaghar, S. B. Jazayeri et al.

ISBN: 978-1-61942-894-2
©2012 Nova Science Publishers, Inc.

*Chapter 2*

# NONTRAUMATIC SPINAL CORD INJURY: ETIOLOGIES AND OUTCOMES

## *William McKinley,[1,*] Camilo Castillo[2] and William Carter[2]*

[1]Department of PM and R, Spinal Cord Injury Medicine, Virginia Commonwealth
University, Richmond, VA, US
[2]Department of PM and R, Virginia Commonwealth University, Richmond, VA, US

## INTRODUCTION:

The pathogenesis of adult nontraumatic (NT) spinal cord injury (SCI) includes such etiologies as vertebral spondylosis (spinal stenosis), neoplastic and infectious-related injury, vascular ischemia, and multiple sclerosis (Table1). [1-4] Other etiologies include inflammatory disease, transverse myelitis, motor neuron disease, radiation myelopathy, syringomyelia, paraneoplastic syndrome, and vitamin B12 deficiency. The clinical presentation and SCI-related medical complications in individuals with nontraumatic SCI warrant an interdisciplinary approach to maximize their medical, functional and psychosocial outcomes. The demographic and clinical comparisons between nontraumatic and traumatic SCI reveal several differences that may be of importance when considering these outcomes. Though they make up a significant percentage of patients with SCI admitted for rehabilitation, their outcomes have not been as thoroughly studied as in those with traumatic etiology. A better understanding of these issues will assist in the medical management, rehabilitation and long-term follow up for individuals with nontraumatic SCI.

## INCIDENCE AND DEMOGRAPHICS

Several studies have revealed a significant incidence of nontraumatic SCI. [5,6] In the United States, a study of patients admitted for SCI inpatient rehabilitation at a Regional SCI Model System center noted that nontraumatic SCI comprised 38% of all SCI admissions with

*E-mail: wmckinley@mcvh-vcu.edu, Phone: 804-828-4233; Fax: 804-828-5074.

the most common etiologies related to spinal stenosis (52%), tumor (26%), ischemia (8%), infection (7%) and transverse myelitis (5%) (Figure 1) .[7-15]

Other studies have reported an overall incidence of between 23%-65% for nontraumatic SCI with common etiologies varying between studies, but including degenerative spine disease/spinal stenosis (6-25%), vascular-related SCI (2-12%), infectious/inflammatory (12-17%), tumor/cancer-related ( 14-32%), multiple sclerosis (15-19%) transverse myelitis (14-33%), and others. A few studies have also noted etiologies related to congenital or pediatric nontraumatic SCI, but this is less well described. The demographic comparison between nontraumatic and traumatic SCI reveals several differences that may be of importance when ultimately considering functional outcome and discharge/community reintegration issues. Individuals with nontraumatic SCI are more likely to be older, female, married and retired when compared to those with traumatic SCI (Table 2).[7-9,13,15-17] In one study, nontraumatic SCI comprised only 31% of patients under 40 years of age, but 87% of those over age 40, with cancer-related (53%) and spondylosis (25%) as the leading causes.[18] The underlying etiology may assist in explaining these differences as spinal stenosis and neoplastic compression of the spinal cord more commonly involve individuals in the fifth decade and beyond. Tumor-related SCI has a peak incidence between 50-70 years of age.[8,10, 19-21] SCI in those younger than 40 years of age is more commonly due to traumatic etiology, such as motor vehicle accidents, acts of violence, or sports. With the likelihood of an increasingly aged population in future decades, an increased incidence of nontraumatic SCI may be expected. Given the likelihood of nontraumatic SCI to affect older individuals, factors such as demographics, neurological presentation, concomitant illness and rehabilitation functional outcome become important issues for consideration. Older age has been shown to affect rehabilitation outcome after SCI. Older individuals may have a decreased functional reserve due to diminished cardiovascular and pulmonary fitness along with muscle weakness. Older individuals with SCI have been reported to have a higher prevalence of co-morbidities and worse outcomes such as increased medical complications, rehospitalization, discharge to nursing homes and need for attendant assistance.[22] Elderly individuals with nontraumatic SCI may present with associated medical complications, such as cardiopulmonary disease or diabetes, which could adversely affect medical and functional outcomes.

### Table 1. Etiologies of Non-traumatic Spinal Cord Injury

| |
| --- |
| Spinal Stenosis |
| Cancer-related Compression |
| Infectious- related Compression |
| Vascular Ischemia |
| Multiple Sclerosis |
| Transverse Myelitis |
| Radiation Myelopathy |
| Paraneoplastic Syndrome |
| Motor Neuron Diseases |
| Syringomyelia |
| Vitamin B12 Deficiency |
| Friedreich's Ataxia |

**Table 2. Demographics: Nontraumatic vs Traumatic SCI**

|  | Nontraumatic (n=86) | Traumatic (n=134) | Significance |
|---|---|---|---|
| Age (years) | 61.2 | 38.6 | P<.01 |
| Gender |  |  |  |
| Male | 50% | 84% | P<.01 |
| Female | 50% | 16% |  |
| Ethnicity |  |  |  |
| Caucasian | 47% | 35% | NS |
| Non-Caucasian | 54% | 65% |  |
| Marital Status |  |  |  |
| Married | 57% | 38% | P<.01 |
| Not Married | 23% | 17% |  |
| Never Married | 12% | 45% |  |
| Work Status |  |  |  |
| Working/Student | 24% | 67% | P<.01 |
| Not Working | 76% | 33% |  |

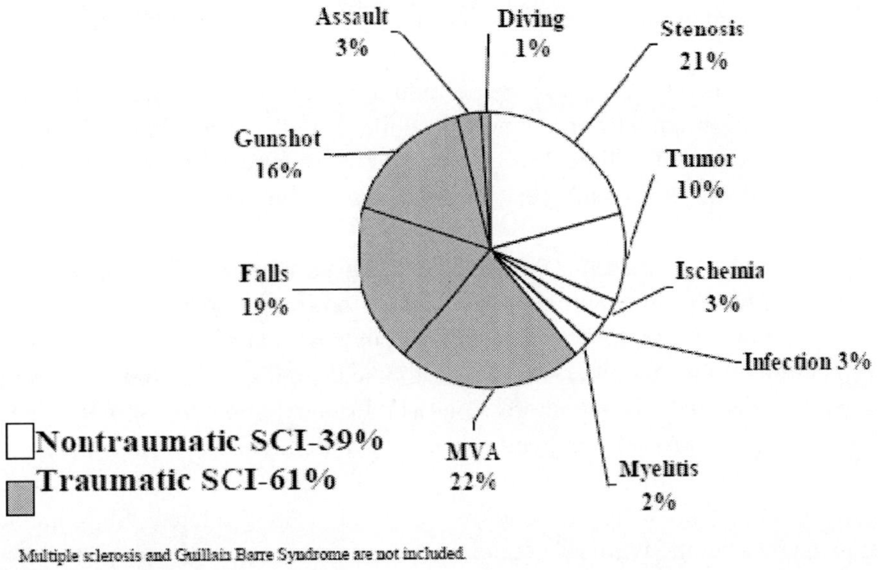

Assault 3% · Diving 1% · Stenosis 21% · Gunshot 16% · Tumor 10% · Falls 19% · Ischemia 3% · Infection 3% · Nontraumatic SCI-39% · Traumatic SCI-61% · MVA 22% · Myelitis 2%

Multiple sclerosis and Guillain Barre Syndrome are not included.

Figure 1. Etiology of SCI Rehabilitation Admissions: Non-traumatic vs. Traumatic SCI.

Additionally, the use of certain medications, in the elderly, must be closely monitored to prevent unintended side effects. Medications used to control spasticity or pain (commonly seen after SCI)) can sometimes cause to sedation along with memory or retention impairments, which can result in diminished rehabilitation efficiency and functional improvement.

## COMMON NONTRAUMATIC SCI ETIOLOGIES

*Spinal stenosis* is a common cause of pain and disability in individuals older than 50 years of age and a common diagnosis in patients over age 65 undergoing lumbar surgery.[23] The degenerative changes that cause progressive narrowing of the spinal canal and the vertebral foramina may give rise to spondylitic myelopathy or cauda equina syndrome. The chronic nature of its onset often leads to a stepwise progression of clinical deterioration with intermittent periods of stability. Spinal cord compression secondary to stenosis can occur with encroachment anteriorly (vertebral body osteophytes), posteriorly (ligamentum flavum), or laterally (intervertebral foramen). Anterior-posterior canal diameters of less than 14 mm in adults have been noted to increase the risk for myelopathy or radiculopathy.[24] The lower cervical (levels C4-7) and lumbar (levels L2-4) regions of the vertebral column are more commonly involved, in part due to their propensity for increased and repetitive vertebral mobility within these regions.

SCI as a result of *tumor-related spinal cord compression* involves several complex medical and quality of life issues stemming from both the direct cancerous effects as well as the neurological complications of the spinal cord involvement. Tumor-related SCI is often classified according to its proximity to the spinal cord and its surrounding meninges. Extramedullary neoplastic compression accounts for over 90% with the majority being epidural (most often neurofibromas and meningiomas).[25] Intramedullary disease account for less than 5% of spinal cord tumors and consists primarily of gliomas (ependymomas and astrocytomas most commonly). Ependymomas represent a primarily benign gliomal tumor involving the ependymal cells, which line the central nervous system. Astrocytomas (the most common intramedullary spinal cord tumors in children) are often graded 1 through 4.[26] Grades 1 and 2 carry the best clinical prognosis for five year survival (greater than 80%) and are seen most commonly.[27] One-year survival rate for grades 3 and 4 astrocytomas are poor.

Vertebral metastasis is seen in 15-40% of individuals with systemic malignancy and has been reported to cause epidural spinal cord compression in up to 5%.[4] The pathogenesis is usually hemodynamic spread to bone marrow through Batson's epidural venous plexus via the pelvic, abdominal and thoracic veins. The thoracic region is the most common site for metastatic epidural spinal cord compression.[21] Primary sites for spinal metastasis are usually breast, lung and prostate in greater than 50%, although nearly 10% have an unknown primary tumor site. In children, the common primary sites include lymphoma, sarcoma and neuroblastomas.[28] The exact pathophysiology of cancer-related SCI includes cord compression and ischemia with subsequent edema, nerve demyelination, hemorrhage and cystic necrosis. Clinical onset is usually days to weeks and often associated with pain (present in over 95%). Paresis is a rare initial clinical finding, but is ultimately present in up to 75% at the time of diagnosis.

In relation to cancer-related SCI, two other issues bear mention, paraneoplastic syndrome and Radiation myelopathy. *Paraneoplastic syndrome* represents myelitis due to the remote effects of systemic cancer and not to direct invasion or compression of the spinal cord. Pathologically, subacute necrosis of spinal cord gray or white matter is seen with no evidence of infection, inflammation or ischemia and is often associated with bronchogenic cancer.[29] *Radiation myelopathy* has an incidence of less than 3% and involves delayed necrosis of the spinal cord gray or white matter. Its onset occurs anywhere from 6 – 48 months (most commonly 12-15 months) following radiation therapy to the vertebral or surrounding region and with total radiation doses exceeding 2500 RADS.[30] This has further demonstrated the importance of the timing and location of radiation treatments and led to recommendations for sites for radiation, along with daily, weekly and total radiation quantities.

*Vascular or ischemic-related SCI* is commonly associated with aortic aneurysms, involving either intraoperative ischemia, systemic hypotension or spinal artery occlusion by the aortic dissection itself.[31, 32] In patients undergoing thoracoabdominal aneurysm repair, there has been an incidence of spinal cord ischemia percentage varying from 4 to 16%, depending on the type of aneurysm and repair. [33] Spinal arteries form an anastamotic chain along the length of the spinal cord, with potential vulnerability in various watershed regions, primarily in the thoracolumbar region, supplied by the great spinal artery of Adamkiewiz. The spinal cord is less vulnerable to ischemia than the brain and can withstand permanent damage with up to 30 minutes of interrupted blood supply (for instance with aortic clamping). [34] The spinal cord gray matter is most susceptible to injuries than the white matter, in part due its higher metabolic rate.

Embolic ischemia to the spinal cord is rare, though one phenomenon involves that of decompression sickness (Caisson disease) seen with embolic occlusion of the venous plexus by nitrogen bubbles during ascension in deep sea diving.[35] Spinal hemorrhage is most often seen as a result of anticoagulation, arteriovenous malformation or coagulopathy.[36, 37] It is often found in the cervical spinal cord region and necessitates prompt evaluation for surgical clot evacuation.

*Infectious-related SCI* is most commonly seen secondary to spinal epidural abscess (SEA) and Pott's disease (spinal tuberculosis), though other causes include vertebral osteomyelitis and intramedullary abscess. [11,38,39] Comorbid risk factors associated with SEA include intravenous drug abuse, pulmonary tuberculosis, endocarditis, cellulitis, alcoholism, chronic steroid use, diabetes mellitus, sepsis and dental abscess. [40,41] The pathophysiology of SEA includes the extension of adjacent vertebral osteomyelitis (most common) or hematogenous spread from distant infectious sites (such as perinephric, pharyngeal or paraspinal) though up to one-third of cases lacks an identifiable cause. [42] SEA is thought to cause SCI by one of three potential mechanisms: direct compression by the abscess on the spinal cord, vertebral collapse associated with osteomyelitis, and vascular occlusion resulting in ischemia. The predominant vertebral level of infection in patients with SEA is thoracic, followed by cervical and lumbosacral. [40,43,44] *Staphylococcus aureus* represents the most common organism for SEA and treatment typically consists of early surgical decompression along with systemic antibiotics. Permanent neurologic deficits are more likely to occur if compression is not relieved within 36-48 hours.

*Acquired Immunodeficiency Syndrome (AIDS) and Human Immunodeficiency Virus (HIV)* can lead to spinal cord involvement in various ways, including compression by associated neoplasm (such as Karposi Sarcoma or lymphoma), direct infection by opportunistic organisms or vacuolar degeneration of the white matter (seen in up to 30% of AIDS patients at autopsy).[45] *Syphilis* represents a rare spinal cord insult by the treponema parasite in the tertiary stages of syphilis. Pathophysiology is that of a chronic inflammatory process involving the dorsal root ganglion and posterior column (tabes dorsalis) or syphilitic meningitis.

Acute *transverse myelitis* represents a heterogenous group of inflammatory disorders that area characterized by acute or subacute spinal cord dysfunction secondary to demyelination (often perivascular), axonal injury, glial cell necrosis and edema within the spinal cord. Although most often idiopathic, it is felt to be autoimmune in origin often with association to connective tissue disorders and metabolic etiologies, and it has been seen in post-viral or post vaccine setting. [46] 1.3 -8 per million are affected with a bimodal age incidence of 10-19 and

30-39.[47] Diagnosis often includes the exclusion of vascular, infectious or multiple sclerosis as an etiology. The prognosis is worse when accompanied by MRI lesions, severe weakness, and electrodiagnostic evidence of denervation.[48]

*Multiple sclerosis* of the spinal cord involves multifocal spinal demyelinative lesions. The usual presentation of chronic spinal multiple sclerosis is that of a slowly progressive, asymmetric spastic paraparesis with variable sensory ataxia. Associated lesions in the cerebrum, brainstem and optic nerves often complicate diagnosis and clinical outcome.

*Syringomyelia,* a cystic cavitation within the spinal cord, is more-often associated with post-traumatic SCI, though is sometimes idiopathic in nature. These longitudinal spinal cavitations, commonly located near the anterior commissure, can lead cord compression or vascular compromise typically resulting in alterations of pain sensation, along with other later-onset sensory or motor abnormalities. They typically occur months to years after initial SCI and may lead to ascending neurological symptoms. Surgical management, if applicable, involves decompression and consideration of shunting of cerebrospinal fluids into the subarachnoid space or peritoneal cavity.

# CLINICAL PRESENTATION AND MANAGEMENT

Spinal cord injury is typically associated with muscle weakness and sensory impairment along with bladder, bowel and sexual dysfunction. The clinical presentation of nontraumatic SCI usually reveals a pattern of less severe neurological impairment as compared to traumatic SCI. Individuals with nontraumatic SCI are much more likely to present with paraplegia (as opposed to tetraplegia) and with motor incomplete (as opposed to complete) lesions. [9,13,15,16,49-51] This is likely related to both location and pathophysiology of spinal cord involvement along with their often insidious progression. Nontraumatic spinal cord involvement is more common in the thoracic level. Pain may be a presenting symptom, especially in cancer-related injury, where it is the initial presenting symptom in about 90% of individuals.[52] Spinal metastasis should be considered with an acute onset of localized back pain (worse at night or when supine) in a patient with cancer.

A comprehensive and detailed neurologic examination preformed early and repeated as necessary is important and can assist with neurologic outcomes prognosis. Key elements of the examination include motor and sensory testing, which allows for the designation of a neurologic level and completeness of injury. Diminished sensation with loss of pinprick, temperature, position, or vibratory sensation may occur early. Perianal and rectal examination is important to assess sacral motor and sensory function. Hyperreflexia, clonus or a positive Babinski sign (upward movement of the toe in response to plantar stimulation) indicate upper motor neuron involvement, though they may be absent early in the course of compression. Provocative physical exam maneuvers (such as straight leg raise or Lhermitte sign) may elicit findings indicative of neural/meningeal irritation. Valsalva maneuvers (induced by coughing or straining) may exacerbate radicular back pain from intradural cord compression.

Some, though not all, studies have noted greater neurological improvement following nontraumatic SCI as compared to traumatic SCI. [15] Greater neurological recovery is often related to a greater degree of initial motor/sensory incompleteness, as seen in those with nontraumatic SCI. Additionally, certain specific etiologies, such as those related to spinal epidural abscess, have been noted to have potential for significant improvement in neurological deficits. [11] Associated medical complications are common following nontraumatic SCI. [12, 14, 16,49,53,54] Some are directly related to SCI itself, while others develop secondarily and are often preventable. Neurogenic bladder/bowel, pain, spasticity, autonomic dysfunction (such as orthostasis or autonomic dysreflexia) are seen as a result of interruption of normal spinal nerve pathways. In addition, secondary SCI-related medical complications consist of infections (commonly genitourinary, respiratory and wound), pain, pressure ulcers, deep venous thrombosis (DVT), contractures, sleep disturbance, depression and heterotopic ossification. These complications can lead to a loss of rehabilitation therapy time, increased hospital length of stay, and ultimately to increased costs of care, re-hospitalization rates, disability and decreased survival. The most frequent complications noted were typically urinary tract infections, pressure ulcers, depression and pain. [14,16,49,54] Those with more severe disability at time of rehabilitation admission had more complications. Less frequently encountered complications were spasticity, orthostasis, DVT, autonomic dysreflexia and pneumonia, possibly related to both the lower neurological levels and greater incompleteness of injury. [54] The most commonly preventable complications include UTI, pressure ulcers, pain, pneumonia, and DVT [12,49,53]. Strategies for prevention (when applicable), early assessment, diagnosis and treatment should be stressed as an ongoing part of their rehabilitation and education. Model system programs for SCI have noted a decline in rehabilitation length of stay and in re-hospitalization rates, citing advances in their prevention of and improved treatment efficacy.[55] Early and comprehensive diagnosis and rehabilitative management are important and have been noted to be related to improved medical and functional outcomes. Although not readily studied, survival rate of patients with non-traumatic SCI has been noted to be similar to those with traumatic SCI, though differences were noted within etiologic groups and for age at SCI onset. Longer survival in patients with paraplegia and less severe neurological involvement (as seen in nontraumatic SCI) might be expected, if not offset by an older age and more comorbidities.

## FUNCTIONAL OUTCOME FOLLOWING NONTRAUMATIC SCI

Rehabilitation intervention utilizing an interdisciplinary team approach can improve mobility, self-care skills, psychological adjustment and community reintegration as well as reduce complications. Individuals with nontraumatic SCI have been shown to achieve functional improvement during rehabilitation, though the overall degree of improvement may be less than in those with traumatic SCI. This may be significant, given that in individuals with SCI, rehabilitative functional outcomes are associated with level of injury, completeness of injury, and age.[22] The Functional Independence Measure (FIM) is a commonly used, valid and reliable measure of disability, often used to measure rehabilitation outcomes. Prior studies have revealed significant FIM improvements in nontraumatic SCI during rehabilitation, though admission functional status has been reported to be lower in nontraumatic SCI and there was greater total FIM change in those with traumatic SCI. [7,9-10,11, 13,15,18,51,56-58] FIM efficiencies (FIM change per day) were often comparable between the two groups, which may indicate similar rates of functional gains. [14,16,17,59]

Decreased overall functional improvements in nontraumatic SCI may be related to their older age or to associated comorbidities (such as cardiovascular disease, diabetes, cognitive issues).

Rehabilitation lengths of stay (LOS) for patients with nontraumatic SCI are typically similar or slightly shorter in duration than those with traumatic injury. [7-10, 57,60] This may reflect an earlier FIM plateau secondary to higher admission motor FIM scores seen in the NT/SCI group.

Additional factors influencing LOS include the level and completeness of SCI. Patients with cancer-related SCI have been noted to have shorter rehabilitation LOS, possibly related to issues such as physical tolerance limitations, pain or quality of life decisions due to reduced life expectancy. [8,58] The majority of patients with nontraumatic SCI return home following rehabilitation and typically with similar rates to those with traumatic SCI.[9,50,53,61] Factors predicting return to home include functional mobility, bladder and bowel status and availability of resources. The impact of managed care has affected LOS and thus discharge disposition, increasing the proportion of patients discharged to nursing homes. In nontraumatic SCI, this tendency may have been offset by more often having less severe neurological impairment and more often being married.

# CONCLUSION

Patients with nontraumatic SCI represent a significant proportion of individuals with SCI admitted to rehabilitation settings. Their incidence and etiologies seem to vary depending on geographic location and study population evaluated. The high cost of overall SCI care, along with clinical and functional outcomes; make further understanding of this issue very important. These individuals tend to be older and have a greater incidence of incomplete and paraplegic injuries compared to those with traumatic injury. During rehabilitation, patients have shown the ability to achieve comparable rates of functional gains, may have a shorter rehabilitation length of stay, and can achieve similar discharge to community rates. This information can assist health care professionals with further decisions regarding rehabilitation along with management and prevention of medical complications. Encouragement should be given to future investigation in this area to more fully address functional outcome, medical complications, cost-of-care, quality of life and survival issues. In addition, clinical and functional outcome differences between the various etiologic groups (such as spinal stenosis, tumor, infection, ischemia, myelitis, etc) of non-traumatic-SCI and these groups should be further evaluated and compared.

# REFERENCES

[1]   Adams RD, Salam-Adams M. Chronic Nontraumatic Diseases of the Spinal Cord. *Neurol. Clin.* 1991; 9:605-23.

[2]   Dawson DM, Potts F. Acute Nontraumatic Myelopathies. *Neurol. Clin.* 1991; 9:585-602.

[3]   Schmidt RD, Markovchick V. Nontraumatic Spinal Cord Compression. *J. Emerg. Med.* 1992; 10:189-99.

[4]     Byrne TN, Waxman SG. Spinal Cord Compression: Diagnosis and Principles of Treatment: Contemporary Neurology Series. Philadelphia, *FA Davis,* 1990.

[5]     Kurtzke JF. Epidemiology of Spinal Cord Injury. *Exp. Neurol.* 1975; 48:163-236.

[6]     Guttman L. Spinal Cord Injuries. Comprehensive Management and Research. *Oxford: Blackwell;* 1973.

[7]     McKinley W, Tellis A, Cifu D, Johnson M, Kubal W, Keyser-Marcus L, et al. Rehabilitation Outcome of Individuals with Nontraumatic Myelopathy Resulting from Spinal Stenosis. *J. Spinal. Cord. Med.* 1998; 21:131-6.

[8]     8. McKinley WO, Conti-Wyneken A, Vokac C, Cifu D. Rehabilitative Functional Outcome of Patients with Neoplastic Spinal Cord Compression. *Arch. Phys. Med. Rehabil.* 1996;77:892-5.

[9]     McKinley W, Hardman J, Seel R. Nontraumatic Spinal Cord Injury: Incidence, Epidemiology and Functional Outcome. *Arch. Phys. Med. Rehab.* 1998; 79:1186-7.

[10]    McKinley WO, Tewksbury MA. Neoplastic vs. Traumatic Spinal Cord Injury: An Inpatient Rehabilitation Comparison. *Am. J. Phys. Med. Rehabil.* 2000; 79:138-144.

[11]    McKinley W, Merrell C, Meade M, Brooke K, DiNicola A. "Rehabilitation Outcomes after Infection-Related SCI/D". *Amer Jnl PMandR* 2008, 87(4):275-80.

[12]    Nair K, Taly A, Maheshwarappa B, Kumar J, Murali T, Rao S. Nontraumatic spinal cord lesions: a prospective study of medical complications during in-patient rehabilitation. *Spinal. Cord.* 2005; 43:558-564.

[13]    Gupta A, Taly A, Srivastava A, Vishal S, Murali T. Traumatic vs non-traumatic spinal cord lesions: comparison of neurological and functional outcome after inpatient rehabilitation. *Spinal. Cord.* 2008; 46:482-487.

[14]    Cosar SN, Yemisci OU, Oztop P, Cetin N, Sarifakioglu B, Yalbuzdag SA, Ustaomer K, Karatas M. Demographic characteristics after traumatic and non-traumatic spinal cord injury: a retrospective comparison study. *Spinal. Cord.* 2010;48:862-866.

[15]    Scivoletto G, Farchi S, Laurenza L, Molinari M. Traumatic and non-traumatic spinal cord lesions: an Italian comparison of neurological and functional outcomes. *Spinal. Cord.* 2011;49:391-396.

[16]    Ones K, Yilmaz E, Beydogan A, Gultekin O, Caglar N. Comparison of functional results in non-traumatic and traumatic spinal cord injury. *Disabil. Rehabil.* 2007;29:1185-1191.

[17]    Guilcher SJ, Munce SE, Couris CM, Fung K, Craven BC, Verrier M. Health care utilization in non-traumatic and traumatic spinal cord injury: a population-based study. *Spinal. Cord.* 2010;48:45-50.

[18]    Murray P. Functional Outcome and Survival in Spinal Cord Injury Secondary to Neoplasia. *Cancer* 1985; 55:197-201.

[19]    Sundaresan N, Galicich J, Bains M, Martini N, Beattie E. Vertebral Body Resection in Treatment of Cancer Involving the Spine. *Cancer* 1984; 53:1393-6.

[20]    Helweg-Larsen S. Clinical Outcome in Metastatic Spinal Cord Compression. A Prospective Study of 153 Patients. *Acta Neurol. Scand.* 1996; 94:269-75.

[21]    Gilbert RW, Kim JH, Posner JB. Epidural Spinal Cord Compression from Metastatic Tumor: Diagnosis and Treatment. *Ann. Neurol.* 1978; 3:40-51.

[22]    DeVivo MJ, Kartus PL, Rutt RD, Stover Sl, Fine PR. The Influence of Age at Time of Spinal Cord Injury on Rehabilitation Outcome. *Arch. Neurol.* 1990; 47:687-91.

[23] Lees F, Turner J. Natural History and Prognosis of Cervical Spondylosis. *Br. Med. J.* 1963; 2:1607-10.

[24] Payne EE, Spillane JD. The Cervical Spine: An Anatomicopathological Study of 70 Specimens (Using a Special Technique) with Particular Reference to the Problems of Cervical Spondylosis. *Brain.* 1957; 80:571-96.

[25] Levy W, Bay J, Dohn D. Spinal Cord Meningioma. *J. Neurosurg.* 1982; 57:804-12.

[26] Epstein F, Epstein N. Intramedullary Tumors of the Spinal Cord. In Shillito J and Matsoin D (eds): *Pediatric Neurosurgery: Surgery of the Developing Nervous System. Grune and Stratton,* New York, 1982. 529-39.

[27] Reimer R, Onofrio BM. Astrocytomas of the Spoinal Cord in Children and Adolescents. *J. Neurosurg.* 1985; 63:669-675.

[28] Lewis D, Packer R, Raney B. Incidence, Presentation, and Outcome of Spinal Cord Disease in Children with Systemic Cancer. *Pediatrics* 1986; 78:438-442.

[29] Henson RA, Urich H. Cancer and the Nervous System. *Blackwell, Oxford* 1982.

[30] Burns BJ, Jones AN, Robertson JS. Pathology of Radiation Myelopathy. *J. Neurol. Neurosurg. Psychiatry* 1972; 35:888.

[31] Blumbergs PC, Byrne E. Hypotensive Central Infarction of the Spinal Cord. *J. Neurol.* 1980; 43:751-3.

[32] Foo D, Rosier AB. Anterior Spinal Artery Syndrome and its Natural History. *Paraplegia* 1983; 21:1-10.

[33] Zvara, D. Thoracoabdominal aneurysm surgery and the risk of paraplegia: contemporary practice and future directions. *J. Extra Corpor. Technol.* 2002; 34 (1): 11-7

[34] Otomo E, VanBuskirk C, Workman JB. Circulation of the Spinal Cord Studied by Autoradiography. *Neurology* 1960; 10:112-20.

[35] Hellenback JM, Bove AA, Elliott DH. Mechanisms Underlying Spinal Cord Damage in Decompression Sickness. *Neurology* 1975; 25:308-16.

[36] Mattle H, Sieb JP, Rohner M, Mumenthaler M. Nontraumatic Spinal Epidural and Subdural Hematomas. *Neurology* 1987; 37:1351-1358.

[37] Foo D, Chang YC, Rossier AB. Spontaneous Cervical Epidural Hemorrhage, Anterior Cord Syndrome and Familial Vascular Malformations: Case Report. *Neurology.* 1980; 30:308-11.

[38] Baker AS, Ojemann RJ, Swartz NM, et al. Spinal Epidural Abscess. *N. Engl. J. Med.* 1975 293:463-468.

[39] Verner E, Musher D. Spinal Epidural Abscess. *Med. Clin. North Am.* 1985; 375-84.

[40] Akalan N, Ozgen T. Infection as a cause of spinal cord compression: a review of 36 spinal epidural abscess cases. *Acta Neurochirurgica* 2000; 142:17-23.

[41] Khanna RK, Malik G, Rock J. Spinal epidural abscess: evaluation of factors influencing outcome. *Neurosurgery* 1996; 39:958-64.

[42] Carey M : Infections of the spine and spinal cord. In: Youmans JR, editor. *Neurological surgery:* 4th ed. Philadelphia: Saunder; 1996. p 3275-3304.

[43] Zafonte R, Ricker J, Hanks R. Spinal epidural abscess: study of early outcome. *J. Spinal Cord. Med.* 2003; 26:345-51.

[44] Morillo-Leco G, Alcaraz-Rousselet M, Díaz-Borrego P. Clinical characteristics of spinal cord injury caused by infection. *Revista de neurología* 2005; 41:205-8.

[45]  Petito, CK, Navio BA, Cho ES. Vaculoar Myelopathy Pathologically Resembling Subacute Combined Degeneration in Patients with Acquired Immunodeficiency Syndrome. *N. Eng. J. Med.* 1985; 312:874-879.

[46]  Brinar VV, Habek M, Zadro I, Barun B, Ozretic D, Vranjes D. Current concepts in the diagnosis of transverse myelopathies. *Clin. Neurol. Neurosurg.* 2008;110 (9):919-27.

[47]  Frohman EM, Wingerchuk DM. Clinical practice Transverse myelitis. *N. Engl. J. Med.* 2010 Aug 5;363(6):564-72.

[48]  Kalita J, Misra UK, Mandal SK. Prognostic Predictors of Acute Transverse Myelitis. *Acta Neurol. Scand.* 1998; 98:60-3.

[49]  New P, Rawicki H, Bailey M. Nontraumatic spinal cord injury: demographic characteristics and complications. *Arch. Phys. Med. Rehabil.* 2002; 83:996-1001.

[50]  New P, Rawicki H, Bailey M. Nontraumatic spinal cord injury rehabilitation: pressure ulcer patterns, prediction, and impact. *Arch. Phys. Med. Rehabil.* 2004; 85:87-93.

[51]  New P. Functional outcomes and disability after nontraumatic spinal cord injury rehabilitation: results from a retrospective study. *Arch. Phys. Med. Rehabil.* 2005;85:250-261.

[52]  Posner J. Spinal Metastases. In: Davis F, ed. *Neurological Complications of Cancer.* Philadelphia, 1995; 111-41.

[53]  New P, Epi M. Influence of age and gender on rehabilitation outcomes in nontraumatic spinal cord injury. *J. Spinal Cord. Med.* 2007; 30:225-237.

[54]  McKinley W, Godbout C, Tewksbury M. "Medical Complications Following Nontraumatic SCI", *Jnl. Spinal Cord. Med.* 2002, 25(2) 88-93.

[55]  DeVivo MJ. Discharge disposition from model spinal cord injury care system rehabilitation programs. *Arch. Phys. Med. Rehabil.* 1999; 80: 785-790

[56]  Hacking HGA, Van As HHJ, Lankhorst GJ. Factors Related to the Outcome of Inpatient Rehabilitation in Patients with Neoplastic Epidural Spinal Cord Compression. *Paraplegia* 1993; 31:367-74.

[57]  McKinley WO, Huang ME, Brunsvold KT. Neoplastic vs Traumatic Spinal Cord Injury: An Outcome Comparison after Inpatient Rehabilitation. *Arch. Phys. Med. Rehab.* 1999, 80:1253-7.

[58]  Fattal C, Fabbro M,Rousays-Mabit H, Verollet C, Bauchet L. Metastatic paraplegia and functional outcomes: perspectives and limitations for rehabilitation care Part 2. *Arch. Phys. Med. Rehabil.* 2001 Jan; 92(1):134-45.

[59]  New PW, Simmonds F, Stevermuer T. A population-based study comparing traumatic spinal cord injury and non-traumatic spinal cord injury using a national rehabilitation database. *Spinal Cord.* 2011 Mar: 49(3):397-403.

[60]  Yokoyama I, Sakuma F, Itoh R, Sashika H. Paraplegia after aortic aneurysm repair versus traumatic spinal cord injury: Functional outcome, complications, and therapy intensity of inpatient rehabilitation. *Arch. Phys. Med. Rehabil.* 2006; 87:1189-1194.

[61]  Citterio A, Franceschini M, Spizzichino L, Reggio A, Rossi B, Stampacchia G. Nontraumatic spinal cord injury: an Italian survey. *Arch. Phys. Med. Rehabil.* 2004; 85:1483-1487.

In: Epidemiology of Spinal Cord Injuries
Editors: V. Rahimi-Movaghar, S. B. Jazayeri et al.

ISBN: 978-1-61942-894-2
©2012 Nova Science Publishers, Inc.

*Chapter 3*

# EPIDEMIOLOGY OF PEDIATRIC-ONSET SPINAL CORD INJURIES IN THE UNITED STATES

## *Kathy Zebracki and Lawrence C. Vogel*
Rush Medical College, Shriners Hospitals
for Children, Chicago, Illinois, US

## ABSTRACT

This chapter provides an overview of the epidemiology of spinal cord injuries (SCIs) in the general United States (U.S.) population, followed by an in-depth discussion of the prevalence, causes, and complications of SCIs in children and adolescents. The annual incidence of SCIs in the U.S. is approximately 40 cases per million population or approximately 12,000 new cases each year. Approximately 20% of traumatic SCIs occur in individuals younger than 21 years of age, with 3% to 5% of injuries occurring in those younger than 15.Compared to adult-onset SCI, individuals with pediatric-onset SCI are unique in several ways. Because of their younger age at injury and longer lifespan, they will be more susceptible to long-term complications such as cardiovascular disease, and overuse syndromes. The pediatric-onset SCI population also has developmental needs and experiences relatively unique complications, such as scoliosis and hip dysplasia, which will impact them throughout their life-span. Moreover, demographic and injury related factors vary as a function of age at injury, including pediatric-specific etiologies and presentations, such as lap-belt injuries, neonatal SCI, transverse myelitis, and SCI associated with Down syndrome, juvenile idiopathic arthritis and skeletal dysplasias as well as SCI without radiographic abnormality.

## DATA ON SCIs IN THE GENERAL POPULATION

The annual incidence of SCIs in the U.S., excluding those who do not survive prior to hospitalization, is approximately 40 cases per million population or approximately 12,000 new cases each year [1]. In 2010, the prevalence of SCIs in the U.S. was estimated to be 265,000 persons, with a range of 232,000 to 316,000 [1].

The National Spinal Cord Injury Database (NSCID) was established in 1973 to study the longitudinal course of traumatic SCIs and to identify trends over time in etiology, demographic, and injury severity characteristics of individuals who sustain a SCI. Since its inception, 26 federally funded SCI Model Systems, specialized programs of care in SCI, have contributed data to the NSCID, capturing approximately 13% of new SCI cases per year in the U.S.. As of October 2010, the database contains information on 27,553 persons who sustained a traumatic SCI.

Over the past four decades, the mean age at injury has increased from 28.7 years in 1973-1979 to 40.7 years in 2005. This trend may be related to several factors, including an increase in the median age of the U.S. population by 9 years during this period, changes in underlying age-specific incidence rates or survival rates of older persons at the scene of the accident, and changes in referral patterns or locations of the model systems centers. Overall, 81% of SCIs have occurred in males; however, recently, this percentage has decreased slightly. Moreover, there have been significant changes in the racial/ethnic distribution of SCIs, with the percentage of injuries increasing among minority populations in recent years. Among those injured between 1973 and 1979, 77% were Caucasian,14% were African American, 6% Hispanic, and 1% were Asian. In comparison for those injured from 2005 to 2010, 66% were Caucasian, 27% African American, 8% Hispanic, and 2% Asian. Similar to age data, these trends reflect racial/ethnic trends in the general U.S. population as well as changing catchment areas and referral patterns of the Model System centers.

Since 2005, the most common causes of SCIs in the U.S. are motor vehicle crashes (40%), falls (28%), violence (15%), and sports (8%). Over the past 40 years, the proportion of injuries due to sports has decreased while the proportion of injuries due to falls has increased. Rates of injuries due to violence peaked between 1990 and 1999 at 25%, but have recently declined to 15%, which is consistent with rates prior to 1980 (13%).

Since 2005, the distribution of neurologic categories at initial discharge of persons from the Model Systems is incomplete tetraplegia (40%), complete paraplegia (22%), incomplete paraplegia (22%) andcomplete tetraplegia (16%), with less than 1% of persons experiencing complete neurologic recovery. Over the last 15 years, the percentage of individuals with incompletetetraplegia has increased while complete injuries, both paraplegia andtetraplegia, have decreased slightly.

Although life expectancies for individuals with a SCI continue to increase, they remain below that of the general population. Mortality rates are significantly higher during the initial year after injury compared to subsequent years, particularly for those with more severely neurologic lesionsor those who are ventilator-dependent. Prior to the 1970s, the leading cause of death among persons with a SCI was renal failure; however, improvements in urologic management have resulted in a significant drop in these deaths. Since 1973,the most common causes of death with the greatest impact on reduced life expectancy are pneumonia and septicemia.

## DATA ON SCIS IN THE PEDIATRIC POPULATION

Approximately 20% cases of traumatic SCIs occur in individuals younger than 21 years of age, with 3% to 5% of injuries occurring in those younger than 15 [2-8]. Despite this relatively low incidence of SCIs in children and adolescents, individuals with pediatric-onset SCI will make up a proportionately greater percentage of those living with a SCI because of their longer life spans. Furthermore, as compared to those with adult-onset SCI, individuals with pediatric-onset SCI are unique in several ways. First, as a result of their younger age at injury and longer lifespan, individuals with pediatric-onset SCI will be particularly susceptible to long-term complications related to a sedentary lifestyle, such as cardiovascular disease, and overuse syndromes, such as upper extremity pain. Second, they experience relatively unique complications, such as scoliosis and hip dysplasia, which may impact them both during childhood and as adults. Persons with pediatric-onset SCI also have unique developmental needs. They not only experiencethe typical ongoing challenges of each developmental stage (e.g., childhood, adolescence) but also changes owing to their SCI. Moreover, normative and SCI-specific changes occur within a larger environmental context that itself undergoes transformation over time. Finally, individuals with pediatric-onset SCI also face health system discontinuities, such as the transition from pediatric medical care to adult care and the transition from parent-controlled health care to self-management.

In 1987, the Shriners Hospitals for Children SCI database was established in conjunction with the NSCISC at University of Alabama at Birmingham. Information about pediatric-onset SCI presented in this section is derived from combining these two databases and includes data from approximately 14,000 individuals injured prior to 21 years of age. Although these databases are not population-based, they have the advantage of having a large sample size and represent a significant geographic diversity in the U.S. The age ranges chosen for descriptive purposes are birth to 5 years, 6 to 12 years, 13 to 15 years, and 16 to 21 years, representing early childhood, middle childhood, early adolescence, and late adolescence/ emerging adulthood, respectively.

**Table 1. Relationship between age at injury and gender and race**

|            | Male | Female | Caucasian |
|------------|------|--------|-----------|
| 0-5 years  | 51%  | 49%    | 63%       |
| 6-12 years | 58%  | 42%    | 60%       |
| 13-15 years| 69%  | 31%    | 70%       |
| 16-21 years| 83%  | 17%    | 66%       |
| 22+ years  | 81%  | 19%    | 64%       |

**Table 2. Etiology of spinal cord injuries as a function of age at injury**

|                  | 0-5 years | 6-12 years | 13-15 years | 16-21 years | 22+ years |
|------------------|-----------|------------|-------------|-------------|-----------|
| Motor Vehicle    | 65%       | 52%        | 41%         | 49%         | 44%       |
| Violence         | 9%        | 22%        | 19%         | 22%         | 16%       |
| Sports           | < 1%      | 11%        | 28%         | 18%         | 8%        |
| Falls            | 6%        | 6%         | 8%          | 8%          | 24%       |
| Medical/surgical | 12%       | 5%         | 3%          | < 1%        | 3%        |
| Other            | 8%        | 5%         | 1.5%        | 2%          | 5%        |

**Table 3. SCI due to violence as a function of age at injury, gender and race**

|  | Male | Female | Caucasian | African American | Hispanic |
|---|---|---|---|---|---|
| 0-5 years | 10% | 7% | 6% | 26% | 9% |
| 6-12 years | 29% | 11% | 17% | 35% | 29% |
| 13-15 years | 21% | 13% | 8.5% | 58% | 36% |
| 16-21 years | 23% | 13% | 6% | 64% | 50% |
| 22+ years | 17% | 12% | 7% | 37% | 34% |

Table 1 illustrates the frequency of injuries per age at injury group. Gender differences have been found in incidence rates. In children 5 years of age and younger, injuries are equally proportional in males and females [9]. Males, however, are more likely to sustain SCIs than females during adolescence, which is consistent withthe adult SCI population (Table 1). With regards to ethnic/ racial distributions, similar to the experience of adults with SCI, minorities are more likely to sustain SCI than Caucasians.

Table 2 demonstrates the etiology of SCI as a function of age at injury. Similar to adults, motor vehicle crashes are the most common cause of SCIs in children and adolescents, followed by violence and sports. Sports–related SCIs primarily occur in the two adolescent age at injury groups, with diving and American football being the leading activities. In comparison to the adolescent groups, sports and violence are less common etiologies of SCIs in those 5 years and younger, whereas the most common are motor vehicle incidents and medical/surgical causes. In contrast to adults, falls are a relatively uncommon etiology of SCI in children and adolescents.

Although it is generally assumedthat violence is a more common cause of SCIs in adolescents and young adults than in younger children, it is a significant cause of injuries for children of all ages. Violence-related SCIs occurred in 9% of children ages 0 to 5 years, 22% of those 6 to 12 years and those 16 to 21. Males and persons in lower socioeconomic groups are more likely to sustain violence-related SCIs (Table 3). Although males in all age groupings were more likely than females to sustain their SCI from violence, this was most marked in those injured at 6 years and above. In all age groupings, violence as a cause of SCI was least common in Caucasians, and more prominent in African-American or Hispanic individuals. This was particularly evident in both of the African American adolescent age groups and the older Hispanic adolescent group where violence caused 50% or more of the SCIs.

# PEDIATRIC-SPECIFIC SCI ETIOLOGIES

There are various SCI etiologies that are unique to the pediatric population, including lap-belt injuries, birth injuries, child abuse [10], and transverse myelitis. Ischemic infarction of the spinal cord as a result of a nucleus pulposus embolism may also be mistakenly diagnosed as transverse myelitis [11]. Additionally, children with skeletal dysplasias, juvenile idiopathic arthritis, and Down syndrome are susceptible to cervical SCIs (ref), and rarely C1-C2 subluxation may result from inflammation related to tonsillophayrngitis [12].

Lap-belt injuries most commonly occur in children weighing between 18.2 to 27.3 kilograms [13]. These injuries ensue from the lap-belt, which rises above the pelvic brim, acting as a fixed anterior fulcrum resulting in flexion/distraction forces in the mid-lumbar spine. There are three manifestations of lap belt injuries: abdominal wall bruising, intra-abdominal injuries and spinal cord damage. The abdominal wall bruising is caused by trauma from the lap-belt and ranges from abrasions and contusions to full-thickness skin loss. Common intra-abdominal injuries include tears or perforations of the small or large intestine, with injuries less frequently occurring to the liver, spleen, pancreas, kidneys, bladder or uterus. With a lap-belt injury, injury forces are localized to the mid-lumbar spine. The most common location for vertebral damage is between L2 to L4, with a Chance fracture, characterized by compression injury to the anterior portion of the vertebral body and a transverse fracture through the posterior elements of the vertebra and the posterior portion of the vertebral body. Twenty-three percent to 30% of patients with lap-belt related injuries have a SCI without radiographic abnormality (SCIWORA, see below). Lastly, it is not uncommon for children with lap belt injuries to have concomitant cervical level injuries that may be related to the shoulder component of a three-point restraint. The neurological level in children with lap belt injuries can vary from conus or cauda equina lesions as a result of the mid-lumbar vertebral damage, to lower thoracic lesions as a result of concomitant damage to the spinal cord immediately cephalad to the conus, or to mid-thoracic levels as a result of vascular damage. In order to reduce the incidence of lap belt injuries, it is recommended that children 2 years or older should use a forward-facing car seat for as long as possible, up to the highest weight (generally above 18.2 kilograms) or height allowed by their car safety seat's manufacturer. All children whose weight or height is above the forward-facing limit for their car safety seat should use a belt-positioning booster seat in the back seat until the vehicle seat belt fits properly, which is typically when they have reached 1.45 meters in height and are between 8 and 12 years of age. Seat belts fit properly when the lap belt lays across the upper thighs and the shoulder belt fits across the chest [14].

SCIs incurred in the newborn period are relatively uncommon with an incidence of approximately 1 per 60,000 births [15]. The most common injury is an upper cervical lesion which is usually caused by torsional forces during delivery. SCIs related to breech deliveries most commonly cause lower cervical or upper thoracic injuries and are due to traction forces during delivery. Thoracic or lumbar lesions are the least common presentation of neonatal SCI and may result from vascular occlusion associated with umbilical artery catheters or paradoxical air embolism through transitional vascular shunts. Neonatal SCI may have associated brachial plexus or phrenic nerve injuries or hypoxic encephalopathy.

Acute transverse myelitis presents with symmetrical motor and sensory deficits with progression over hours to several days [16]. Initial symptoms may include paresthesias or back pain. The severity of the neurologic deficits range from complete to various degrees of sensory, motor, bladder and bowel preservation. In addition, the degree of recovery ranges from significant recovery to persistent neurologic deficits. For the vast majority of pediatric-onset cases, there are no identifiable causes of transverse myelitis; however, some cases may be associated with viral infections such as Epstein-Barr, cytomegalovirus, varicella-zoster or herpes simplex. Although transverse myelitis in adults is not infrequently related to neuromyelitis optica or autoimmune diseases such as systemic lupus erythematosus, this is uncommon in children or adolescents.

Children with Down syndrome may be at an increased risk of sustaining a SCI secondary to atlanto-axial instability, which is related to ligamentous laxity [17,18]. An atlanto-dens interval (ADI) greater than 4.5 mm is considered abnormal and occurs in approximately 15% to 20% of individuals with Down syndrome; however, the majority of those affected are asymptomatic. Additionally, occipital-atlanto instability can occur in children with Down syndrome [17].

Children with juvenile idiopathic arthritis may develop C1-C2 instability due to synovitis of the facet and synovial joints surrounding the odontoid process and from destruction of the odontoid process as a result of inflammation [19]. Children with polyarticular juvenile idiopathic arthritis may also experience fusion of the cervical vertebra, particularly C2-C3, which may progress to further fusion of the cervical spine, placing the patient at risk of a cervical fracture and possible tetraplegia from relatively minor trauma [20].

Cervical myelopathy may be associated with Larson's syndrome and skeletal dysplasias, such as achondroplasia and Morquio syndrome [21]. Infants with achondroplasia may experience compression of the upper cervical cord and the caudal medulla as a result of a small foramen magnum [22]. In addition, individuals with achondroplasia, particularly males, are at risk of developing spinal stenosis and associated spastic paraplegia [21]. Children with dwarfing syndromes with odontoid dysplasia, such as Morquio's mucopolysaccharidosis IV, may develop atlantoaxial instability with resultant myelopathy [21].

SCIWORA occurs most commonly in children injured prior to puberty. Approximately two-thirds of children injured at 5 years of age and younger and one-third of children injured between 6 and 12 years of age will have SCIWORA. It occurs in about 20% of adolescents and adults with SCI. SCIWORA results from unique anatomic and biomechanical characteristics of the spine [23], including increased elasticity of the spine in relation to a less flexible spinal cord, shallow and horizontally oriented facet joints, anterior wedging of the vertebral bodies, vulnerability of the growth zone of vertebral end plates, and poorly developed uncinate processes [24].

## UNIQUE COMPLICATIONS IN PEDIATRIC-ONSET SCI

In addition to complications that commonly affect individuals with adult-onset SCI, those with pediatric-onset SCI also may experience relatively unique complications such as hypercalcemia, scoliosis and hip dysplasia.

Hypercalcemia affects 10% to 23% of individuals with SCI. It occurs most commonly in adolescent and young adult males and usually during the first 3 months after injury [25,26]. Hypercalcemia presumably occurs as a result of increased bone resorption as a consequence of the immobilization associated with SCI. The increased incidence of hypercalcemia in the pediatric SCI population is caused by the increased bone turnover in growing children and their large and active bone mass, particularly in adolescent males.

Spine deformities are an extremely common problem in pediatric SCI, especially if the injury is sustained prior to skeletal maturity [27,28]. For children injured prior to skeletal maturity, 98% will develop scoliosis with 67% requiring surgery. In contrast, for those whose SCI occurred after skeletal maturity, the risk of scoliosis isreduced to 20%, with approximately 5% requiring surgical correction. Spine deformities may be a result of muscle weakness or imbalance, residual deformity, or may be iatrogenic [29].

Hip dysplasia is a very common complication in children injured at a young age. In one series, hip dysplasia was observed in 100% of those injured when they were less than 5 years of age [30].

## NEUROLOGICAL LEVEL AND SEVERITY OF INJURY

Neurological level and degree of completeness vary as a function of age (Table 4) [9]. Children injured at 12 years or younger are more likely to have paraplegia and complete lesions. In contrast, similar to adults, adolescents are slightly more likely to have tetraplegia than paraplegia. Adolescents, however, are slightly more likely to have complete injuries than adults. The prevalence of paraplegia in the two youngest age at injury groups may be related to the fact that the most common etiologies of their SCI are motor vehicle crashes and medical/surgical, whereas the prevalence of tetraplegia in adolescents may be related to sports-related injuries, which are more likely cervical. The greater prevalence of violence-related SCIs, which tend to cause complete injuries, in adolescents may account for the greater occurrence of complete lesions in this age group compared to adults. Furthermore, there is a greater prevalence of falls in older adults, which more commonly cause incomplete injuries, than in adolescents. Younger children are more likely to sustain upper cervical injuries and less likely to have C4 to C6 injuries. Among children who sustained their SCI at 12 years of age or younger, 8 to 10% have C1 to C3 lesions compared to 4% of those injured as adolescents. This higher risk for upper cervical injuries in children compared to adolescents is probably due to a proportionately larger head and underdeveloped neck musculature in infants and younger children.

The accuracy of epidemiological studies in pediatric-onset SCI may be reduced by limitations in the neurological examination and classification in children under 8 years of age, particularly those 5 years of age or younger [31-33]. The utility of the International Standards for Neurological Classification of Spinal Cord Injury (ISNCSCI) in young children is significantly limited and thus, interpretation of examination results and designation of neurological level, motor level and injury severity (ASIA Impairment Scale) must be made with prudence, particularly in children under 8 years of age. In contrast, the reliability of the ISNCSCI motor, sensory and anorectal examinations is acceptable for children and youths 8 years of age and older.

**Table 4. Neurologic level and injury severity as a function of age at injury**

|            | Paraplegia | Tetraplegia | Complete | Incomplete |
|------------|------------|-------------|----------|------------|
| 0-5 years  | 66%        | 33%         | 68%      | 30%        |
| 6-12 years | 64%        | 34%         | 62%      | 36%        |
| 13-15 years| 44%        | 54%         | 55%      | 43%        |
| 16-21 years| 47%        | 52%         | 56%      | 42%        |
| 22+ years  | 45%        | 54%         | 47%      | 51%        |

**Table 5. Cervical injuries as a function of age at injury**

|       | 0-5 years | 6-12 years | 13-15 years | 16-21 years | 22+ years |
|-------|-----------|------------|-------------|-------------|-----------|
| C1-C3 | 8%        | 10%        | 4%          | 4%          | 6%        |
| C4-C8 | 26%       | 25%        | 50%         | 47%         | 48%       |

## LIFE EXPECTANCY

The life expectancy of children and adolescents with SCI is a function of neurological level and category with longer survival with less severe lesions [34]. In addition, those injured prior to 16 years of age have a slightly lower life expectancy than that of otherwise comparably injured person who suffered their SCI as adults.

## CONCLUSION

Understanding the epidemiology of pediatric-onset SCI is important for several reasons. Long-term management of individuals with pediatric-onset SCI must take into account their susceptibility to long-term complications related to a sedentary lifestyle, such as cardiovascular disease, and overuse syndromes, such as upper extremity pain, because of their relatively long life span. Additionally relatively unique complications, such as scoliosis and hip dysplasia, may impact them during childhood as well as adulthood. Although pediatric-onset SCI are relatively uncommon, this population will make up a proportionately greater percentage of those living with a SCI because of their longer life spans.Lastly, SCI prevention programs for children and adolescents must take into account the unique epidemiologic features of pediatric-onset SCI.

## REFERENCES

[1]   DeVivo M. J. Epidemiology of Spinal Cord Injury. In: Lin V, ed. Spinal Cord Medicine Textbook, Second Edition. *Spinal.* Demos, New York, New York, 2010, 78-84.

[2]   Nobunaga A. I, Go B. K, Karunas R. B. Recent demographic and injury trends in people served by the Model Spinal Cord Injury Care Systems. *Arch Phys Med Rehabil,* 1999;80:1372-1382.

[3]   Price C., Makintubee S., Herndon W., et al. Epidemiology of traumatic spinal cord injury and acute hospitalization and rehabilitation charges for spinal cord injuries in Oklahoma, 1988-1990. *Am J Epidemiol,* 1994; 139:37-47.

[4]   Bracken M. B., Freeman D. H., Hellenbrand K., Incidence of acute traumatic hospitalized spinal cord injury in the United States, 1970-1977. *Am J Epidemiol,* 1981;113:615-622.

[5]   Colorado Department of Public Health and Environment. 1995 *Annual Report of the Spinal Cord Injury Early Notification System.* Denver: Colorado Department of Transportation Printing Office; 1996.

[6]    Hadley M. N., Zabramski J. M., Browner C. M., et al. Pediatric spinal trauma. Review of 122 cases of spinal cord and vertebral column injuries. *J Neurosurg*, 1988;68:18-24.

[7]    Hamilton M. G., Myles S. T., Pediatric spinal injury: Review of 174 hospital admissions. *J Neurosurg*, 1992;77:700-704.

[8]    Kewalramani L. S., Kraus J. F., Sterling H. M., Acute spinal-cord lesions in a pediatric population: Epidemiological and clinical features. *Paraplegia,* 1980;18:206-219.

[9]    Vogel L. C., DeVivo M. J., Pediatric spinal cord injury issues: etiology, demographics, and pathophysiology. *Top Spinal Cord Inj Rehabil,* 1997; 3:1-8.

[10]   Gabos P. G., Tuten H. R., Leet A., et al. Fracture-dislocation of the lumbar spine in an abused child. *Pediatrics*, 1998;101:473-477.

[11]   Toro G., Roman G. C., Navarro-Roman L., Cantillo J., Serrano B., Vergara I., Natural history of spinal cord infarction caused by nucleus pulposus embolism. *Spine* 1994; 19:360-366.

[12]   Wilberger J. E. Jr., Clinical aspects of specific spinal injuries. In: Wilberger JE Jr, ed. Spinal Cord Injuries in Children. *Mount Kisco: Futura Publishers*, 1986;69-95.

[13]   Apple D. F., Murray H. H., Lap belt injuries in children. In: Betz RR, Mulcahey MJ, eds. The Child With a Spinal Cord Injury. *Rosemont: American Academy of Orthopaedic Surgeons*, 1996; 169-177.

[14]   National Highway Traffic Safety Administration. *http://www.nhtsa.dot.gov/portal/site /nhtsa/menuitem.9f8c7d6359e0e9bbbf30811060008a0c/.* Accessed October 6, 2011.

[15]   Ruggieri M., Smarason A. K., Pike M., Spinal cord insults in the prenatal, perinatal, and neonatal periods. *Dev Med Child Neurol*, 1999;41:311-317.

[16]   Knebusch M., Strassburg H. M., Reiners K., Acute transverse myelitis in childhood: Nine cases and review of the literature. *Dev Med Child Neurol*, 1998:40;631-639.

[17]   Tredwell S. J., Newman D. E., Lockith G., Instability of the upper cervical spine in Down syndrome. *J Pediatr Orthop.*, 1990;10:602-606.

[18]   Ward W. T., Atlanto-axial instability in children with Down syndrome. In: Betz RR, Mulcahey MJ, eds. The Child with a Spinal Cord Injury. *Rosemont: American Academy of Orthopaedic Surgeons*, 1996;89-96.

[19]   Nathan F. F., Bickel W. H., Spontaneous axial subluxation in a child as the first sign of juvenile rheumatoid arthritis. *J Bone Joint Surg*, 1968; 50A:1675-1678.

[20]   Vogel L. C., Lubicky J. P., Cervical spine fusion not protective of cervical spine injury and tetraplegia. *Am J Orthopaedics*, 1997;26:636-640.

[21]   Goldberg M. J., Orthopedic aspects of bone dysplasias. *Orthop Clin of N Am*, 1976;7:445-455.

[22]   Yang S. S., Corbett D. P., Brough A. J., et al. Upper cervical myelopathy in achondroplasia. *Am J Clin Path*, 1977;68:68-72.

[23]   Pang D., Wilberger J. E., Spinal cord injury without radiographic abnormalities in children. *J Neurosurg*, 1982;57:114-129.

[24]   Osenbach R. K., Menezes A. H., Spinal cord injury without radiographic abnormality in children. *Pediatr Neurosci,* 1989;15:168-175.

[25]   Maynard F. M., Immobilization hypercalcemia following spinal cord injury. *Arch Phys Med Rehabil.* 1986;67:41-44.

[26]   Tori J. A., Hill L. L., Hypercalcemia in children with spinal cord injury. *Arch Phys Med Rehabil*, 1978;59:443-447.

[27] Dearolf W. W. III, Betz R. R., Vogel L. C., et al. Scoliosis in pediatric spinal cord-injured patients. *J Pediatr Orthop*, 1990;10:214-218.

[28] Lancourt J. E., Dickson J. H., Carter R. E., Paralytic spinal deformity following traumatic spinal-cord injury in children and adolescents. *J Bone Joint Surg.* 1981;63A:47-53.

[29] Betz R. R., Orthopaedic problems in the child with spinal cord injury. *Top Spinal Cord Inj Rehabil*, 1997;3:9-19.

[30] Miller F., Betz R. R., Hip joint instability. In: Betz RR, Mulcahey MJ, eds. The Child with a Spinal Cord Injury. *Rosemont: American Academy of Orthopaedic Surgeons*, 1996;353-361.

[31] Mulcahey M. J., Gaughan J., Betz R. R., Johansen K. J., The international standards for neurological classification of spinal cord injury: reliability of data when applied to children and youth. *Spinal Cord* 2007;45: 452-459.

[32] Mulcahey M. J., Gaughan J., Betz R. R., Vogel LC. Rater reliability on the ISCSCI motor and sensory scores obtained before and after formal training in testing technique. *J Spinal Cord Med* 2007;30: S146-S149.

[33] Vogel L. C., Samdani A., Chafetz R., Gaughan J., Betz R. R., Mulcahey M. J., Intra-rater agreement of the anorectal exam and classification of injury severity in children withspinal cord injury. *Spinal Cord,* in press.

[34] Shavelle R. M., DeVivo M. J., Vogel L. C., Strauss D. J., Paculdo D. R., Long-term survival after childhood spinal cord injury. *J Spinal Cord Med*, 2007; 30:S48-54.

In: Epidemiology of Spinal Cord Injuries
Editors: V. Rahimi-Movaghar, S. B. Jazayeri et al.

ISBN: 978-1-61942-894-2
©2012 Nova Science Publishers, Inc.

*Chapter 4*

# THE EPIDEMIOLOGY OF TRAUMATIC SPINAL CORD INJURY IN CANADA

## *Jefferson R. Wilson and Michael G. Fehlings[1]*

University of Toronto Department of Surgery, Canada

## ABSTRACT

An understanding of region specific spinal cord injury(SCI) epidemiology is important for the targeting of primary preventive efforts and to understand deficiencies in current clinical care practices. The epidemiology of traumatic SCI in Canada appears similar to data published from other developed countries throughout the world such as the United States and the United Kingdom. Current estimates of SCI incidence in Canada range from approximately 23 to 52 per million per year with prevalence estimated at 1290 per million. As the Canadian population continues to age, we anticipate a greater number of elderly patients presenting to acute care centers predominately with cervical SCI. Throughout this chapter we will explore in detail the available Canadian epidemiologic data for traumatic SCI while making comparisons to data from countries around the world.

## INTRODUCTION

Although the devastating effects of spinal cord injury (SCI) have been described for centuries, a proven therapy, highly effective in preserving neurological tissue and maintaining function, remains elusive [1-3]. While we wait for the arrival of such a therapy, a different but complementary strategy to reducing the burden of SCI at a societal level, is primary prevention [4,5]. Such prevention strategies require an accurate and up to date description of injury epidemiology in the region of interest, including specific information on injury

---

[1] Corresponding Author: Michael G. Fehlings MD PhD FRCSC FACS Professor of Neurosurgery Krembil Chair in Neural Repair and Regeneration McLaughlin Scholar in Molecular Medicine University of Toronto Medical Director Krembil Neuroscience Center Head Spinal Program 399 Bathurst St. Toronto Western Hospital, Toronto, Ontario Canada. Email: *Michael.Fehlings@uhn.on.ca*.

incidence, the age and demographic characteristics of individuals affected, as well as the level, severity and etiology of new cases. An understanding of these details allows for targeted allocation of resources, with an overall aim of reducing the number of new injuries amongst population subgroups deemed to be at the highest risk. In addition to acute injury epidemiology, obtaining information on SCI prevalence and details surrounding non-acute features such as secondary complications and hospital length of stay, is necessary to characterize current deficiencies in the chronic care of SCI patients and to optimize outcomes in the long-term.

Although certain similarities exist, SCI epidemiology has been shown to vary considerably between countries, depending on the geographic, demographic and economic characteristics of the region examined6-8. Our goal in the current chapter is to summarize the available Canadian epidemiologic data for traumatic SCI. When relevant, we will make comparisons with other countries, to create an international contextual framework.

## CANADIAN GEOGRAPHY AND POPULATION CHARACTERISTICS

With a total landmass area of almost 10,000,000 km$^2$, geographically, Canada is the second largest country in the world [9] (Table 1). However, with a total population of approximately 34,000,000 (36th largest in the world), the population density is low with many communities separated by long distances from the larger urban centers [10]. Canada's geographical and population characteristics pose significant challenges to delivery of health care, especially to those injured in trauma. Since level 1 trauma centers almost exclusively exist within the larger urban centers, trauma patients often require transport across long distances which can lead to delays in obtaining definitive medical and surgical care. Fortunately, large trauma triage networks, combined with dynamic medical transport systems, help to mitigate such barriers to care.

Canada is divided into 10 provinces and 3 northern territories, with the eastern provinces of Ontario and Quebec harboring over half of the country's total population. According to reports of the World Bank, Canada is considered a "High-Income" country, with a Gross Domestic Product of approximately 1.5 trillion USD and an average annual family income of 74,000 USD [11]. The nation's health care system is publically funded and administered primarily at a provincial level. Sole governmental healthcare administration within Canada facilitates the accurate tracking of health epidemiologic patterns and statistics. However, since administration proceeds primarily from individual provincial governments, healthcare databases and trauma registries exist predominately at a provincial as opposed to a national level.

## INCIDENCE

Published incidence rates of SCI in Canada are variable depending on the region and specific study examined. Four studies form the basis for existing Canadian estimates, with 3 providing data from the province of Ontario and 1 based on Alberta data [12-15] (Table 2). At present, there is no published study of the epidemiology of SCI at a national level.

**Table 1. Important Canadian Statistics**

| Characteristic | Value |
|---|---|
| Population | 34 million (36th in world) |
| Land Mass Area | 10 million km2 (2nd in world) |
| Population Density | 3.41/km2 (228th in world) |
| Gross Domestic Product | 1.5 Trillion USD |
| Annual Family Income | 74,000 USD |
| Health Care System | Publically funded and administered |

**Table 2. Canadian SCI Incidence Estimates**

| Study Author | Incidence Estimate |
|---|---|
| Pickett et al, 2003 | 37.2 – 46.2 per million |
| Dryden et al, 2003 | 44.3 – 52.5 per million |
| Pickett et al, 2006 | 41.9 per million |
| Couris et al, 2010 | 23.1 – 24.2 per million |

Based on analysis of the Ontario Trauma Registry between 1994 and 1999, Picket et al calculated the annual age adjusted incidence rate to range from 37.2 to 46.2 per million [15]. These results are commensurate with the findings of another Ontario study which employed injury codes within a hospital medical records database and found the annual incidence rate for individuals age 15-65 years to be 41.9 per million [14]. Children less than 14 years old and elderly individuals older than 65 had different annual incidences of 3.4 per million and 50.9 per million respectively. Couris et al estimated the annual incidence of SCI in Ontario through use of a province wide hospital discharge registry [13]. From 2003-2006 the age adjusted incidence ranged from 23.1 per million to 24.2 per million. A single study has evaluated SCI incidence outside of Ontario, within the province of Alberta [12]. Between 1997 to 2000, Dryden et al gathered injury event data from three sources including a provincial dataset, the provincial trauma registry and the Office of the Medical Examiner.

Coalescing information from these sources, the annual incidence rate was determined to be 44.3 per million. This estimate rose to 52.5 per million once SCI patients who died prior to hospital admission were considered.

Summarizing the existing Canadian literature, it appears that incidence rates of SCI range from approximately 23 to 52 per million per year. This figures falls within international incidence estimates ranging from 10 to 85 per million [16-29]. The variation in estimates from Canadian studies is likely the result of several factors including regional variation in demographics and injury patterns, differences in data sources and diagnostic coding, as well as differences in inclusion criteria and study methodology.

# GENDER

In all of the Canadian studies examined, males experienced a higher incidence of SCI as compared to females, across all age groups considered [12-15]. Depending on the specific study, the overall male to female injury ratio rate ranged from 2.5 to 3.0:1. Dryden et al showed the magnitude of this ratio varies depending on the specific age category considered: approximately 1.5:1 in children and elderly patients, and 2.2 to 3.5:1 in patients aged 10 to 69 [12]. As regards etiology, falls and motor vehicle accidents were the predominant mechanisms amongst both sexes however, injuries resulting from violence or those wherein individuals were struck by or against an object, were most commonly experienced by men [15]. Amongst existing Canadian studies there have been no specific differences noted between males and females with respect to presenting neurological level or injury severity.

## AGE

Regardless of gender, the distribution of SCI incidence rates in Canada appear bimodal with the first peak occurring in adolescence and younger adulthood (between 15 and 30 years old) and the second peak occurring in the older adult stage (greater than 70 years old) [12]. The first peak is related to an increase in injuries secondary to violence, sports accidents, and motor vehicle accidents, whereas the second peak is related to an increase in fall related SCI in the elderly [12,13,15]. As regards neurological level of injury, for older adults and elderly patients, 95% of injuries occurred in the cervical region as compared to 75% when all age groups are considered [14]. The high proportion of cervical injuries amongst the elderly likely reflects their increased fall risk combined with their higher background risk for cervical spondylosis with concomitant spinal canal narrowing. The latter point is supported by the fact that the majority of the SCI cases without a fracture were observed in older patients suggesting a pre-existing degree of spinal stenosis in these patients. In spite of documented differences in injury etiology and level , there has been no report of differences in injury severity depending on age. Based on the information above, we can summarize that as the incidence of SCI changes across the lifecycle it is apparent that injury specific characteristics also evolve. In younger age groups we observe cervical, thoracic and lumbar injuries resulting primarily from motor vehicle accidents and other high energy mechanisms which often result in bony spinal injuries in concert with neurological tissue injuries. In contrast, the prototypical elderly SCI patient presents with a cervical injury, after a fall, typically in the absence of significant bony spinal column disruption.

As the average life expectancy continues to increase, the demographic structure within Canada changes also, with individuals older than 65 expected to comprise 16% of the national population by 2016 [30]. This demographic restructuring will undoubtedly change the face of SCI epidemiology in the country and lead to a greater number of elderly patients presenting with SCI. Based on what we know at present, primary preventive efforts, specifically aimed at fall prevention, are urgently needed to reduce the burden of SCI in the coming years [31].

## LEVEL/SEVERITY

Commensurate with the findings of previous international studies, Canadian data support the observation that cervical injuries are the most common, accounting for 61 to 75% depending on study examined [7,12-15]. Thoracic and lumbosacral injuries are substantially less common, and account for 15% and 10% of all SCI respectively. As noted previously, cervical SCI occurs at a proportionately higher rate amongst older patients(>60 years old), whereas thoracic and lumbosacral injuries are more frequent in the younger population(<60 years old). Spinal fractures were noted to occur commonly with thoracic and lumbar injuries, however only 56% of cervical injuries were associated with a concurrent bony injury [14].

Unfortunately, of Canadian epidemiologic SCI studies only 2 report on initial injury severity [12,14], with only one of these articles using the internationally accepted American Spinal Injury Association classification system for reporting SCI severity [14,32]. This likely reflects the fact that the majority of these studies rely on large administrative datasets or province wide registries, many of which would not incorporate system specific injury details. Pickett et al reported that ASIA Impairment Severity (AIS) grade A injuries (motor sensory complete) were most common followed by AIS grade D (incomplete injury with distal motor power greater than 3/5 in at least 50% of muscles), ASIA grade C (incomplete injury with distal motor power greater than 3/5 in less than 50% of muscles) and AIS grade B (incomplete with distal sensory preservation but no distal motor function) injuries, in order of decreasing frequency [14]. There was a significant association between complete injuries and the presence of spinal column fractures, particularly burst fractures and bilateral facet fracture-dislocations. Central cord syndrome was the most commonly observed syndrome amongst patients with incomplete injuries, with anterior cord syndrome and Brown-Sequard syndrome observed less frequently.

# ETIOLOGY

Motor vehicle accidents and falls are the 2 most common causes of traumatic SCI in Canada with motor vehicle accidents accounting for 25-56% of injuries and falls accounting for 19-47% of injuries, depending on the study examined [12-15]. Other common causes of SCI include sport injuries (9.3-11%), assault (2.2-5%), and self inflicted injuries (1.3-2.0%). One of the ongoing problems with performing a comparative analysis of SCI etiology between studies, is the lack of uniformity in the classification of etiology [7]. Not only do individual studies use different etiology categories, additional difficulty lies in understanding what is included in the categories utilized. For instance, are diving accidents included with sport injuries? Are falls from a height included with falls from standing, or, should they be separated? Are off road vehicle accidents considered motor vehicle accidents? Such questions need to be addressed before a methodologically sound comparison can take place. In spite of these issues, results from Canadian studies are in agreement with international studies, supporting motor vehicle accidents and falls as the 2 most common injury etiologies [6,7,33].

# EARLY MORTALITY

For purposes of this chapter, we define early mortality as death occurring between the time of injury and the time of acute care discharge. Two separate time windows can be considered in this period: 1) the pre-hospital time and 2) the acute hospital admission period, between admission and patient discharge to home or rehabilitation. In Canada the pre-hospital case fatality rate for SCI has been reported at 15.8% [12]. Amongst those who died in the pre-hospital setting the median age was 27, 63% were male, with the vast majority of injuries (87%) occurring at the cervical level. In addition, 68% of these patients had evidence of co-existent traumatic brain injuries or poly-system trauma. Once admitted, the case fatality rate for SCI patients during acute hospital stay ranges from 7-11%. These estimates are in agreement with previous population-based studies from the United States that have reported in-hospital SCI fatality rates to range from 3.6 to 21.5%34-39. Risk factors for in-hospital mortality gleaned from the Canadian literature include age over 60, male sex, cervical neurological level of injury and injury from a fall.

## ACUTE HOSPITAL STAY

The average length of time between acute hospital admission and acute care discharge for patients with traumatic SCI in Canada ranges from 10 to 22 days [14,15]. Picket et al reported longer acute hospitalization with a progressively worse degree of injury severity with AIS grade A patients staying an average of 25 days, AIS grade B patients an average of 16 days, AIS grade C patients an average of 17.9 days and AIS grade D patients an average of 7.4 days [14]. Other factors associated with longer duration of hospital stay included cervical level of injury, self inflicted injuries and injuries related to gunshot wounds and motorcycle accidents. Canadian length of stay figures are in agreement with US data from 24 Model Systems centers indicating that the average length of stay for SCI patients in the acute care unit in 1999 was 16 days [6]. In Canada, approximate 50% of SCI patients are discharged directly to rehabilitation units with the remainder going to long term care facilities or home [14].

## PREVALENCE

In the absence of any population based epidemiologic data, a precise estimate of SCI prevalence in Canada is lacking. However, there has been an attempt to estimate prevalence using known epidemiologic parameters. In unpublished research coordinated by the Rick Hansen Institute, investigators used age-specific discharge incidence rates and average life expectancies from previous US and Canadian studies to calculate the expected number of Canadians alive with a diagnosis of SCI [40,41]. Using these techniques they estimated that there are 43,974 patients living with SCI as a result of trauma; 19,232 with paraplegia and 24,742 with quadriplegia. This would translate into a Canadian prevalence rate of approximately 1,290 per million, using 2010 population statistics. Interestingly, this prevalence figure is substantially higher than recent reports from Australia and the United States in which estimates ranged from 681 to 750 per million [8,42]. The explanation for this discrepancy likely rests in differences in study methodology and in the significant assumptions made when generating this Canadian estimate. Nonetheless, this serves as a starting point and as a point of reference for future epidemiologic studies attempting to answer this question.

## COMPLICATIONS AND HEALTH CARE UTILIZATION

Complications occur with a high frequency after SCI leading to increased length of hospitalization, higher rates of mortality and diminished functional recovery. In our own unpublished series of 435 SCI patients, 137 (39.1%) experienced 245 complications. Of these, 96 were cardio-pulmonary (39.2%), 89 were infectious (36.3%), 28 were surgical (11.4%), 21 were thrombotic (8.6%) and 11 involved decubitus ulcer development (4.5%). Previous published research from the Fehlings group has indicated a trend towards an increased incidence of secondary complications amongst the elderly, however in the same study, preexisting co-morbidities were more common amongst the elderly, a factor which may have contributed to a higher rate of complications amongst these individuals [43]. The incidence of complications after SCI in other developed countries ranges from 20% to 35% across the literature [7]. Obviously these comparisons are inherently challenging given the heterogeneity in complication categorization and depending on the specific time period considered after injury.

As regards long-term complications, Dryden et al followed 233 SCI patients in Alberta over a 6 year period and reported that 47.6% were treated for a urinary tract infection, 33.8% for pneumonia, 27.5% for depression and 19.7% for decubitus ulcer development [44]. In the same study, patients with SCI were randomly matched to controls from the general population to gauge relative utilization of healthcare resources. The authors found that SCI patients were hospitalized 2.6 times more often, had 2.7 times the number of physician office visits and required 30 times the amount of home care services as compared to the control group. The median length of stay for the initial period of hospitalization, including acute care and inpatient rehabilitation, was 139 days for patients with complete injuries and 50 days for patients with incomplete injuries. In a follow-up study from the same group and based on the same patient population, the average healthcare costs in the first year for a patient with a complete injury was 121,600 CDN dollars, whereas the average costs in the first year for a patient with an incomplete injury was found to be 42,100 CDN dollars [45].

## CONCLUSION

To summarize, Canadian SCI epidemiology appears consistent with data published from other developed countries throughout the world such as the United States and the United Kingdom. As the Canadian population continues to age, we expect a concurrent change in SCI epidemiology and anticipate a greater number of elderly patients presenting to acute care centers predominately with cervical SCI. One major drawback of existing Canadian SCI studies is that they are primarily based on data obtained from a single province or from a specific region within a province, with a national perspective largely absent at present. As such, our knowledge of SCI prevalence within Canada is based largely on approximated figures, from estimation models, with a number of attendant assumptions. One major step forward would be the creation of a unified Canadian SCI registry which would enable a much more rigorous and comprehensive evaluation of national epidemiologic parameters.

# REFERENCES

[1]    Wilkins R, ed. Neurosurgical Classics. Chicago: American Association of Neurological Surgeons; 1992.

[2]    Hawryluk G, Roland J, Kwon B, Fehlings M. Protection and repair of the injured spinal cord: a review of completed, ongoing, and planned clinical trials for acute spinal cord injury. *Neurosurgical Focus* 2008;25:E14.

[3]    Rowland J, Hawryluk G, Kwon B, Fehlings M. Current status of acute spinal cord injury pathophysiology and emerging therapies: promise on the horizon. *Neurosurgical Focus* 2008;25:E2.

[4]    Wigglesworth E. Towards prevention of spinal cord injury: the role of a national register. *Paraplegia* 1988;26:389-92.

[5]    Bedbrook G. Update on spinal cord paralysis. A preventable injury, a surgical challenge? *Aust N Z J Surg* 1991;61:478-81.

[6]    Sekhon L, Fehlings M. Epidemiology,demographics, and pathophysiology of acute spinal cord injury. *Spine* 2001;26:S1-12.

[7]    Ackery A, Tator C, Krassioukov A. A global perspective on spinal cord injury epidemiology. *J Neurotrauma* 2004;21:1355-70.

[8]    Wyndaele M, Wyndaele J. Incidence, prevalence, and epidemiology of spinal cord injury: what learns a worldwide literature survey? *Spinal Cord* 2006;44:523-9.

[9]    Significant Canadian Facts. 2011. (Accessed June 15, 2011, at *http://atlas.nrcan.gc.ca/auth/english/learningresources/facts/supergeneral.html*.)

[10]   Canada's population clock. 2011. (Accessed June 15, 2011, at *http://www.statcan.gc.ca/pub/82-003-x/pop/pop-h-clock-eng.htm*.)

[11]   Open Data. 2003. (Accessed at *www.worldbank.org/data*.)

[12]   Dryden D, Saunders L, Rowe B, et al. The Epidemiology of Traumatic Spinal Cord Injury in Alberta, Canada. *Canadian Journal of Neurological Sciences* 2003;30:113-21.

[13]   Couris C, Guilcher S, Munce S, et al. Characteristics of adults with incident traumatic spinal cord injury in Ontario Canada. *Spinal Cord* 2010;48:40-4.

[14]   Pickett G, Campos-Benitez M, Keller J, Duggal N. Epidemiology of Traumatic Spinal Cord Injury in Canada. *Spine* 2006;31:799-805.

[15]   Pickett W, Simpson K, Walker J, Brison R. Traumatic Spinal Cord Injury in Ontario, Canada. *J Trauma* 2003;55:1070-6.

[16]   Albert T, Ravaud J. Rehabilitation of spinal cord injury in France: a nationwide multicentre study of incidence and regional disparities. *Spinal Cord* 2005;43:357-65.

[17]   Surkin J, Gilbert B, Harkey H, Sniezek J, Currier M. Spinal Cord Injury in Mississippi. Findings and evaluation, 1992-1994. *Spine* 2000;25:716-21.

[18]   O'Connor P. Incidence and patterns of spinal cord injury in Australia. *Accid Anal Prev* 2002;34:405-15.

[19]   Burke D, Linden R, Zhang Y, Maiste A, Shields C. Incidence rates and populations at risk for spinal cord injury: A regional study. *Spinal Cord* 2001;39:274-8.

[20]   Karacan I. Traumatic spinal cord injuries in Turkey: a nation-wide epidemiological study. *Spinal Cord* 2000;38:697-701.

[21]  Warren S, Moore M, Johnson M. Traumatic head and spinal cord injuries in Alaska (1991-1993). *Alaska Medicine* 1995;37:11-9.

[22]  Martins F, Freitas F, Martins L, Dartigues J, Barat M. Spinal cord injuries epidemiology in Portugal's central region. *Spinal Cord* 1998;36:574-8.

[23]  Chen Y, Chen S, Chiu W, et al. A nationwide epidemiological study of spinal cord injury in geriatric patients in Taiwan. *Neuroepidemiology* 1997;18:241-7.

[24]  Maharaj J. Epidemiology of spinal cord paralysis in Fiji. *Spinal Cord* 1996;34:549-59.

[25]  Silberstein B, Rabinovich S. Epidemiology of spinal cord injuries in Novosibirsk, Russia. *Paraplegia* 1995;33:183-8.

[26]  van Asbeck F, Post M, Pangalila R. An epidemiological description of spinal cord injuries in The Netherlands in 1994. *Spinal Cord* 2000;38:420-4.

[27]  Otom A, Doughan A, Kawar J, Hattar E. Traumatic spinal cord injuries in Jordan - an epidemiological study. *Spinal Cord* 1997;35:253-5.

[28]  Karamehmetoglu S. Traumatic spinal cord injuries in southeast Turkey: an epidemiological study. *Spinal Cord* 1997;35:531-3.

[29]  Karamehmetoglu S. Traumatic spinal cord injuries in Istanbul, Turkey. An epidemiological study. *Paraplegia* 1995;33:469-71.

[30]  Canada's Aging Population. 2004. (Accessed June 15, 2011, at *http://www.sustreport.org/signals/canpop_age.html.*)

[31]  O'Connor P. Trends in spinal cord injury. *Accid Anal Prev* 2006;38:71-7.

[32]  AmericanSpinalInjuryAssociation, ed. International Standards for Neurological Classification of Spinal Cord Injury. Chicago IL; 2000.

[33]  DeVivo M. Causes and costs of spinal cord injury in the United States. *Spinal Cord* 1997;35:809-13.

[34]  Gerhart K. Spinal cord injury outcomes in a population-based sample. *J Trauma* 1991;31:1529-35.

[35]  Griffin M, Optiz J, Kurland L, al e. Traumatic spinal cord injury in Olmstead County, Minnesota. *Am J Epidemiology* 1985;121:884-95.

[36]  Krause J, Sternberb M, Lottes S, Maides J. Mortality after Spinal Cord Injury: An 11-year prospective study. *Arch Phys Med Rehab* 1997;78:815-21.

[37]  Thurman D, Burnett C, Jeppson L. Surveillance of spinal cord injuries in Utah, USA. *Paraplegia* 1994;32:665-9.

[38]  Surkin J, Smith M, Penman A. Spinal cord injury incidence in Mississippi: a capture-recapture approach. *J Trauma* 1998;45:502-4.

[39]  Price C, Makintubee S, Herndon W, Istre G. Epidemiology of traumatic spinal cord injury and acute hospitalization and rehabilitation charges for spinal cord injuries in Oklahoma, 1988-1990. *Am J Epidemiology* 1994; 139:37-47.

[40]  Noonan V, Fingas M, Farry A, et al. The incidence and prevalence of spinal cord injury in Canada: A National Perspective. in press 2011.

[41]  The Incidence and Prevalence of Spinal Cord Injury in Canada Overview and estimates based on current evidence. Rick Hansen Institue, 2010. (Accessed June 15, 2011, at *http://www.urbanfutures.com/reports/Report%2080.pdf.*)

[42]  O'Connor P. Prevalence of spinal cord injury in Australia. *Spinal Cord* 2005;43:42-6.

[43] Krassioukov A, Furlan J, Fehlings M. Medical Co-Morbidities, Secondary Complications, and Mortality in Elderly with Acute Spinal Cord Injury. *J Neurotrauma* 2003;20:391-9.

[44] Dryden D, Saunders L, Rowe B, et al. Utilization of health services following spinal cord injury: a 6-year follow-up study. *Spinal Cord* 2004; 42:513-25.

[45] Dryden D, Saunders L, Jacobs P, et al. Direct health care costs after traumatic spinal cord injury. *J Trauma* 2005;59:443-9.

In: Epidemiology of Spinal Cord Injuries
Editors: V. Rahimi-Movaghar, S. B. Jazayeri et al.

ISBN: 978-1-61942-894-2
©2012 Nova Science Publishers, Inc.

*Chapter 5*

# EPIDEMIOLOGY OF SPINAL CORD INJURIES ON BRAZIL

*Ana Cristina Ferreira Garcia*

Dr. Henrique Santillo Rehabilitation and Readaptation
Center, CRER- Goiânia, Goiás, Brazil

## INTRODUCTION

Spinal cord injury (SCI) occurrence is more common in recent years due to increasing urban violence. The sequelae of spinal cord injury leads to a health problem as many cases are irreparable.

About 15 to 20% of people who suffer a spinal fracture have an associated spinal cord injury [2]. In such cases, greater complexity and length of hospital stay contribute to an increased hospitalization cost. Overall, the average time of hospitalization for SCI is 9.2 days, twice the time of natural causes [3]. Hospitalizations for injuries resulting from trauma generated a cost of $102 million; this represents the third largest expense and the sixth leading cause of hospitalizations.

### SUS admissions for trauma, Brazil, 2000 to 2005

| SUS admissions for trauma, Brazil, 2000 to 2005:Year | Patients Number |
|---|---|
| 2000 | 12.962 |
| 2001 | 12.156 |
| 2002 | 17.650 |
| 2003 | 19.537 |
| 2004 | 20.717 |
| 2005 | 21.684 |

In Brazil, there are several published studies on the epidemiology of spinal cord injury, but there is no general data on the incidence and prevalence, since this is a nonreportable condition. Therefore, the data presented here are from several studies published in the country.

The study of spinal cord injury in this population is important since the results of this work could enable the development of preventive and educational campaigns. These campaigns could be effective in reducing the incidence, and preventing the disabilities of spinal cord injury.

Brazil is the fifth largest country, with about 8.500.000 Km$^2$, which portends important regional differences, both geographic and cultural [4]. In 2001, a study was published which demonstrated the diversity of characteristics for spinal cord injury in the country (figure 1). [5] Twenty percent of Brazilian hospitals were selected in the DATASUS (National Information System and Data of the Ministry of Health). They received 80 (9%) of survey responses and the data was analyzed and distributed according to geographic region (North, Northeast, Southeast, Midwest and South). The survey was conducted in January 1997 and repeated in January 1998 for confirmation.

The calculation of the incidence of SCI in Brazil resulted in an annual value of 71 cases/million inhabitants [3]. Literature data has shown the annual incidence of new patients hospitalizations range from 9.2 to 53.4 per million 6,7,8,910,11. This survey showed 71 new cases per million inhabitants, a higher incidence when compared to other countries. Certain regions have higher incidences, as seen in regional analysis (Figure 1). This is mainly explained by the irregular distribution of population, resources and developmental lines in Brazil.

Also according to this survey the most frequent causes were traffic accidents, followed by falls, dives and gunshot wounds [5], as shown in Figure 2.

The male to female ratio was nine to one. The average age was 30.4 ± 15.5 years [5] . In Brazil, similar to other developed countries, young adult males are the most common patients. These subjects often put themselves in risky situations that culminate in an accident that may injure the spine. [12]

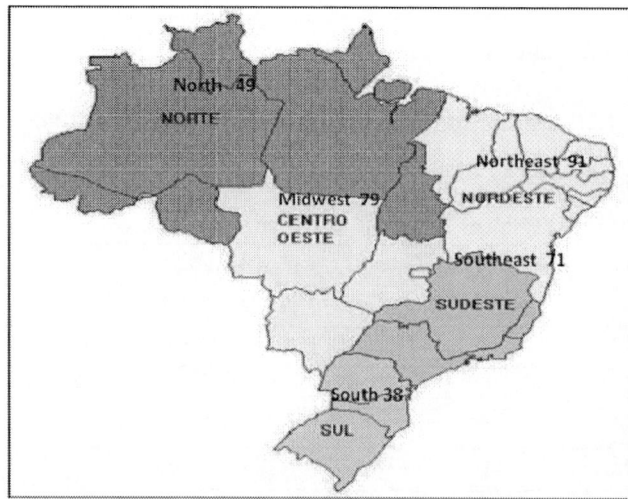

Figure 1. Distribution of the incidence rate of spinal cord injury in Brazil by geographic regions.

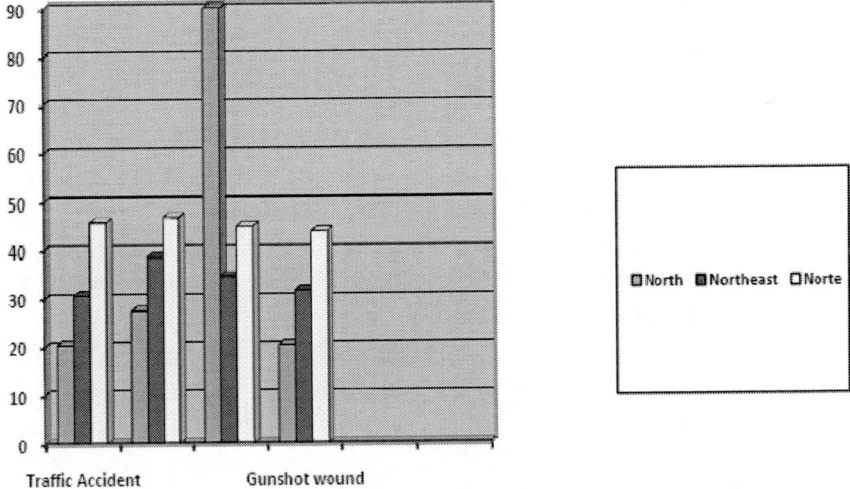

Figure 2. Causes of spinal Cord injury in Brazil ( Masini, 2001).

The following describes some of the regional differences in the epidemiological data. A study in Belem, northern Brazil, between January 2002 and August 2003 showed clear predominance of male patients (89.20%) with peak incidence between 20 and 40 years. The most common causes of SCI were falls (39.60%), followed by acts of violence (24.40%), traffic accidents (8.40%) and diving (7.20%). The most commonly affected spinal region was thoracic (35.60%), with higher incidence of fractures (55.20%). Most cases had some degree of neurological deficit [13].

In the Midwest of Brazil, data was analyzed from the Dr Henrique Santillo Rehabilitation Center, Goiania, Goias, from March 2007 to March 2009. There was a predominence of males (78.85%) with average age of 35.3 years. Paraplegia was the neurological deficit more prevalent (64.90%), 54.33% classified as ASIA A (complete lesion). The cervical and thoracolumbar transitions were the most affected spinal segments [14,15]. The average time from injury to admission was 129.72 days and the mean length of hospitalization for rehabilitation of these patients was 44.9 days. Hospitalization time for rehabilitation is still difficult to compare in Brazil because of the low number of rehabilitation centers that capture data. It is known that the rehabilitation process in most of the country still occurs later than ideal.

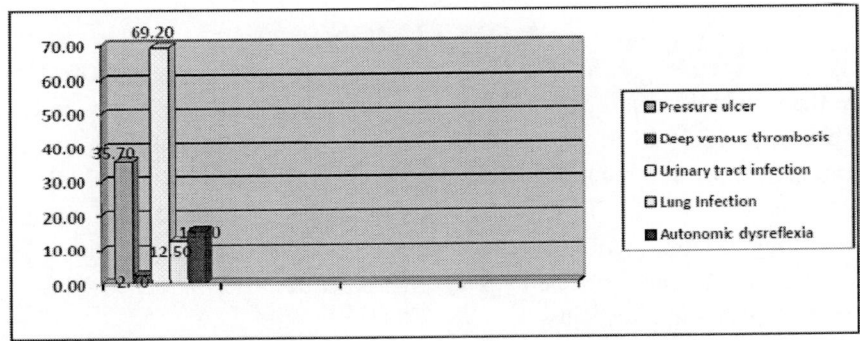

Figura 3. Complications.

Regarding the etiology, the principal cause was traumatic, 44.70% (motorcycle accidents 26.92%, and car accidents 17.78%). The second leading cause was gunshot injury. Among the complications caused by the SCI, urinary tract infection was the most prevalent, as shown Figure 3 [16].

A total of 61% used urinary catheter at admission and 83.1% performed intermittent catheterization during hospitalization. The majority of patients were admitted with an indwelling urinary catheter, which explains the high number of urinary tract infections16. Gaspar et al. [17] noted pressure ulcers were the next most common complication, present in 36%4. The prevalence of these complications in the literature varies widely from 2.7 to 29.5% [18]. The high incidence of pressure ulcers and other complications may be responsible for the high average length of hospital stay, delaying the onset of rehabilitation. This data reveals that Brazilian hospitals have difficulties with the care of SCI, with indwelling urinary catheter left for too long, and few or no protocols for prevention of pressure ulcers.

Sociodemographic status is another important aspect, along with educational level and occupation. In a study in Brasília, midwest Brazil, the most common patients were single men, since they undergo more risky situations. Most patients (53%) had only elementary school education.

The major occupation (52%) was represented by manual laborers, workers in the steel industry and farms [19].

There are regional etiology differences for spinal cord injury. Large cities have the biggest variance, as in the city of São Paulo, southeastern Brazil. A study in a rehabilitation center showed the highest etiology prevalence was gunhot injury. This may be explained by great violence in young males within the city [17]. Another study, also conducted in São Paulo, showed falling slab was the main cause of spinal cord injury. Falling slab constitutes an etiology related to areas of high population density, with pockets of poverty. This phenomenon occurs due to remodeling of buildings near brick shacks. While waiting for resources to complete house construction, the slab is transformed into a space for functional flexibility (leisure and work). This etiology requires preventive action,as well-targeted information can educate the population about the danger [20].

This condition causes high costs for health care and the irreparable damage to individuals requires preventive measures. Since the main cause is traumatic, prevention campaigns and guidance to the population is needed.

# CONCLUSION

Despite the regional variations in Brazil, automobile accidents are the main cause. There is a higher prevalence of SCI in young males, between 16 and 30 years old, and the cervical and thoracolumbar transition are most affected.

The high incidence of SCI in Brazil exceeds most published statistics from other countries, requiring careful attention. As the major etiology is preventable trauma, prevention campaigns represent the most efficient treatment to reduce the incidence of SCI and their resultant disabilities and impairments.

# REFERENCES

[1]     Greve JMA; Ares MJ. Reabilitação da lesão da medula espinhal. In: Greve JMA, Amatezzi MM. Medicina de reabilitação aplicada à ortopedia e traumatologia. *São Paulo: Roca*; 1999. p.323-24.

[2]     Delfino HLA. Trauma raquimedular. *Medicina, Ribeirão Preto*, 32: 388-400, out./dez. 1999.

[3]     Tuono, V. L. Traumas de coluna no Brasil: análise das internações hospitalares. 2008, 214f. Dissertação (Mestrado em Saúde Pública), Faculdade de Saúde Pública da Universidade de São Paulo USP: São Paulo, 2008.

[4]     IBGE, Instituto Brasileiro de Geografia e Estatística.

[5]     MASINI M – Estimativa da incidência e prevalência de lesão medular no Brasil. *J Bras Neurocirurg*, 2001 12 (2): 97-100.

[6]     Braken MB; Freeman DH; Hellenbrand K: Incidence of acute traumatic hospitalized spinal cord injury in the United States, 1970-1977. *Am J Epidemiol*, 1981 113: 615-22.

[7]     Burke DC; Toscano J: Incidence and distribution of spinal cord injury. *Menzies Foundation Technical Report*, 1987 1: 13-47.

[8]     Campos, ADP; Beraldo PSS; Almeida MCRR; Neves EGC; Alaves CMF; Khan P: Traumatic injury tothe spinal cord. Prevalence in Brazilian Hospitals. *Paraplegia*, 1992 30: 636-40.

[9]     Celani MG; Spizzichino L; Ricci S; Zampolini M; Franceschini M: Spinal cord injury in Italy: a multicenter retrospective study. *Arch Phys Med Rehabil*, 82: 589-96, 2001.

[10]    Chen CF; Lien IN: Spinal cord injuries in Taipei, Taiwan, 1978-1981. *Paraplegia*, 23: 364-70, 1985.

[11]    Delilla T: Spinal Cord Injury Program. Central registry statistics. Five-year summary January 1984-December 1988. Division of Vocation Rehabilitation, Department of Labor and Employment Security: Florida.

[12]    HCFMRP-USP. Pesquisa de incidência e comportamento sobre o trauma raquimedular, 2009.

[13]    Souza M FJ; Neves, A C A; Medeiros, A A A; Jallageas, D N. Epidemiological characteristics of spinal cord injury in the Amazon region: Prospective analysis of 250 cases. *J. Bras. Neurocir*, 2003;14(3):97-104.

[14]    Green BA; David C; Falcone S; Razack N; Klose K. Spinal Cord Injuries in Adults. In: Youmans JR. Neurological Surgery: a comprehensive reference guide to the diagnosis and management of neurosurgical. 4th ed. Philadelphia: W.B. *Saunders Company*; 1996. p.1972.

[15]    Brain L. Traumatismos de la médula espinal. In: Enfermedades del Sistema Nervioso. 2 ed. *Buenos Aires: El Ateneo*; 1965. p. 460.

[16]    Garcia ACF; Custódio NRO; Carneiro MR; Feres CC; Lima GHS; Jubé MRR; Watanabe LE; Saliba LGRSO; Daher S;. Spinal Cord Injury In Dr. *Henrique Santillo Rehabilitation And Readaptation Center* (Crer- Go) Coluna/Columna. 2009;8(3):265-268.

[17]    Gaspar AP; Ingham SJM; Vianna PCP; Santos FPE; Chamlian TR; Puertas EB. Avaliação epidemiológica dos pacientes com lesão medular atendidos no Lar de São Francisco. *Acta Fisiátrica*. 2003;10(2):73-7.

[18]  Taricco MA. Etiologia das lesões medulares. In: Greve JMA, Casalis MEP, Barros
      TEP, editores. Diagnóstico e tratamento da lesão da medula espinal. *São Paulo: Roca*;
      2001. p. 1-8.

[19]  Neves, Luciana da S. Bampi.Perceived quality of life of people with traumatic spinal
      cord injury: a way to study the experience of disability. Brasilia University, 2007.

[20]  Borelli, M; Gonlaves, AMT; Rosa,LN; D'Angelo, CT; Savordelli, CL; Bonin, GL;
      Squarcino, IM. Epidemiological features of spinal cord injury in the reference area of
      Hospital Estadual Mário Covas. *Arq Med ABC*. 2007;32(2):64-6.

In: Epidemiology of Spinal Cord Injuries
Editors: V. Rahimi-Movaghar, S. B. Jazayeri et al.

ISBN: 978-1-61942-894-2
©2012 Nova Science Publishers, Inc.

*Chapter 6*

# BRAZILIAN EPIDEMIOLOGY OF SPINAL AND SPINAL CORD INJURY

## *Ricardo Vieira Botelho, Emilio Afonso França Fontoura and Marcos Masini*

[1]Brazilian Neurosurgical Society Guidelines Director, Brazil
[2]Neurosurgery Service Director.Conjunto Hospitalar do Mandaqui. São Paulo, Brazil
[3]Honorary President of Latin American Federation of Neurosurgical Societies.
Vice Chairman, WFNS Spine Committee, Brazil

## INTRODUCTION

In 2010, Brazil had almost 200 million inhabitants. It is a large country that has a population with a varied economic and development distribution. The population's age has changed in recent years with a smaller proportion of people younger than 25 years-old and a greater proportion of older people then 65 years old (7,4%) (http://www.ibge.gov.br/home).

The country is geographically divided into five different regions: South, Southeast, Middle-east, North and Northeast. There is currently no existing literature that that describes the national epidemiology of spinal and spinal cord (SCI) study but several regional smaller studies.

To reveal the current SCI epidemiologic status , an electronic search using the LILACS database (Latinoamerican and Caribean electronic database in health sciences) was performed. The following MESH TERMS in Portuguese Language were used: Traumatismos da Medula Espinal AND "Estudos de Incidência" OR Estudos de Prevalência OR Epidemiologia. Twelve papers described the epidemiologic status with regards to SCI in the country [1-12]. The majority of papers were based on regional hospital registry data. One paper was based on a questionnaire response by all Hospitals in the National public health system [9]. One other paper was a cross-sectional study revealing the prevalence of hospitalized SCI patients [4]. One paper described specifically the epidemiology related to diving in shallow water in the City of Ribeirão Preto. Data from this later work, because of its specificity, was not polled together with other papers [12].

## STUDIED REGIONS

All regions had at least one study describing SCI patients. One study described the epidemiology in the state of Goias, city of Goiania (middle east region) [7]. Two papers were published about the same city (Belém) by the same group. This is probably revealing a continuation of the same study with one year difference, in the north region state of Para [1,11]. The other two papers were in regards to the northeast region states of Piaui [6] and Pernanbuco [2].

Two papers were based on National information: One of them was based on spinal cord injured patients hospitalized in the hospitals from the National system of public health (SUS)[9]. The other was based on SCI patients from rehabilitation Hospitals throughout the country [4]. Five papers studied the epidemiology in the state of São Paulo, in the southeast region [3,4,5,8,10].

### Table 1. Causes of SCI injury by states in studies based on direct hospital database samples. X=mean

| State/City | | | | | | |
|---|---|---|---|---|---|---|
| Causes % | Falls | Auto | Moto | Gunshot | Diving | Other |
| Pernanbuco/Recife | 1.91 | 4,76 | 19.05 | 4.76 | ___ | 9.52 |
| Goias/Goiania | 31 | 44 | 17 | 13 | 9 | 8 |
| SãoPaulo/SP (Downtown) | 14.8 | * | * | 26.9 | 9.3 | ___ |
| Pará/Belém (2002) | 41.25 | 23.15 | | 23.75 (violence) | 5 | 13 |
| Pará/Belém (2003) | 39,6 | 8.4 | | 24.4 (violence) | 7.12 | 3.6 |
| São Paulo/Fco Morato | 45.1 | 18.72 | | | | |
| São Paulo/SP (South) | 63 | 10 | 14 | 18 | ___ | ___ |
| Piauí/Terezina | 39.6 | 24.4 | | 24.4 | 7.12 | 3.6 |
| São Paulo/Sto André | 47 | 14 | 10 | 18 | ___ | ___ |
| São Paulo/SP (North) | 39 | 20 | 4 | 2.3 | 10 | 24.7 |
| X | 44 | 18.55 | 11.25 | 16.33 | 24.54 | 15.23 |

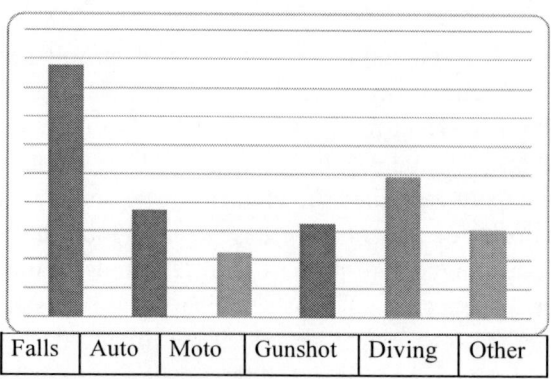

Figure 1. Distribution of SCI causes among all papers.

## SCI INCIDENCE

In three hospital based studies, the population estimate permitted a regional incidence calculation of 17 to 37 cases of SCI per million per year[3,6,10].

## CAUSES

In six studies [1,3,6,8,10,12] the most frequent cause of injury was a fall from height, primarily from rooftops. There is a unique kind of habitation in the suburbs of large urban centers in which the rooftop is often compatible with leisure activities. As a result, falls from these rooftops are relatively frequent. For this reason, rooftop falls have become a national public health problem. The described causes of SCI (rates) and their distribution are described in the table 1 and figure 1.

## AFFECTED SPINE SEGMENTS

The most commonly affected spine region was the cervical spine. Eight studies revealed that cervical spine injuries occurred 41 % of times (Table 2). *Complete SCI rates*: The average rate of Asia A and B patients (among all studies) were calculated as 26.6 percent (Table 2). This rate may have been inflated due to one study that evaluated only hospitalized SCI patients [1].

*Mortality rate*. Only two papers reported the in-hospital mortality rate. The work by Barros et al. [5] and by Souza et al.[10] reported rates of 21% and 15.2%, respectively. The first study was conducted exclusively with spinal cord injured patients and the second with severe cervical spinal trauma.

*Epidemiology in the State of Sao Paulo*. Six papers [3,4,5,8,10,13] studied the epidemiology in the state of São Paulo, the southeast country region. Three of these were based on hospitals in the Capital, São Paulo city, in three different regions of the city. Two other papers were conducted in regions described as "Great São Paulo", a larger region around the capital. One paper was described in the central part of state [13].

## EPIDEMIOLOGY OF SEVERE CERVICAL SCI

One study was conducted prospectively during 10 years in the north Zone of São Paulo city [10]. This study selected for analysis only unstable or neurologically damaged patients with Cervical spine lesions. All patients with severe CST in the north area of São Paulo City were studied. 217 hospitalized patients were evaluated. The average incidence was 21.6 cases annually or 1.8 cases monthly. The mean patient age was 36.75 years. The 20–40-year-old age bracket was found to have the highest rat of injury, corresponding to 52.6% of total patients. Patients were predominantly male; 191 patients (88.01%) were male compared with only 26 female patients (11.99%).

**Table 2. Characteristics of all epidemiological studies. Auto:automobile accidents. Moto:motorcycle accidents**

| Place | Year | Spine segment | Author | Method | N | Estimated Studied Population | Mean Age | % male | Causes | ASIA |
|---|---|---|---|---|---|---|---|---|---|---|
| Recife | 2009 | L1 38,9% T1218,5% L2 11,1% | Pereira | Specific Hospital data base | 42 | -------- | 39±15(17-70) | 73,8% | Fall from height1,91% motorcycle 19,05% auto 4,76% gun shot 4,76% others 9,52% | A=2,3% B=4,7% C=2,3% D=4,7% E=85,7% |
| Goiás | 2005 | TL 51% C=45% 1% C+T 3%SCIWORA | Barros Melissa | Rehabilitation clinic | 632 | -------- | 27 | 86,2 | Auto26% Moto 19% Fall 31% Gunshot13% 9%Diving 8%Others | 44% E 17% tetraplegia 26% paraplegia 4% tetraparesis 2% paraparesis 7% others |
| São Paulo | 1992 | cervical | Barros FIlho | Retrospective chart search.Hospital database | 428 | -------- | 0-10 -0,6% 11-20=15,7% 21-30=20,8% 31-40=27,1% 41-50=7,7% 51-60=1,9%. 61-70=1,3% | 91,8% | FAF 36,7% Traffic aciddents. 26,9% falls 22,4% diving 7,7% others 2,3% | Only Cord injured patients |
| Brazilian Hospitals | 1992 | | Campos da paz | Hospitalized cord injuried patients prevalence study | 138 | | 30,3±1,1 (6-56) | 80,6% | Traffic acidents=41,7% Firearm=26,9% Falls from heights=14,8% Shallow diving=9,3% Nknife wounds=0,9% 21,3% work accidents | A=87% (61 paraplegico and 33 quadriplegic) |

| Place | Year | Spine segment | Author | Method | N | Estimated Studied Population | Mean Age | % male | Causes | ASIA |
|---|---|---|---|---|---|---|---|---|---|---|
| Belem Para | 2002 | C=36,25 T=38,75 L=25% | Souza Junior | Prospective. Hospital based | 80 | -------- | <10=0 11-20=17 21-30=21 31-40=19 41-50=8 51-60=11 >60=4 | 83,75 | Falls=33 Auto=19 Violences=13 Diving=4 Others=10 | A=26 B=7 C=13 D=11 E=23 |
| Brasil | 2001 | Only cord injuriesr | Masini | Questionaries to public hospital of National insurance system | 93 | 159.884.278 | 30,4 ± 15,5 | | Transit acacidentes, Divings,falls, gunshot injury | -------- |
| São Paulo | 2009 | Cervical SPine | SIlva | bank data of Reference based hospital | 217 | 2.148.835 | 36.53 ± 1.06 (20-40) | | falls, motor vehicle accidents, and diving into shallow water. | A=28% B=5% C=6% D=10% E=43% Centro medular=6% |
| Francisco Morato | 2010 Maio 2005 a dezembro de 2008 | C0C3: 1,4% C3-C7: 34,7% Thoracic 14,4% TL40,5% Lumbar 8,6% | Anderli | Retrospective chart evaluation Of Hospital Based reference | 69 | 519969 | 10-20=5,8% 20-30=23,2% 30-40=29% 40-50=23,2% 50-60=7,2% | 73% | Fall from rooftop:36,4% 11,6% Car accidents 8,7% fall from heights 7,2% motorcicle | E=56,5% A=26,1% |
| São Paulo Heliópolis | ------- | C=39,5% TL=60,5% | Campos | Cross-sectional data bank study of a reference based hospital | 100 | -------- | >60=11,6% | 86% | Falls 63% Auto 20,9% Gunshot 8,1% | -------- |

**Table 2. (Continued)**

| Place | Year | Spine segment | Author | Method | N | Estimated Studied Population | Mean Age | % male | Causes | ASIA |
|-------|------|---------------|--------|--------|---|------------------------------|----------|--------|--------|------|
| Santo Andre | Set 2003 a nov 2006 | C=50% T=24% L=24% | Gonçalves | Chart retrospective study of Reference hospital based | 100 | ---------- | >21 A 40%. | 83% | Falls=47% Moto=14% FAF=18% Auto=10% | ---------- |
| Terezina | 2008 Jan 95 a dez 2002 | Cs=51% TS=30% LS=22% | Leal-Fillho | Prospective Reference Based Hospital | 386 | 3000000 | <17=9,6% 18-59=84,4% >60=6% | 86,3 | Falls=38,3% Auto=22% 11,9%=fgunshot 9,1%=moto 6,5%=diving 6,2%=local diving 3,9%=Run over 1,3% Physical aggression 0,8%=knife | A=50% B=3,4% C=16,3% D=14,8% E=15,5% |
| Belem | 2003 Jan sto200320 02 a ag | C=30,4 | Souza JR. | Reference based hospitals | | | | 89,2 | | |

The ratio of men to women was 7.35:1. Injuries in the craniocervical region corresponded to 43 (19.8%) of the cases; injuries in the subaxial cervical region corresponded to 174 (80.2%) of the cases and were associated with worse neurological lesions. Additionally, 40.6% of patients presented with complications in other organ systems; several patients presented with multiple complications, and 33 patients (15.02%) died. During the hospitalization period, 4 patients presenting as Grade A on the American Spinal Injury Association (ASIA) Scale evolved to Grade C, 1 patient presenting as ASIA Grade A evolved to Grade B, and 2 patients evolved to Grade E. Two patients who had been admitted without neurological lesions evolved to ASIA Grade C (1 patient postsurgery and 1 patient post-traction). Two patients presenting initially as ASIA Grade E evolved to Grade D, and another to a central cord syndrome clinical picture. On average, patients with incomplete lesions improved 1 grade in ASIA classification during hospitalization.

## NATIONAL BASED STUDIES

Two studies were performed using national samples of patients [9,12]. In 2001, Masini and cols. [9] conducted a one year study based on public health national information system (DataSus). Only SCI patients were studied. Data from 92 patients was collected. A total of 23% of 872 associated hospitals responded to the questionnaire.

In 1992, Campos da Paz conducted a study based on hospitalized patents interviewed by nurses, revealing the prevalence of Hospitalized SCI patients [12]. The average patients' age was 30,3±1,1 (6-56), 80,6% of them were males, 87% had complete cord lesions (ASIA A), 61 paraplegic and 33 quadriplegic patients.

A total of 138 patients were evaluated and injuries were caused by Traffic accidents (41,7%), gunshot wounds (26,9%), falls from heights(14,8%), shallow diving (9,3%) and others. This was an in-hospital SCI prevalence study.

## DISCUSSION

Spinal Cord injury is one of the most disabling injuries . Epidemiological data are fundamental to prevention programs and to estimate the amount of resources needed for primary treatment strategies.

In the majority of countries, the incidence varies from 30 to 70 new cases per year. Prevalence rate varies between 11 to 112 persons per million/year.

Brazil is a large Country with a heterogeneous population density with a diverse human development index across its several states. In this way, local or regional data tend to reveal the epidemiology more precisely than national data. As an example, in Ribeirão Preto, a central city in the State of São Paulo, one important cause of SCI is diving in shallow water.

There was an outstanding difference among the studies based on directly retrieved data from referral hospitals and those acquired by data registries or questionnaire responses. Brazilian incidence of SCI is similar to the previously published incidence in other countries, with outstanding differences related to the causes, with falls resulting in SCI in the majority of studies.

# REFERENCES

[1]   Souza Jr, MF; Neves, ACA; Medeiros A AA; Jallageas,DN.Características epidemiológicas do trauma raquimedular na Amazônia: Análise prospectiva de 250 casos. *J Bras Neurocirurg.* 2003; 14(3): 97-104.

[2]   Pereira, AFF; Portela, LED; Lima, GDA; Carneiro, WCG; Ferreira, MAC; Rangel, TAM; Santos, RBM. Avaliação epidemiológica das fraturas da coluna torácica e lombar dos pacientes atendidos no Serviço de Ortopedia e Traumatologia do Hospital Getúlio Vargas em Recife/PE. *COLUNA/COLUMNA.* 2009; 8(4):395-400.

[3]   Anderle, DV;Joaquim, AF; Soares, MS; Miura FK; Silva, FL; Veiga, JCE; Milagres, AC;.Daniel, JW; Souza, AH; Mudo, ML. Avaliação epidemiológica dos pacientes com traumatismo raquimedular operados no Hospital Estadual "Professor Carlos da Silva Lacaz". *COLUNA/COLUMNA.* 2010;9(1):58-61.

[4]   Campos, MF; Ribeiro, AT;Listik, S; Pereira, CAB; Sobrinho, JÁ; Rapaport, A. Epidemiologia Do Traumatismo Da Coluna Vertebral. *Rev. Col. Bras. Cir.* 2008; 35(2),88-93.

[5]   Barros, TEP;Taricco, MA;Oliveira, RP;Greve, JMA; SANTOS, LCR;Napoli, MMM. Estudo epidemiológico dos pacientes com traumatismo da coluna vertebral e déficit neurológico, internados no Instituto de Ortopedia e Traumatologia do Hospital das Clinicas da Faculdade d Medicina da USP. *Rev. Hosp. Clin. Fac. Med.* S. Paulo. 1990; 45(3): 123-126.

[6]   Leal-Filho, MB; Borges, B; Almeida, BR; Aguiar, AAX; Vieira, MACS; Dantas, KS; Morais, RKP; Santos, CRN; Mendes, SS; Pinheiro, LM. Spinal Cord Injury. Epidemiologycal study of 386 cases with emphasis on those patients admitted more than four hours after the trauma. *Arq Neuropsiquiatr.* 2008; 66(2-B):365-368.

[7]   Barros, MN; Basso, RC. Trauma raquimedular-Perfil epidemiológico dos pacientes atendidos pelo serviço público do estado de Goiás nos anos de 2000 a 2003. *Fisioterapia Brasil.* 2005; 6(2):141-144.

[8]   Gonçalves, AMT;Rosa LN. D'ângelo CT.Savordelli CL. Bonin GL. Squarcino IM. Borrelli M. Aspectos epidemiológicos da lesão medular traumatica na área de referência do Hospital Estadual Mario Covas. *Arq Med ABC.* 2007; 32(2):64-6.

[9]   Masini M.Estimativa da incidência e prevalência de lesão medular no Brasil. *J Bras Neurocirurg.* 2001; 12 (2): 97-100.

[10]  Santos, EAS; Santos Filho, WJ; Possatti, LL; Bittencourt, LRA; Fontoura, EAF; Botelho, RV. Epidemiology of severe cervical spinal trauma in the north area of São Paulo City: a 10-year prospective study. *J Neurosurg Spine.* 2009;,11:34–41.

[11]  Júnior, MFS; Bastos, BPR; Jallageas, DN; Medeiros, AAA. Perfil epidemiológico de 80 pacientes com traumatismo raquimedular, internados no Hospital do Pronto-Socorro Municipal de Belém, PA, noperíodo de janeiro a setembro de 2002. *J Bras Neurocirurg.* 2002; 13(3): 92-98.

[12]  Paz, AC; Beraldo, PSS; Almeida, MCRR; Neves, EGC; Alves, EMF; Khan, P. Traumatic injury to the spinal cord. Prevalence in Brazilian hospitals. *Paraplegia.*1992; 30: 636-640

[13]  Silva, CLC; Defino, HLA. Estudo epidemiológico das fraturas da coluna cervical por mergulho na cidade de Ribeirão Preto-SP. *Medicina, Ribeirão Preto.* 2002; 35:41-47.

# SECTION II: EPIDEMIOLOGY OF SPINAL CORD INJURIES IN EUROPE

In: Epidemiology of Spinal Cord Injuries
Editors: V. Rahimi-Movaghar, S. B. Jazayeri et al.

ISBN: 978-1-61942-894-2
©2012 Nova Science Publishers, Inc.

*Chapter 7*

# FALL-INDUCED CERVICAL SPINE INJURIES AMONG OLDER FINNS

## *Pekka Kannus*[1,2,*] *and Seppo Niemi*[1]

[1] Injury and Osteoporosis Research Center, UKK Institute for Health Promotion Research, Tampere, Finland
[2] Medical School, University of Tampere, and Division of Orthopaedics and Traumatology, Department of Trauma, Musculoskeletal Surgery and Rehabilitation, Tampere University Hospital, Tampere, Finland

## ABSTRACT

Although fall-induced injuries among older adults are said to be a major public health concern in modern societies with aging populations, reliable epidemiologic information on their secular trends is limited.

We assessed the secular trend in the number and incidence (per 100 000 persons) of fall-induced severe cervical spine injuries (fracture, cord injury, or both) of older adults in Finland, an EU-country with a well-defined white population of 5.3 million, by taking into account all persons 60 years of age or older who were admitted to Finnish hospitals for primary treatment of such injuries in 1970-2009. Similar patients aged 20 through 49 years served as a reference group.

The number and raw incidence of fall-induced cervical spine injury among Finns 60 years of age or older rose considerably between the years 1970 and 2009, from 37 (number) and 5.7 (incidence) in 1970 to 280 and 21.7 in 2009. The relative increases were 657% and 280%, respectively. Throughout the study period, the age-adjusted incidence of injury was higher in men than women and showed a clear increase in both sexes in 1970-2009: from 9.7 to 30.0 in men, and from 3.0 to 13.2 in women. A similar finding was observed in the age-specific incidences of the study group. In the reference group, the annual number and incidence of injury decreased somewhat over time. Assuming that the observed increase in the age-adjusted or age-specific injury incidence continues in the 60-year-old or older Finns and the size of this population increases as

* Correspondence to: Prof. Pekka Kannus, MD, PhD. UKK Institute, P.O. Box 30. FIN-33501 Tampere, Finland. email: *Pekka.Kannus@uta.fi.*

predicted, the annual number of fall-induced cervical spine injuries in this population will be almost two-times higher in the year 2030 than it was in 2009.

In Finnish persons aged 60 years or older, the number of fall-induced severe cervical spine injuries seems to show an alarming rise with a rate that cannot be explained merely by demographic changes. The finding underscores an increasing influence of falls and subsequent injuries on health and well-being of our older adults, and therefore, wide-scale fall-prevention measures should be urgently adopted to control this development.

# INTRODUCTION

Falls and fall-induced injuries in elderly people are a serious public health concern in contemporary societies with aging populations.[1-5] Approximately one-third of community-dwelling persons aged 65 years and older, and more than a half of those living in residential care facilities or nursing homes, fall every year. Furthermore, about one half of those individuals who fall do so repeatedly.[4-7] The risk of falling increases with age, functional impairment, and disability. Fall risk is highest in the frail elderly aged 90 years and older.[1]

Not all falls of older adults result in injury, but about 20% require medical attention, 5% result in a fracture, and 5-10% lead to other serious injuries, such as severe head and spine injuries, dislocations, and severe soft tissue bruises, contusions, and lacerations.[1,8-10] Of these injury categories, a fall-induced spinal cord injury or fracture to the cervical spine, alone or in combination, is relatively rare but one of the most severe and disabling conditions for the victim.[11-15].

# OBJECTIVES

Very little epidemiologic information on fall-induced cervical spine injuries in older persons is available, especially concerning their secular trends. Therefore, we assessed trends in the absolute number and incidence of fall-induced cervical spine injuries, and the gender-specific age-adjusted and age-specific incidence rates of these injuries, in the 60-year-old or older population in Finland between 1970 and 2009. Finland is an EU-country having a well-defined white population of 5.3 million inhabitants in 2009 (4.6 million in 1970).

# METHODS

The data of the fall-induced cervical spine injuries occuring in Finland from 1970-2009 originates from the National Hospital Discharge Register (NHDR). This statutory, computer-based register is the oldest nationwide discharge register in the world (in operation since 1967), and provides reliable data for severe injuries and their causes among the Finnish population.[1,16-18] The Finnish NHDR contains data on age, sex, place of residence, hospital number and department, place and cause of injury, diagnosis, day of admission and discharge, and place of further treatment. Its injury diagnoses at discharge of the patient are based on all the available clinical and radiological information obtained from the patient during the hospital stay. Concerning hospital treated acute cervical spine injuries, the final diagnosis is always based on both of these methods. The annual midyear populations were taken from the Official Statistics of Finland, the statutory, computer-based population register of the country.[19]

This epidemiologic study defined a fall-induced cervical spine injury of an older adult to be an injury (fracture, cord injury, or their combination) that occurred in a person aged 60 years or older as a consequence of a fall from standing height of 1 m or less (that is, all falls from a raised surface up to 1 m were included) that resulted in hospitalization of the victim. Thus, all patients aged 60 years or older, and for a younger reference group all patients aged between 20 and 49 years, who were admitted to hospitals in Finland for primary treatment of an acute above noted injury between January 1, 1970, through December 31, 2009, were selected from the NHDR. Cervical spine injuries caused by vehicular crashes or other high energy traumas were excluded, as were cases with codes identifying sequalae of previous injuries or their orthopedic or neurologic aftercare. The fall-induced severe cervical spine injuries were recorded from the NHDR by evaluating the primary and secondary diagnoses. According to the directives given by the Finnish National Board of Health, the first diagnosis describes the main reason for the hospital stay. The second, third and fourth diagnoses indicate other possible diseases or injuries. In calculating the gender-specific age-adjusted injury incidence (per 100 000 persons), the age adjustment was done by direct standardization using the mean population of persons aged 60 years or older between 1970 and 2009 as the standard population or reference point (a point to which each annual injury incidence was adjusted for). In this way, the population and its injury rates became comparable across the study years and allowed annual assessment of the average individual risk for fall-induced cervical spine injury. The age-specific incidences (per 100 000 persons) were calculated for three 10-year age groups (60-69, 70-79, and >80 years). For data validation and comparison, the incidence of injury was also studied in a younger reference group (patients aged 20-49 years) to determine whether possible epidemiologic changes in the study groups were specific to the older population. In each of the above noted study groups, the future incidence prediction was assessed using a linear regression model, and then, within each age and sex group, the predicted absolute number of injuries in 2030 was obtained by multiplying the incidence by the estimated number of inhabitants. This estimation was obtained from the Finnish Population Projections 2010-2030.[20]

The injury data was drawn from the entire population of Finland, thus covering completely the intended study population.. In other words, the absolute numbers and incidences of fall-induced cervical spine injuries were not cohort-based estimates but complete population results, and therefore the study, in full agreement with previous investigations, [1,2] did not use statistical analyses with confidence intervals characteristically needed in cohort or sample-based estimations.

# RESULTS

The number and raw incidence of a fall-induced cervical spine injury among 60-year-old or older Finns rose considerably between the years 1970 and 2009, from 37 (number) and 5.7 (incidence) in 1970 to 280 and 21.7 in 2009 (Figure, Panel A). The relative increases were 657% and 280%, respectively.

Throughout the study period, the age-adjusted incidence of injury was higher in men than women and showed a clear increase from 1970 to 2009: from 9.7 to 30.0 in men, and from 3.0 to 13.2 in women (Figure, Panel B). A similar finding was observed in age-specific incidences. In men, the injury incidence rates in 1970 were 10.0, 12.9, and 0.0 in the age groups of 60-69, 70-79, and 80 years or older, respectively, vs. 18.3, 38.1, and 67.7 in 2009. In women, these incidence rates were 2.1, 3.2, and 5.6 in 1970, vs. 8.7, 10.5, and 31.6 in 2009. In the younger reference group aged 20 through 49 years, the annual number and incidence of injury decreased somewhat over time: in 1970, the number and incidence were 85 and 4.5, respectively, and 58 and 2.8 in 2009 (Figure, Panels A And B). Across the study years, male predominance was clear in this age group, too: 79% and 86% of the patients were men in 1970 and 2009, respectively. If the aforementioned increase in the elderly people's age-adjusted and age-specific injury incidence continues at the same rate as in 1970-2009 and the size of the 60-year-old or older population of Finland increases as predicted (approximately 45% increase during the coming 20 years), [19] the number of fall-induced cervical spine injuries in this population will be almost two-times higher in the year 2030 (about 550 injuries) than it was in 2009 (280 injuries) (Figure, Panel C).

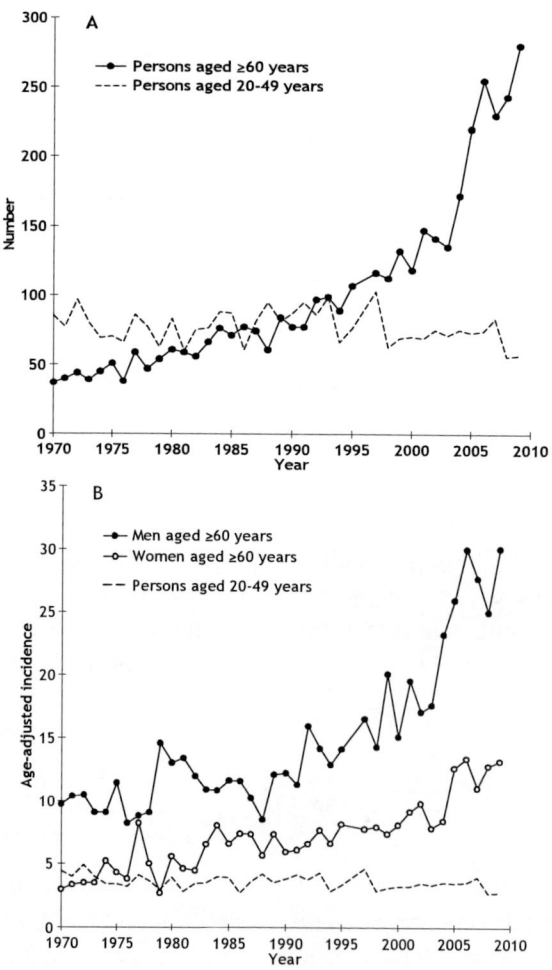

Figure 1. (Continued).

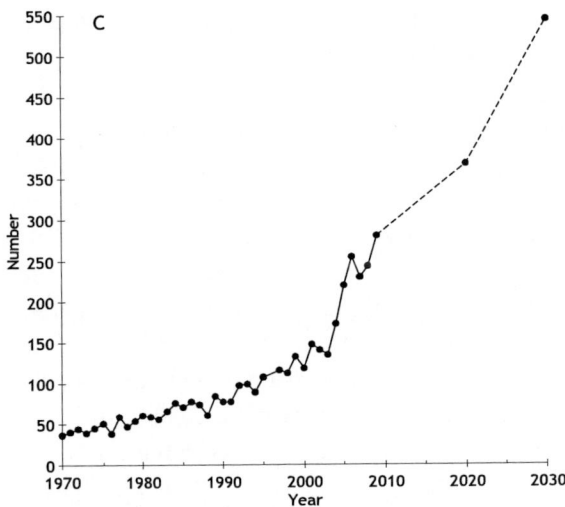

Figure 1. Number (A) and age-adjusted incidence (per 100 000 persons) (B) of fall-induced severe cervical spine injuries in Finland in people 60 years of age or older between 1970 and 2009, and prediction of the number of injuries until 2030, as calculated with a regression model (C). The number of people in this age group was 0.65 million in 1970 and 1.29 million in 2009, and is estimated to increase to 1.86 million in 2030. For comparison, the number and incidence of similar injuries in patients aged 20-49 years are shown with a dotted line in panels A and B.

## DISCUSSION

In this nationwide epidemiologic study we used the entire Finnish population aged 60 years or older to describe the trends between 1970 and 2009 for the absolute number and incidence of fall-induced cervical spine injuries in the older population. Our findings suggest that the injury incidence increases with age, is higher in men than women, and that overall number as well as the age-adjusted and age-specific incidence of these injuries clearly rose from 1970 to 2009 without signs of leveling off during the most recent years of observation. In the reference group of younger adults, such a rise was not seen. Thus, fall-induced cervical spine injuries, among other fall-related traumas, seem to represent an alarming epidemic in older populations, and the predicted growth among this group will soon accentuate the burden on our health care systems.[1,20] Our results confirm previous observations in Finland and elsewhere that various fall-induced injuries and related deaths of older adults have been a rapidly growing problem during recent decades.[1-11,21-25] They suggest further that this undesirable trend has not stopped in the new millennium. Even worse is that the further aging of the population is likely to increase the problem so that by the year 2030, Finland may face approximately 550 fall-induced injuries of the cervical spine among persons 60 years of age or older each year. This prediction requires, however, that the observed development in the incidence rates of these injuries in 1970-2009 continues between 2010 and 2030. If not, the above noted injury scenario is an overestimation. On the other hand, our assumptions on the continuously rising number of elderly adults in Finland during the coming 20 years is very robust and likely reliable. This is because all individuals who will be 60 years or older in the year 2030 have already been born. In light of these findings, Finland may have great difficulties providing the necessary standard treatments and coping with the financial burden of the fall-induced injuries of elderly adults.[7,21] Many other developed countries are likely to face a similar dilemma, although detailed, injury-specific epidemiologic data from other countries are largely lacking.

The exact reasons for the rise in the elderly people's age-adjusted or age-specific incidence of fall-induced injuries are unknown.[1,2,4,7,9] An increase in the average risk of falling - caused by impaired muscle strength, balance, and reaction time - may partly explain the phenomenon. The decrease in these domains of musculoskeletal performance have been explained by such factors as poorer physical condition, less-active lifestyle, poorer nutritional status (vitamin D and calcium), increased comsumption of cigarettes and alcohol, greater occurrence of coexisting medical problems, and the increased use of balance-affecting drugs.[1,9] On the other hand, today's older people may have more serious consequences of falling than their predecessors; that is, an increasing number of less-healthy and functionally less-capable elderly people are, among others, now surviving to older ages (e.g. due to more effective health care and life-expanding treatments and medication) and this may result in an increase in severe falls.[4,7,9]

In this study of fall-induced severe cervical spine injuries, the age-adjusted injury incidence was higher in men than women. We have made a similar finding in another group of older adults' severe falls or fall-induced deaths.[21] Since the general incidence of falling is higher in elderly women than elderly men,[1,4,7,9,22] it can be hypothesized that elderly men have an increased risk for severe falls than their female counterparts. Further studies are, however, needed to confirm these observations and examine the reasons for this gender difference.

# CONCLUSION

Because the increased number and incidence of fall-induced severe cervical spine injuries among Finnish persons 60 years of age or older between 1970 and 2009 cannot be explained merely by demographic changes, fall-prevention programs are urgently needed to control this alarming development. For older people, effective fall prevention has the potential to reduce serious fall-related injuries, emergency department visits, hospitalizations, nursing home placements, functional decline, and mortality.[7,26,27] Multifactorial interventions aimed at reducing the number of falls of elderly persons by simultaneously modifying many of the predisposing and situational risk factors for falls have shown promising results.[4,5,7,10,26,27] Also, interventions, such as strength and balance training, withdrawal of psychotropic medication, calcium and vitamin D supplementation, and home-hazard assessment and modification, have reduced the risk of falling.[7,10,26-29] We feel that now it is time for their wide-scale implementation.

# ACKNOWLEDGMENTS

This study was funded by the Competitive Research Funding of the Tampere University Hospital, Tampere, Finland, and, the Juho Vainio Foundation, the Paulo Foundation, and the Finnish Ministry of Social Affairs and Health, Helsinki, Finland.

# REFERENCES

[1]     Kannus P, Parkkari J, Koskinen S, et al. Fall-induced injuries and deaths among older adults. *JAMA*. 1999;281:1895-1899.

[2]     Kannus P, Niemi S, Palvanen M, Parkkari J. Continuously increasing number and incidence of fall-induced, fracture-associated spinal cord injuries in elderly persons. *Arch Intern Med*. 2000;160:2145-2149.

[3]     Adekoya N, Thurman DJ, White DD, Webb KW. Surveillance for traumatic brain injury deaths United States, 1989-1998. *MMWR Surveill Summ*. 2002;51:1-14.

[4]     Tinetti ME. Preventing falls in elderly persons. *N Engl J Med*. 2003;348:42-49.

[5]     Gillespie L. Editorial. Preventing falls in elderly people. *BMJ*. 2004;328:653-654.

[6]     Bergland A, Wyller TB. Risk factors for serious fall related injury in elderly women living at home. *Inj Prev* 2004;10:308-313.

[7]     Kannus P, Sievänen H, Palvanen M, Järvinen T, Parkkari J. Prevention of falls and consequent injuries in elderly people. *Lancet*. 2005;366:1885-1993.

[8]     Rivara FP, Grossman DC, Cummings P. Injury prevention. *N Engl J Med*. 1997;337:543- 547.

[9]     Kannus P, Niemi S, Parkkari J, et al. Why is the age-standardized incidence of low-trauma fractures rising in many elderly populations? *J Bone Miner Res* 2002;17:1363-67.

[10]    Gillespie LD, Robertson MC, Gillespie WJ, Lamb SE, Gates S, Cumming RG, Rowe BH.\Interventions for preventing falls in older people living in the community. Cochrane Database of Systematic Reviews 2009, Issue 2.

[11]    Liang HW, Wang YH, Lin YN, Wang JD, Jang Y. Impact of age on the injury pattern and survival of people with cervical cord injuries. *Spinal Cord*. 2001;39:375-380.

[12]    Lomoschitz FM, Blackmore CC, Mirza SK, Mann FA. Cervical spine injuries in patients 65 years old and older: epidemiologic analysis regarding the effects of age and injury mechanism on distribution, type, and stability of injuries. *Am J Roentgenol*. 2002;178:573-577.

[13]    Brolin K. Neck injuries among the elderly in Sweden. *Inj Control Saf Promot*. 2003;10:155-164.

[14]    Hagen EM, Aarli JA, Gronning M. The clinical significance of spinal cord injuries in patients older than 60 years of age. *Acta Neurol Scand*. 2005;112:42-47.

[15]    Almehmi A, Deliri H, Dameron J, Pfister AK. Fracture of the osteoporotic cervical spine from a low-level trauma. *West Virg Med J* 2005;101:71-72.

[16]    Salmela R, Koistinen V. Coverage and accuracy of the Hospital Discharge Register (Finnish) *Hospital*. 1987;49:480-482.

[17]    Keskimäki I, Aro S. Accuracy of data on diagnosis, procedures and accidents in the Finnish hospital discharge register. *Int J Health Sci*. 1991;2:15-21.

[18]    Luthje P, Nurmi I, Kataja M, Heliövaara M, Santavirta S. Incidence of pelvic fractures in Finland in 1988. *Acta Orthop Scand*. 1995;66:245-248.

[19]    Official Statistics of Finland. Structure of Population and Vital Statistics: Whole Country and Provinces, 1970-2009. Helsinki, Finland: Statistics Finland; 2010.

[20]    Official Statistics of Finland. Population Projections by Municipalities 2010-2030. Helsinki, Finland: Statistics Finland, 2009.

[21] Kannus P, Parkkari J, Niemi S, Palvanen M. Fall-induced deaths among elderly people. *Am J Public Health*. 2005;95:422-424.

[22] Shinoda-Tagawa T, Clark DE. Trends in hospitalization after injury: older women are displacing young men. *Injury Prev*. 2003;9:214-219.

[23] Cummings SR, Melton III LJ. Epidemiology and outcomes of osteoporotic fractures. *Lancet*. 2002;359:1761-1767.

[24] Langlois JA, Kegler SR, Butler JA, Gotsch KE, Johnson RL, Reichard AA et al. Traumatic brain injury-related hospital discharges. Results from a 14-state surveillance system, 1997. *MMWR Surveill Summ*. 2003;52:1-20.

[25] Kannus P, Niemi S, Parkkari J, Palvanen M, Vuori I, Järvinen M. Hip fractures in Finland between 1970-1997 and predictions for the future. *Lancet*. 1999;353:802-805.

[26] Chang JT, Morton SC, Rubenstein LZ, et al. Interventions for the prevention of falls in older adults: systematic review and meta-analysis of randomised clinical trials. *BMJ*. 2004;328:680-683.

[27] Panel on Prevention of Falls in Older Persons, American Geriatrics Society and British Geriatrics Society. Summary of the Updated American Geriatrics Society/British Geriatrics Society Clinical Practice Guideline for Prevention of Falls in Older Persons. *J Am Geriatr Soc*. 2011;59:148-157.

[28] Sherrington C, Whitney JC, Lord SR, et al. Effective Exercise for the prevention of falls: a systematic review and meta-analysis. *J Am Geriatr Soc*. 2008;56:2234-2243.

[29] Karinkanta S, Piirtola M, Sievänen H, Uusi-Rasi K, Kannus P. Physical therapy approaches to reduce fall and fracture risk among older adults. *Nat Rev Endocrinol*. 2010;6:396-407.

In: Epidemiology of Spinal Cord Injuries
Editors: V. Rahimi-Movaghar, S. B. Jazayeri et al.

ISBN: 978-1-61942-894-2
©2012 Nova Science Publishers, Inc.

*Chapter 8*

# TRAUMATIC SPINAL CORD INJURIES IN NORWAY

## *Ellen Merete Hagen*

Department of Neurology, Haukeland University Hospital, Bergen and Department of
Clinical Medicine, University of Bergen, Bergen, Norway

## ABSTRACT

The mean annual incidence of traumatic spinal cord injuries (TSCI) increased from
5.9 per million inhabitants in the period 1952–1961 to 21.2 per million inhabitants in the
period 1992–2001 based on hospital data from two counties in western Norway. On
January 1st, 2002, the total prevalence of TSCI was 365 per million inhabitants.

The mean age at time of injury was 42.9 years, and the male: female ratio was 4.7:1.
The most frequent cause of injury was falls (45.5 %), followed by traffic accidents (34.2
%). The frequency of TSCI due to traffic accidents has increased especially among men
less than 30 years of age. The frequency of TSCI due to falls and the frequency of
incomplete cervical lesions have increased especially among men over the age of 60 at
the time of injury.

In our study the level of injury was cervical in 52.4 %, thoracic in 29.5 % and
lumbar/sacral in 18.2 %. The lesion was clinically incomplete in 58.6 % and complete in
41.4 %.

Among patients with TSCI, 3.9 % were age 0–14 years at the time of injury, and
13.1 % were 15–19 years at time of injury. The average age-adjusted incidence was 2.4
per million children, and 25.1 per million adolescences. The age-adjusted incidence of
TSCI among adolescents has increased, while the age-adjusted incidence among children
has remained low. TSCI was highly associated with car and pedestrian accidents among
children. Among adolescents, TSCI was most often associated with car and motorcycle
accidents.

Among patients with TSCI, 46.7 % had a clinical concomitant traumatic brain injury
(TBI). Clinical TBI was classified as mild in 30.1 %, moderate in 11.0 % and severe in
5.7 %. Alcohol was the strongest risk factor for clinical TBI (OR = 3.69) followed by
completeness of TSCI (OR = 2.18).

There is an increasing number of elderly patients sustaining TSCI in Norway. In a
study of TSCI in patients older than 60, fall from height was the most common mode of
injury (77%). The cervical spine was the most common region of the spine injured (71%).

Cervical spinal stenosis increases the risk of TSCI caused by minor trauma. Patients older than 60 years of age at the time of injury benefitted significantly from rehabilitation.

TSCI patients have a 1.85 increase in mortality rate relative to the Norwegian population, with the first ten years after injury being associated with the highest. Complete injury is associated with reduced survival regardless of the level of injury (4.23 versus 1.25). Women have reduced survival compared to men (2.88 versus 1.72). Median survival time was 7.4 years. The cause specific standardized mortality ratio for respiratory disease was 1.96, and for suicide including 3.70 for men and 37.59 for women.

# INTRODUCTION

There are large epidemiological differences in TSCI throughout the world [1-5]. The annual incidence is reported to be from 3.4/million in West Africa to 83/million in Alaska. This is due to differences in definition, classification and procedures to identify patients with TSCI. Geographical and cultural differences also play important roles [1,6]. Most published studies include only patients who are alive upon arrival at the hospital. The incidence and prevalence of TSCI have not changed substantially over the past 30 years [5,7,8]. It is estimated that the annual incidence of TSCI, not including those who die at the scene of the accident, is approximately 40 cases/million/year in USA, or approximately 12,000 new cases each year [9]. Alaska has the highest reported incidence with 83 cases/million/year, and the incidence is especially high among Alaska Natives [10]. In Canada, rural residents were 2.5 times more likely to be injured than urban residents [11]. There are also large differences within Europe, with the highest incidence reported in Portugal (57.8/mill) [12] and the lowest in Denmark (9.2/mill) [13]. This chapter describes the epidemiology of TSCI in Norway. There are three incidence studies from Norway [14-16].

## Definition of Traumatic Spinal Cord Injury

Traumatic spinal cord injury is defined in accordance with Kraus et al [17] as an acute, traumatic lesion of the spinal cord with a varying degree of motor and/or sensory deficit or paralysis. Although injuries of the cauda equina were included, the definition excluded isolated injuries of other nerve roots [18]. In our studies from western Norway, transient paresis or impermanent deficits lasting less than one week were excluded.

## Identification of TSCI

We performed a population-based study in the years 1952–2001 from two counties in western Norway [16]. We initially identified all hospital admissions with discharge codes suggesting a TSCI from ICD-8 to ICD-10 obtained from the electronic database at Haukeland University Hospital. The hospital records from these cases were subsequently reviewed [6].

The International Classification of Diseases (ICD) has become the standard diagnostic classification for epidemiological and health management purposes, and has been subjected to continuous update and revision. We found a low diagnostic accuracy for TSCI using searches of discharge diagnoses in ICD-8, 9 and 10. A combination of 7 codes from ICD-10 gave the highest sensitivity (0.83), specificity (0.97), PPV (0.88) and LR+ (30.23) [6]. Obtaining hospital discharge diagnoses solely from electronic databases overestimates the incidence of TSCI. Identification of patients using ICD-10 codes is more complicated because acute TSCI and TSCI sequelae are listed with several codes. The latest ICD version proved to be most reliable when identifying patients with TSCI. However, ICD data cannot be trusted without extensive validation from research from healthcare planning or administration [6].

## Incidence

Incidence is defined as the number of patients who develop TSCI within a specified period and is expressed as the number of new cases per one million populations per year. Gjone and Nordlie found an incidence of 16.5/mill in 1974–1975 based on information from 62 Norwegian hospitals [14]. Lidal et al found an incidence of 4.5/mill in the period from 1961–1982 based on data from Sunnaas Rehabilitation Hospital [15]. A population-based study from two counties in Western Norway including all age-groups found an incidence of 13.9/mill in the period 1952–2001 [16]. The average annual incidence increased from 5.9/mill in 1952–1961 to 21.2/mill in 1992–2001 (Table 1) [16]. The incidence of TSCI in western Norway showed an increasing trend during the study period. Reviews have recalculated the incidence of TSCI in Europe to be 13.9/mill in 1975–1995 [8], increasing to 19.4/mill in 1995–2005 [5], comparable to our data [16]. Data from other Nordic countries have found an annual incidence of TSCI of 19.5/mill for the Stockholm region [19], 13.8/mill in Finland [20], and 9.2/mill in Denmark [13].

**Table 1. Incidence of TSCI in Hordaland and Sogn og Fjordane Counties, Norway during 1952–2011: Number of cases and crude annual incidence rates per 1 million inhabitants [16]**

| Years | Cases | Average population | Incidence[a] 95% CI[b] |
|---|---|---|---|
|  |  |  |  |
| 1952–1956 | 13 | 418625 | 6.2 ( 3.3, 10.6) |
| 1957–1961 | 12 | 435286 | 5.5 ( 2.9, 9.6) |
| 1962–1966 | 18 | 451137 | 8.0 ( 4.7, 12.6) |
| 1967–1971 | 29 | 468243 | 12.4 ( 8.3, 17.8) |
| 1972–1976 | 33 | 484556 | 13.6 ( 9.4, 19.1) |
| 1977–1981 | 40 | 494553 | 16.2 (11.6, 22.0) |
| 1982–1986 | 45 | 502298 | 17.9 (13.1, 24.0) |
| 1987–1991 | 33 | 513367 | 12.9 ( 8.9, 18.1) |
| 1992–1996 | 42 | 527079 | 15.9 (11.5, 21.5) |
| 1997–2001 | 71 | 539969 | 26.3 (20.5, 33.2) |

a) p < 0.001 for increasing trend from 1952–2001 b) Confidence intervals (CIs) based on the Poisson distribution.

## Prevalence

The prevalence of TSCI is by definition the total number of TSCI in a population at a given time, divided by the total number of individuals in that population. Prevalence is expressed as the number of cases per 100,000 or 1 million population. Data on the prevalence of TSCI is much more limited than incidence. There are few prevalence studies of TSCI. The lowest prevalence was found in India (236/mill) [21], and the highest in Canada (1,173/mill) (estimated) [22]. A review by Wyndaele found a prevalence of 755/mill in Northern America [5].

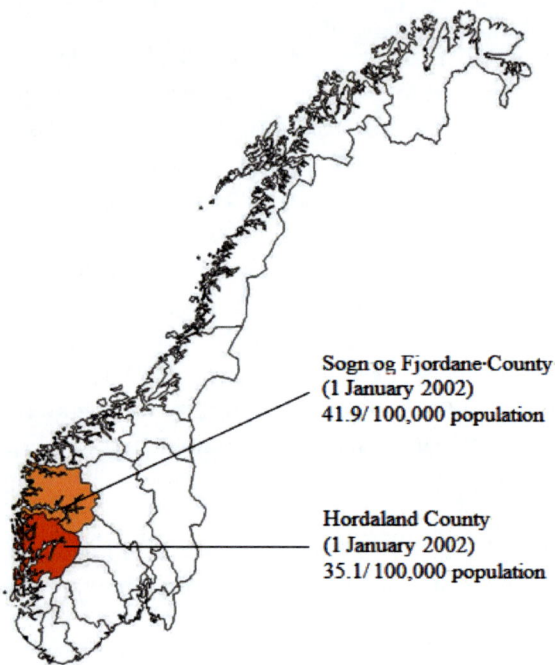

Figure 1. Reported prevalence of TSCI in Hordaland and Sogn og Fjordane counties in Norway on 1 January 2002 per 100,000 populations [25].

There are only three prevalence studies from Europe, all from Scandinavia. Dahlberg found a prevalence of 280/mill in Helsinki in 1999, [23] and Knutsdottir found a prevalence of 316/mill in Iceland in 1989 [24]. A study from western Norway found a prevalence of 365/mill inhabitants in the counties of Sogn og Fjordane and Hordaland in 2002; 419/mill in Sogn og Fjordane county and 351/mill in Hordaland county [16]. This is higher compared to previous reports from Finland and Iceland [23,24]. These studies were hospital based, and underreporting is a potential problem.

Figure 1 shows the age-specific prevalence rates of TSCI in two counties in western Norway by gender on 1 January 2002.

The crude prevalence rate was 365/mill: 120/mill among women and 610/mill among men. The male excess was highest in the age groups over 60 years as shown in Figure 2.

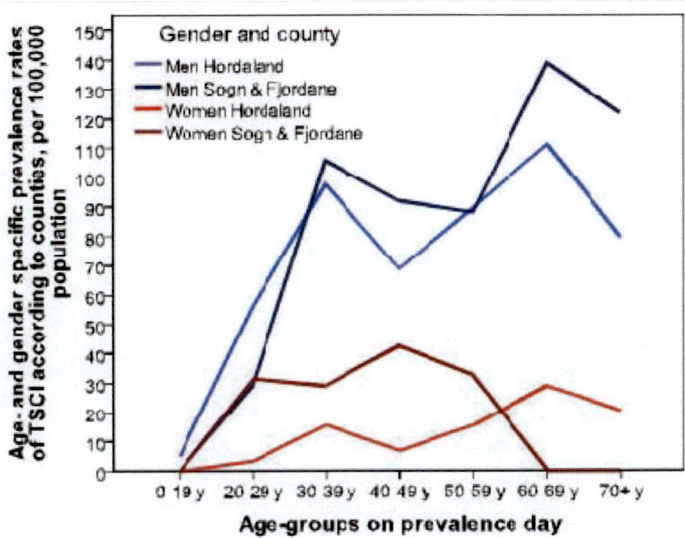

Figure 2. Age and gender-specific prevalence rates of TSCI according to age-groups, in Hordaland and Sogn og Fjordane counties, Norway on 1 January 2002, per 100,000 populations [25].

## Age and Gender

Based on a worldwide literature survey, the mean age at the time of injury is 33 years [5]. However, international studies show a significantly increased mean age at injury over the last decades, and especially an increasing number of people older than 60 years of age at time of injury.

The highest incidences of TSCI are generally reported in persons between 20 and 40 years of age [9;26]. Based on The National Spinal Cord Injury Statistical Center database, the average age at the time of injury was 29 years in 1970 and 37 years in 2005 [26].

The proportion of persons injured by age 60 has increased from 5 % to 13 % over the same period in western Norway [16]. The mean age at the time of injury in Norway was 42.9 years in the period 1952–2001 (42 years for men and 48 years for women) [16]. The average age at the time of injury increased from 40.2 years (1952–1956) to 48.9 years (1997–2001); (women: 24.7 to 57.7 years, men: 41.5 to 46.3 years).

Data from Norway (Figure 3) show an increase in age- and gender-specific incidence primarily among men and especially among men older than 60 years of age at time of injury [16]. This is similar to a study from Canada which found incidence rates for males to be consistently higher than for females in all age groups. The highest incidence of TSCI was found in patients between the ages of 15 and 29 years and in those 70 years and older [11].

There are large variations with regard to gender distribution. Most studies show a predominance of men. Data from the National Spinal Cord Injury Statistical Center database have found a slight trend toward a decreasing proportion of men from 80 % to 78 % in the period 1970–2008 [9].

In Norway, studies have found a male: female ratio of 4.7-5.0:1 [14-16]. The proportion of women increased during a 50 year period, from 15 % in the first decade to 21 % in the last decade [16].

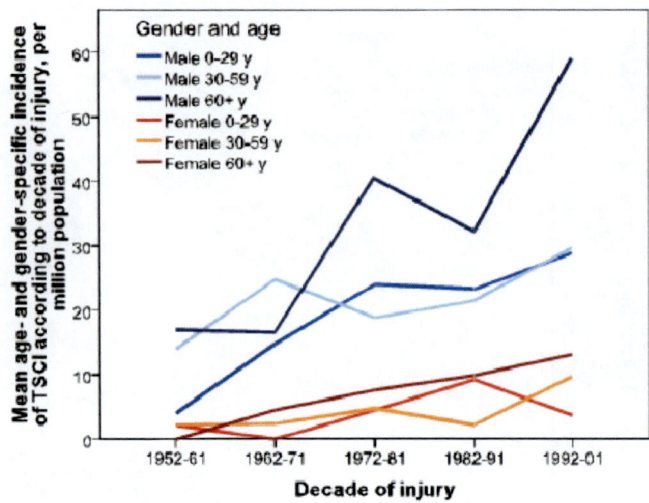

Figure 3. Mean age- and gender-specific incidences of TSCI according to decade of injury, in Hordaland and Sogn og Fjordane counties, Norway 1952 –2001, per million populations [25].

## Cause of TSCI

The causes of TSCI vary because of differences in geography and culture, but differences in data collection may explain part of this variation. The most common cause of TSCI worldwide is motor vehicle accidents (TA) [4]. In the USA, traffic accidents account for 41 % of reported TSCI, followed by fall in 27 %, assault in 15 % (primarily gunshot wounds), and recreational sporting activities in 8 % [9].Traffic accidents account for 56.4% of TSCI in Canada [11]. The highest incidence of traffic accident-related TSCI occurred in the age group 15 to 29 years (60 per million per year).

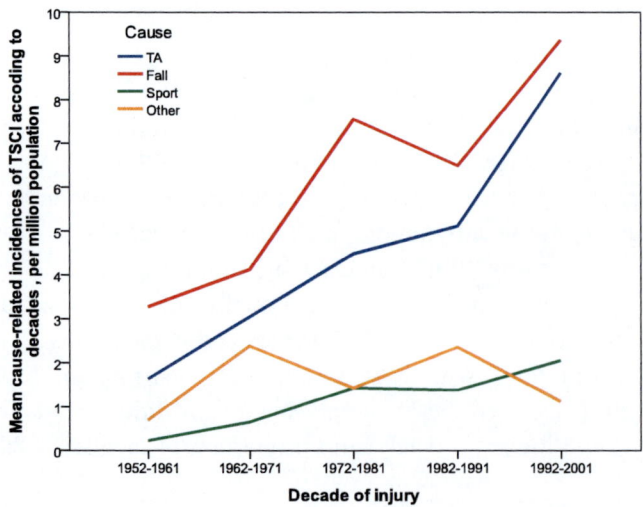

Figure 4. Mean cause-specific incidence of TSCI according to decade of injury, in Hordaland and Sogn og Fjordane counties, Norway 1952–2001, per million populations (n=336) [25].

Figure 4 shows the mean annual incidence per million populations per year according to causes of TSCI during five decades in western Norway. Fall was the most common cause of TSCI in all decades, followed by traffic accidents, and the incidence of both increased during the observation period [25].

The incidence of traffic accident related injuries increased during the observation period, especially among people younger than 30 years (Table 2) [16]. A fall is the second most common cause of TSCI in the US [9]. The proportion of fall-related injuries has increased over time in the US, and among older patients, falling from low heights in combination with spinal canal stenosis is the major cause of cervical TSCI [9].

**Table 2. Mean annual age and gender specific incidence of different causes of TSCI according to decade 1952–2001, in Hordaland and Sogn og Fjordane Counties, Norway, per million inhabitants [16]**

| | 1952-1961 | | 1962-1971 | | 1972-1981 | | 1982-1991 | | 1992-2001 | |
|---|---|---|---|---|---|---|---|---|---|---|
| | Female | Male | Female | Male | Female | Male | Female | Male | Female | Male |
| **TA [a)]** | | | | | | | | | | |
| 0-29 years | 1.08 | 2.05 | 0.00 | 7.39 | 2.72 | 11.18 | 5.63 | 14.31 | 2.84 | 19.87 |
| 30-59 years | 1.15 | 3.51 | 0.00 | 5.91 | 1.20 | 1.18 | 1.12 | 2.15 | 3.87 | 9.30 |
| 60+ years | 0.00 | 0.00 | 0.00 | 2.77 | 0.00 | 9.52 | 0.00 | 2.15 | 1.65 | 13.13 |
| **Falls** | | | | | | | | | | |
| 0-29 years | 0.00 | 2.05 | 0.00 | 4.62 | 1.89 | 7.74 | 1.65 | 3.58 | 0.00 | 2.71 |
| 30-59 years | 1.15 | 7.01 | 1.19 | 9.46 | 1.20 | 12.97 | 1.12 | 14.00 | 5.80 | 13.02 |
| 60+ years | 0.00 | 17.03 | 4.58 | 8.31 | 7.57 | 26.18 | 8.26 | 19.36 | 11.57 | 43.77 |
| **Sports** | | | | | | | | | | |
| 0-29 years | 1.08 | 0.00 | 0.00 | 1.85 | 0.00 | 3.44 | 1.88 | 3.58 | 0.95 | 5.42 |
| 30-59 years | 0.00 | 0.00 | 1.19 | 0.00 | 2.40 | 0.00 | 0.00 | 0.00 | 0.00 | 3.72 |
| 60+ years | 0.00 | 0.00 | 0.00 | 0.00 | 0.00 | 2.38 | 1.65 | 0.00 | 0.00 | 0.00 |
| **Other [b)]** | | | | | | | | | | |
| 0-29 years | 0.00 | 0.00 | 0.00 | 0.92 | 0.00 | 1.72 | 0.00 | 1.79 | 0.00 | 0.90 |
| 30-59 years | 0.00 | 3.51 | 0.00 | 9.46 | 0.00 | 4.72 | 0.00 | 5.39 | 0.00 | 3.72 |
| 60+ years | 0.00 | 0.00 | 0.00 | 5.54 | 0.00 | 2.38 | 0.00 | 10.76 | 0.00 | 2.19 |
| Total | 1.87 | 9.88 | 1.73 | 18.79 | 4.87 | 25.10 | 6.62 | 24.29 | 8.16 | 34.48 |

a) TA = Traffic accidents. b) Other injuries include violence and work-related accidents.

In younger patients, the dominant etiology is traffic accidents, followed by diving injuries and other sport-related injuries. Sports, especially diving in shallow water are a common cause in the US [9]. The proportion of injuries due to sports has decreased over time [9]. While gunshots are a frequent cause of TSCI among young patients in the US [16], only 1.5 % of TSCI in our study from western Norway were due to assault, including gunshot injuries [16].

The incidence of fall related injuries also increased during the observation period, especially among people older than 60 years (Table 2) [16].

## Cause Specific Age- and Gender-Incidences

The age- and gender-incidences of the two main causes of TSCI show two trends. The incidence of fall-related injuries among males older than 60 years increased, and the incidence of injuries due to traffic accidents in males younger than 30 increased during the observational period [16].

Table 3 shows the incidence ratio of injury from each cause obtained from multiple Poisson regression analyses. Injuries caused by motorcycles were significantly associated with decreasing age, whereas fall ≤ 1m and fall 1–5m were significantly associated with increasing age at time of injury [16].

The incidence risk for fall ≤ 1m increased 1.08 per age decade [16]. The incidence of these three causes and car accidents showed a significantly increased trend over time. The incidence risk for car accidents increased 1.67 per decade in the period 1952–2001, whereas the incidence risk of motorcycle accidents increased 1.47 per decade and fall ≤ 1m 1.66 per decade.

Men had a statistically significant increased risk of TSCI from all causes compared with women, except from pedestrian accidents, skiing accidents and other sports accidents (Table 3) [16].

## Fall-Related TSCI

The incidence of fall-related TSCI among patients older than 60 years at time of injury increased from 7.8/mill in 1952–1961 to 25.4/mill in 1992–2001 [16]. Fall-related TSCI rates are high in Western Europe (17–49 %, median 32 %) [3].

Figure 5 shows the mean age- and gender specific incidences of fall-related TSCI according to the decade of injury. There has been an increasing incidence of fall-induced TSCI in western Norway.

Increasing incidence of fall-induced, fracture-associated TSCI among persons aged older than 60 years has also been found in other studies [11;27-29], and is explained merely by an aging population [30]. Europe also has one of the highest proportions of older persons (age >60 years) in the world [3].

A recent study from Australia found a 10 % increase in number of hospitalised fall-related injuries in people aged 65 years and older from 2003–2004 to 2005–2006 [31]. Similar trends have also been found in Canada [32].

For unknown reasons the age-standardized incidence (average individual risk) of fractures in general has risen in many populations during the last decades. Studies from both Finland and Sweden have found a similar increase in fractures of the proximal humerus and hip among elderly [27,30,33]. Possible reasons include a birth cohort effect, deterioration in the average bone strength, or increased risk and severity of falls [34]. Elderly people are vulnerable to TSCI due to osteoporosis, cervical spinal stenosis, sensory loss due to polyneuropathy and side effects of medication causing postural instability [35].

Norway and the other Scandinavian countries have the highest hip fracture rates ever reported [36]. These data supports our findings of an increasing incidence of elderly men sustaining an injury from falling from a low height [25].

**Table 3. Multiple Poisson regression analyses [a] of cause-specific TSCI with respect to age at injury in decades, decade of injury and gender in Hordaland and Sogn og Fjordane Counties, Norway 1952–2001 [16]**

| Cause | Age in decade at injury | | | Decade of injury | | | Gender [b] | | |
|---|---|---|---|---|---|---|---|---|---|
| | IR | 95% CI | p-value | IR | 95% CI | p-value | IR | 95% CI | p-value |
| TA car | 0.99 | (0.98, 1.00) | 0.396 | 1.69 | (1.38, 2.10) | < 0.001 | 4.12 | (2.22, 8.24) | < 0.001 |
| TA motorcycle | 0.98 | (0.96, 1.00) | 0.027 | 1.47 | (1.06, 2.10) | 0.018 | 6.51 | (1.93, 34.19) | < 0.001 |
| TA bicycle | 1.02 | (1.00, 1.04) | 0.122 | 1.16 | (0.78, 1.77) | 0.499 | 6.41 | (1.42, 59.07) | 0.009 |
| TA pedestrian | 0.98 | (0.95, 1.01) | 0.265 | 0.92 | (0.58, 1.43) | 0.766 | 2.62 | (0.63, 15.33) | 0.239 |
| Falls $\leq$ 1 m | 1.08 | (1.06, 1.10) | < 0.001 | 1.66 | (1.25, 2.28) | < 0.001 | 3.18 | (1.51, 7.17) | 0.001 |
| Falls 1 - 5 m | 1.02 | (1.01, 1.03) | < 0.001 | 1.20 | (1.01, 1.42) | 0.035 | 2.02[c] | (1.27, 3.24) | 0.003 |
| Falls > 5 m | 1.00 | (0.99, 1.02) | 0.605 | 1.11 | (0.88, 1.40) | 0.418 | 5.64 | (2.33, 16.46) | < 0.001 |
| Swimming injuries | 0.97 | (0.93, 1.00) | 0.078 | 1.59 | (0.93, 2.99) | 0.099 | 7.72 | (1.04, 342.64) | 0.044 |
| Skiing injuries | 1.00 | (0.97, 1.02) | 0.911 | 1.39 | (0.92, 2.19) | 0.126 | 1.35 | (0.41, 4.71) | 0.777 |
| Other sports injuries | 1.00 | (0.91, 1.01) | 0.123 | 1.72 | (0.87, 4.07) | 0.136 | 4.80 | (0.54, 227.22) | 0.238 |
| Violence | 1.00 | (0.95, 1.04) | 0.923 | 0.95 | (0.48, 1.90) | 0.995 | 6.70 | (0.91, +INF) | 0.063 |
| Other injuries | 1.02 | (1.01, 1.04) | 0.004 | 1.04 | (0.81, 1.33) | 0.829 | 52.40 | (9.41, +INF) | < 0.001 |
| Total | 1.01[c] | (1.01, 1.02) | < 0.001 | 1.31[c] | (1.21, 1.42) | < 0.001 | 3.77[c] | (2.91, 4.89) | < 0.001 |

a) Exact estimates from Cytel LogXact. b) Gender: female = 0, male = 1. c) Asymptotic estimates due to lack of convergence for exact method. Abbreviations: CI = Confidence interval; IR = Incidence ratio; TA = Traffic accident; INF = Infinity.

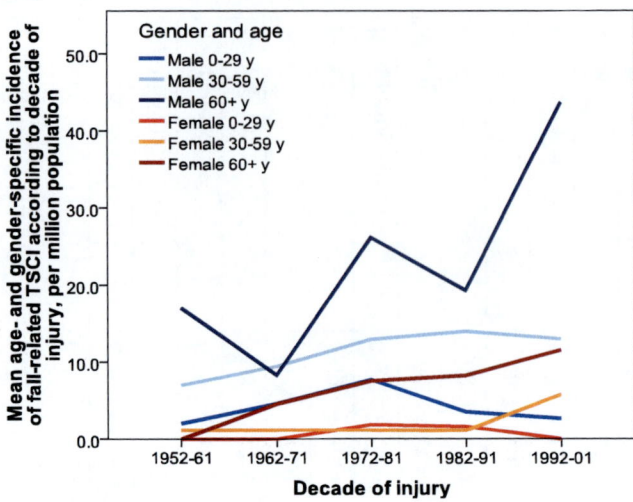

Figure 5. Mean age- and gender-specific incidences of fall-related TSCI according to decade of injury, in Hordaland and Sogn og Fjordane counties, Norway 1952 –2001, per million populations [25].

## Traffic Accident-Related TSCI

We found an increasing incidence of traffic accident-related injuries among men younger than 30 years as shown in Figure 6 [16]. Young men are less cautious and have less driving experience.

Traffic accidents are a leading global cause of injury. It is estimated that nearly 1.2 million people are killed and 20–50 million people are injured or disabled due to traffic accidents worldwide each year [37]. The incidence of TSCI is estimated to be 1.4 % of all non-fatal traffic accidents [37].

Traffic accidents accounted for 56.4 % of injuries in Canada. The highest incidence of traffic accidents related TSCI occurred between the ages of 15 and 29 years (60/mill) [32].

Traffic accidents have a multi-factorial aetiology. One of the most important factors is driver behaviour. Other factors include vehicle safety and improvements in road infrastructure.

## Level and Completeness

Level of injury varies in different regions of the world. The frequency of tetraplegia varies from 5 % in China [38] to 92 % in Turkey [39]. These differences between countries can partially be explained based on different causal patterns, but the hospital availability both geographically and economically contribute to under-reporting of TSCI in many countries. Greenland has the lowest reported frequency of tetraplegia of 33 % among the Nordic countries [40], while Iceland has the highest rate of 56 % [41].In western Norway the lesion was cervical in 52.4 %, thoracic in 29.5 % and lumbar/sacral in 18.2 %. The neurological level of lesion was clinically incomplete in 58.6 % and complete in 41.4 % of the cases [16].

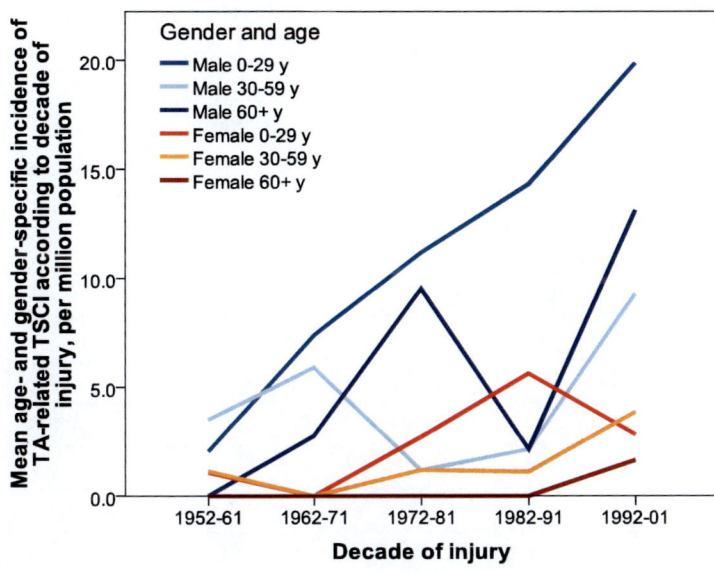

Figure 6. Mean age- and gender-specific incidences of traffic accident-related TSCI according to decade of injury, in Hordaland and Sogn og Fjordane counties, Norway 1952–2001, per million populations [25].

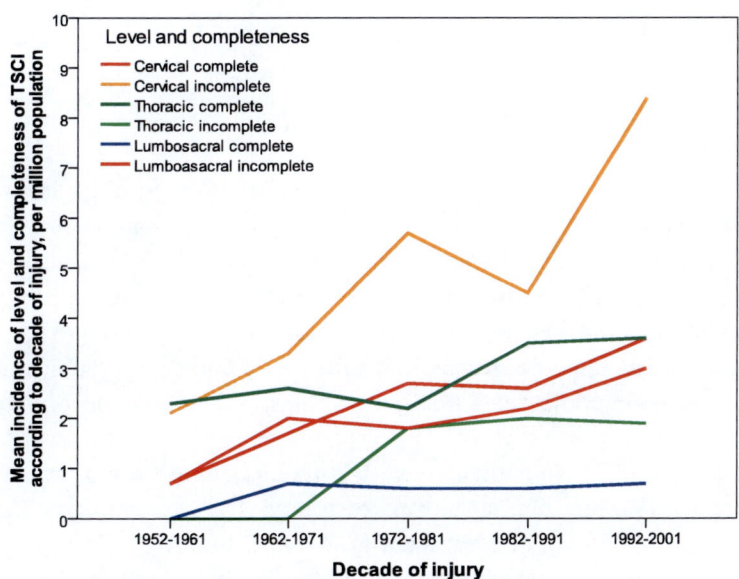

Figure 7. Mean incidence of level and completeness of TSCI according to decade of injury, in Hordaland and Sogn og Fjordane counties, Norway 1952–2001, per million populations [25].

There was an increased incidence of incomplete cervical injuries, particularly in the last decade (Figure 7) [16]. During the last 15 years, the percentage of persons with incomplete tetraplegia has increased slightly while complete paraplegia has decreased slightly [16]. The incidence of incomplete cervical lesions was highest among patients older than 50 years in our population [16].

**Table 4. Causes of trauma according to level and completeness of TSCI [16]**

| Causes | | Cervical | | Thoracic | | Lumbar-sacral | |
|---|---|---|---|---|---|---|---|
| | | Complete | Incomplete | Complete | Incomplete | Complete | Incomplete |
| | n | % | % | % | % | % | % |
| TA car | 67 | 23.9 | 25.4 | 20.9 | 13.4 | 4.5 | 11.9 |
| TA motorcycle | 23 | 13.0 | 17.4 | 43.5 | 17.4 | 0.0 | 8.7 |
| TA bicycle | 14 | 7.1 | 57.1 | 28.6 | 0.0 | 7.1 | 0.0 |
| TA pedestrian | 11 | 27.3 | 45.5 | 18.2 | 0.0 | 0.0 | 9.1 |
| Falls ≤ 1 m | 37 | 10.8 | 78.4 | 2.7 | 5.4 | 0.0 | 2.7 |
| Falls 1 - 5 m | 77 | 15.6 | 41.6 | 15.6 | 9.1 | 2.6 | 15.6 |
| Falls > 5 m | 39 | 7.7 | 10.3 | 30.8 | 7.7 | 7.7 | 35.9 |
| Swimming injuries | 9 | 44.4 | 44.4 | 11.1 | 0.0 | 0.0 | 0.0 |
| Skiing injuries | 14 | 0.0 | 14.3 | 21.4 | 14.3 | 7.1 | 42.9 |
| Other sports injuries | 6 | 16.7 | 33.3 | 16.7 | 0.0 | 16.7 | 16.7 |
| Violence | 5 | 20.0 | 40.0 | 20.0 | 20.0 | 0.0 | 0.0 |
| Other injuries | 34 | 23.5 | 32.4 | 26.5 | 2.9 | 5.9 | 8.8 |
| Total | 336 | 16.7 | 35.7 | 20.8 | 8.6 | 3.9 | 14.3 |

Abbreviation: TA = Traffic accident.

## Children and TSCI

TSCI is rare among children. Only a few population-based estimates of pediatric TSCI exist [42;43]. The incidence of SCI was 1.9/mill among children aged 0–18 years in Finland in the period 1997–2006 [42]. A study from Sweden found an incidence of 4.6/mill children [43]. If pre-hospital fatalities were excluded, the incidence was 2.4/mill [43].

We have assessed the temporal trends in the incidence and demographic characteristics of TSCI among children and adolescents in a geographically defined cohort in western Norway during 1952–2001 [44].

Of 336 patients, 13 (3.9 %) patients were 0–14 years old at time of injury, and 44 (13.1 %) patients were 15–19 years old at the time of injury. The average age-adjusted incidence was 2.4/mill children and 25.1/mill adolescences (Table 5, Figure 8). Children were injured in car and pedestrian accidents, whereas adolescences were injured in car and motorcycle accidents (Table 5) [44].

The population of children younger than 15 years in the two counties was 104 234 on January 1st 1952, and 108 336 on January 1st 2002 [45]. The population of adolescence between 15 and 19 years in the two counties was 24 966 on – January 1st 1952, and 32 563 on January 1st 2002 [45].

The average annual incidence of TSCI among children increased from 0.0/mill in the first decade (1952–1961) to 1.9/mill in the last decade (1992–2001), and for adolescents from 3.7/mill in the first decade to 39.1/mill in the last decade. The average annual incidence for all patients under the age of 20 years was 0.7/mill in the first decade increasing to 10.9/mill in the last decade (Table 5, Figure 8) [44].

**Table 5. Incidence of TSCI in children and adolescents 1952–2001, in Hordaland and Sogn og Fjordane counties, Norway: Number of cases and age-adjusted annual incidence rates per 1 million inhabitants less than 20 years of age [44]**

| Years | Age 0-19 years | | | Age 0-14 years | | | Age 15-19 years | | |
| --- | --- | --- | --- | --- | --- | --- | --- | --- | --- |
| | n | Incidence | 95 % CI | n | Incidence | 95 % CI | n | Incidence | 95 % CI |
| 1952 – 1961 | 1 | 0.7 | (0.0, 4.1) | 0 | 0.0 | (0.0, 3.4) | 1 | 3.7 | ( 0.1, 20.4) |
| 1962 – 1971 | 11 | 7.3 | (3.6, 13.0) | 1 | 0.9 | (0.0, 4.9) | 10 | 26.7 | (12.8, 49.1) |
| 1972 – 1981 | 16 | 10.5 | (6.0, 17.1) | 10 | 8.7 | (4.2, 16.1) | 6 | 15.9 | ( 5.9, 34.7) |
| 1982 – 1991 | 14 | 10.0 | (5.4, 16.7) | 0 | 0.0 | (0.0, 3.7) | 14 | 35.1 | (19.2, 59.0) |
| 1992 – 2001 | 15 | 10.9 | (6.1, 18.0) | 2 | 1.9 | (0.2, 6.9) | 13 | 39.1 | (20.8, 66.9) |
| Total | 57 | 7.9 | | 13 | 2.4 | | 44 | 25.1 | |
| P-value for trend | 0.126 | | | 0.004 | | | 0.013 | | |

Abbreviations: CI: Confidence interval based on the Poisson distribution.

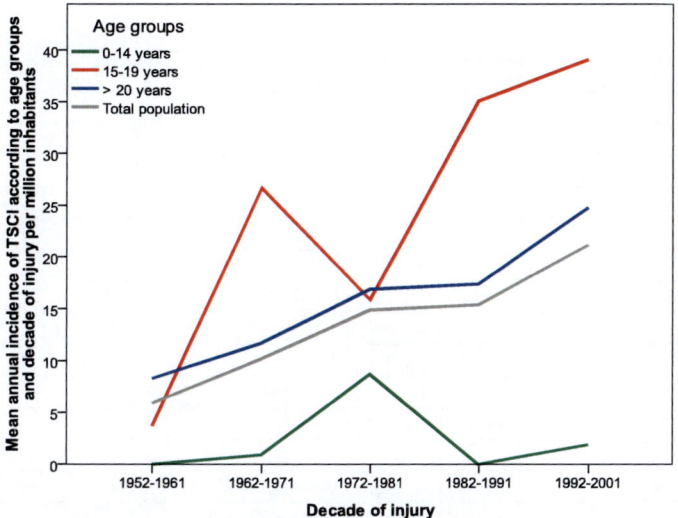

Figure 8. Incidence of TSCI according age groups at time of injury and decade of injury, per million populations in Hordaland and Sogn og Fjordane counties (n = 336) [44].

The average age-adjusted incidence of TSCI among children and adolescence in the 1990's was 13 per million in Norway [44], compared to 20 per million in the United States [46]. The higher incidence in the US is explained by TSCI caused by firearms, which did not occur in the Norwegian population. The average incidence for children was however identical to the incidence of SCI in Sweden [47].

Among the children, 53.9 % were injured in car accidents or in pedestrian accidents; whereas adolescents were more likely to be injured in car or motorcycle accidents (56.8 %) (Table 6) [44]. Eight children were under the age of 10 years at time of injury. Of these, four were injured due to pedestrian accidents and two were injured due to car accidents [44].

**Table 6. TSCI in children and adolescence 1952–2001, in Hordaland and Sogn og Fjordane counties, Norway (n = 57) [44]**

| | Age 0-19 n = 57 (%) | Age 0-14 n = 13 (%) | Age 15-19 n = 44 (%) | p-value |
|---|---|---|---|---|
| Gender | | | | 0.288[a] |
| Female | 10 (17.5) | 1 ( 7.7) | 9 (20.5) | |
| Male | 47 (82.5) | 12 (92.3) | 35 (79.5) | |
| Period of injury | | | | 0.001[a] |
| 1952–1961 | 1 ( 1.8) | 0 ( 0.0) | 1 ( 2.3) | |
| 1962–1971 | 11 (19.3) | 1 ( 7.7) | 10 (22.7) | |
| 1972–1981 | 16 (28.1) | 10 (76.9) | 6 (13.6) | |
| 1982–1991 | 14 (24.6) | 0 ( 0.0) | 14 (31.8) | |
| 1992–2001 | 15 (26.3) | 2 (15.4) | 13 (29.5) | |
| Level of TSCI | | | | 0.204[b] |
| Cervical | 22 (38.6) | 7 (53.8) | 15 (34.1) | |
| Thoracic | 21 (36.8) | 4 (30.8) | 17 (38.6) | |
| Lumbosacral | 14 (24.6) | 2 (15.4) | 12 (27.3) | |
| Completeness of TSCI | | | | 0.114[a] |
| Complete | 33 (57.9) | 10 (76.9) | 23 (52.3) | |
| Incomplete | 24 (42.1) | 3 (23.1) | 21 (47.7) | |
| Traumatic brain injury | | | | 0.068[a] |
| None | 29 (50.9) | 5 (38.5) | 24 (54.5) | |
| Mild/ Moderate | 23 (36.8) | 4 (30.8) | 17 (38.6) | |
| Severe | 7 (12.3) | 4 (30.8) | 3 ( 6.8) | |
| Causes | | | | 0.023[a] |
| Car accidents | 18 (31.6) | 3 (23.1) | 15 (34.1) | |
| Motorcycle accidents | 10 (17.5) | 0 ( 0.0) | 10 (22.7) | |
| Bicycle accidents | 3 ( 5.3) | 1 ( 7.7) | 2 ( 4.5) | |
| Pedestrian accidents | 5 ( 8.8) | 4 (30.8) | 1 ( 2.3) | |
| Falls | 10 (17.5) | 2 (15.4) | 8 (18.2) | |
| Swimming accidents | 4 ( 7.0) | 1 ( 7.7) | 3 ( 6.8) | |
| Skiing accidents | 2 ( 3.5) | 0 ( 0.0) | 2 ( 4.5) | |
| Other sport accidents | 2 ( 3.5) | 0 ( 0.0) | 2 ( 4.5) | |
| Other injuries | 3 ( 5.3) | 2 (15.4) | 1 ( 2.3) | |
| Status | | | | 0.001[a] |
| Alive[c] | 52 (91.2) | 9 (69.2) | 43 (97.7) | |
| Dead | 4 ( 7.0) | 4 (30.8) | 1 ( 2.3) | |

a) Pearson's chi-square test between the two groups.
b) Linear-by-linear chi-square test.
c) One patient injured at the age of 18.5 years emigrated 16.9 years after the injury.

In our study, 14 patients were younger than 16 years at time of injury (4.2 % of the population, n=336) [44]. Among the children, 85.7 % was male. Our data is comparable to data from the US covering the period 1973–2002, where 3.9 % of patients were below 16 years at time of injury [48]. Of these, 63.6 % were male.

Boys dominate the injuries among children which was higher than previous studies [48-50]. In the present study the only girl in the child-population was injured as a pedestrian, while the cause of injury was more diverse among the boys [44].

There was no statistical significant difference in the level of injury between children and adolescents, although there was a tendency for more cervical injuries in the children as was previously found by Bilston and Brown [51].

In the Norwegian study there were more complete injuries among the children compared to adolescents, which is in accordance with findings from the US [48].

Mild/moderate traumatic brain injury (TBI) was recorded in eight of 13 children, and four had severe TBI (Table 6).

Among the adolescents, almost half were recorded having mild/ moderate TBI, and only one of fifteen had a severe TBI. The differences between children and adolescence regarding TBI severity are most likely explained by differences in the cause of injury. This was, however, not statistically significant (Table 6) [44].

The proportion of severe TBI was higher among children as a result of the higher incidence of traffic accidents. These resulted in complete cervical injuries and concomitant TBI, which is in accordance with data from Australia [51].

Traffic accidents were the primary cause of paediatric TSCI in our population, 64.3 %, compared to 47.4 % in the US [48]. The level of injury was cervical in 50 % of the population (Table 6), compared to 47 % in the US. In our population, 71.4 % had complete injuries, higher than the 59.8 % found in the US [48].

## Age and Outcome

Historically, rehabilitation of elderly people with TSCI has been a low priority. TSCI in elderly patients has been associated with increased frequency of complications, higher mortality and poorer prognosis in this group, compared to younger patients [52,53]. Rehabilitation goals with lower-intensity treatment and lower charges for older patients were proposed as a more efficacious use of resources [54].

As the general population is aging and the mean age at the time of TSCI increases [55,56], the potential for rehabilitation is now considered a very important issue, and will even be more so in the future.

In Norway there has been an increasing number of elderly sustaining a TSCI. We studied the causes and the rehabilitation outcome of TSCI in patients older than 60 years at the time of injury [56]. We included 44 patients and calculated retrospectively the American Spinal Injury Association (ASIA) Motor score both on admission and at discharge according to patient records.

A total of 34 patients (77 %) were injured after falling from a height (24 with cervical injuries). Thirty-five patients (80 %) had incomplete lesions and had the best outcome with regard to functional level [56].

During the primary rehabilitation, 28 patients improved, two patients had declined funcion, and six patients remained unchanged as shown in Figure 9. Similar finding have later been reported from other studies [56].

MR images of 15 patients with cervical lesions revealed pre-existing cervical stenosis in 80 % [56]. A high proportion of the patients had cervical spinal stenosis and incomplete TSCI and most of them regained good function.

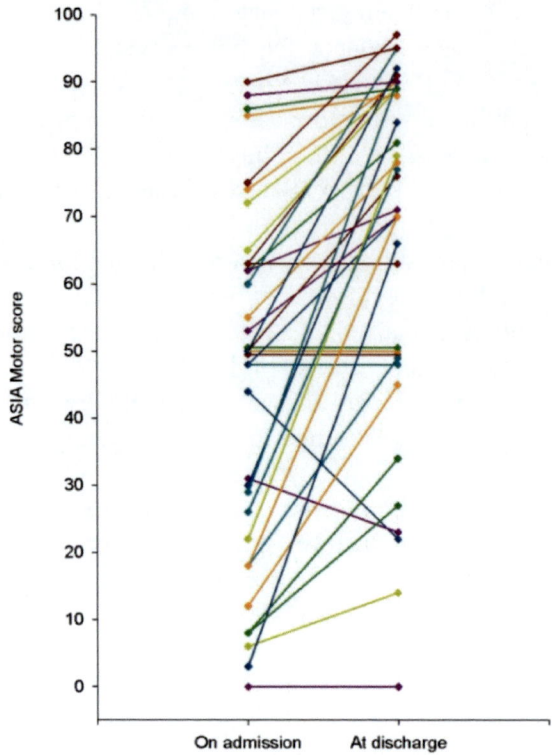

Figure 9. Change in ASIA Motor score from admission to discharge (mean time 0.4 years) among patients aged 60 years or older at time of injury, Haukeland University Hospital, Norway 1952–2001 (n = 36) [56].

Twenty-six patients (62 %) were discharged to home, 8 (19 %) to nursing homes, and 8 (19 %) to local hospitals. Three (27 %) patients with complete lesions and 23 (70 %) with incomplete lesions were discharged to home [56].

We found that patients older than 60 years of age at the time of injury also benefited significantly from rehabilitation. Cervical spinal stenosis seems to increase the risk of TSCI caused by minor trauma. This group of patients will pose a great challenge for rehabilitation [56].

## TSCI and Concomitant Traumatic Brain Injury

Patients with TSCI and a concomitant traumatic brain injury (TBI) have increased morbidity and need complex rehabilitation [57]. The incidence of head injury varies from 26 % to 74 % in different patient materials with traumatic spinal cord injury [58,59].

A prospective study found that 34 % of patients with TSCI had a mild head injury while 26 % had a severe head injury [58]. Traffic accidents and falls increased the risk of having a concomitant TBI; also cervical injuries were associated with TBI.

We assessed the temporal trends in the incidence and demographic characteristics of TSCI with clinical concomitant TBI during the period 1952–2001 [60].

Clinical traumatic brain injury (TBI) was defined as; a) no TBI where no head injury could be identified, b) mild/ moderate head injury, and c) severe head injury defined as an unconscious patient. The Glasgow Coma Scale was introduced in 1974 [61], and therefore not available in the present retrospective study. By using additional clinical information like duration of loss of consciousness or amnesia, impaired alertness or memory, we classified the patients retrospectively [60].

Of 336 patients, 157 (46.7 %) had a concomitant TBI. Clinical TBI was classified as mild in 30.1 %, moderate in 11.0 % and severe in 5.7 %. The average annual incidence increased from 3.3 per million in the first decade to 10.7 per million in the last. Alcohol was the strongest risk factor for clinical TBI (OR = 3.69) followed by completeness of TSCI (OR = 2.18) [60].

Demographic and injury characteristics of 336 patients with TSCI with or without clinical TBI are shown in Table 7. Patients with severe TBI were significantly younger than patients with mild TBI or no TBI [60].

**Table 7. Demographic and injury characteristics of 336 patients with TSCI with or without clinical TBI [60]**

| Characteristic | No TBI | Mild TBI | Moderate TBI | Severe TBI | Total | p-value |
|---|---|---|---|---|---|---|
| | n = 179 (53.3 %) | n = 101 (30.1 %) | n = 37 (11.0 %) | n = 19 (5.7 %) | n = 336 (100 %) | |
| Age (years) | | | | | | $0.009^a$ |
| Mean (SD) | 43.9 (20.7) | 45.1 (23.1) | 40.9 (20.2) | 25.7 (18.6) | 42.9 (21.6) | |
| Age-groups | | | | | | $0.003^b$ |
| Age 0-29 | 58 (46.0) | 38 (30.2) | 15 (11.9) | 15 (11.9) | 126 (37.5) | |
| Age 30-59 | 73 (60.8) | 30 (25.0) | 15 (12.5) | 2 ( 1.7) | 120 (35.7) | |
| Age 60 + | 48 (53.3) | 33 (36.7) | 7 ( 7.8) | 2 ( 2.2) | 90 (26.8) | |
| Sex, $n$ (%) | | | | | | $0.525^c$ |
| Female | 33 (55.9) | 19 (32.2) | 6 (10.2) | 1 ( 1.7) | 59 (17.6) | |
| Male | 146 (52.7) | 82 (29.6) | 31 (11.2) | 18 ( 6.5) | 277 (82.4) | |
| Alcohol, $n$ (%) | | | | | | $< 0.001^c$ |
| Yes | 19 (29.7) | 23 (35.9) | 16 (25.0) | 6 ( 9.4) | 64 (19.0) | |
| No | 160 (58.8) | 78 (28.7) | 21 ( 7.7) | 13 ( 4.8) | 272 (81.0) | |
| Status, $n$ (%) | | | | | | $0.880^c$ |
| Alive | 99 (55.9) | 51 (28.8) | 18 (10.2) | 9 ( 5.1) | 177 (52.7) | |
| Dead | 77 (50.0) | 48 (31.2) | 18 (12.3) | 0 ( 0.0) | 154 (45.8) | |
| Emigrated | 3 (60.2) | 2 (40.0) | 0 ( 0.0) | 0 ( 0.0) | 5 ( 1.5) | |
| Level of TSCI, $n$ (%) | | | | | | $0.068^a$ |
| Cervical | 86 (48.9) | 60 (34.1) | 22 (12.5) | 8 ( 4.5) | 176 (52.4) | |
| Thoracic | 51 (51.5) | 27 (27.3) | 12 (12.1) | 9 (9.1) | 99 (29.5) | |
| Lumbosacral | 42 (68.9) | 14 (23.0) | 3 ( 4.9) | 2 ( 3.3) | 61 (18.2) | |
| Completeness of TSCI, $n$ (%) | | | | | | $< 0.001^c$ |
| Incomplete | 117 (59.4) | 60 (30.5) | 16 ( 8.1) | 4 ( 2.0) | 197 (58.6) | |
| Complete | 62 (44.6) | 41 (29.5) | 21 (15.1) | 15 (10.8) | 139 (41.4) | |

[a] Linear-by-linear chi-square test.

[b] Analysis of variance.

[c] Pearson's chi-square test.

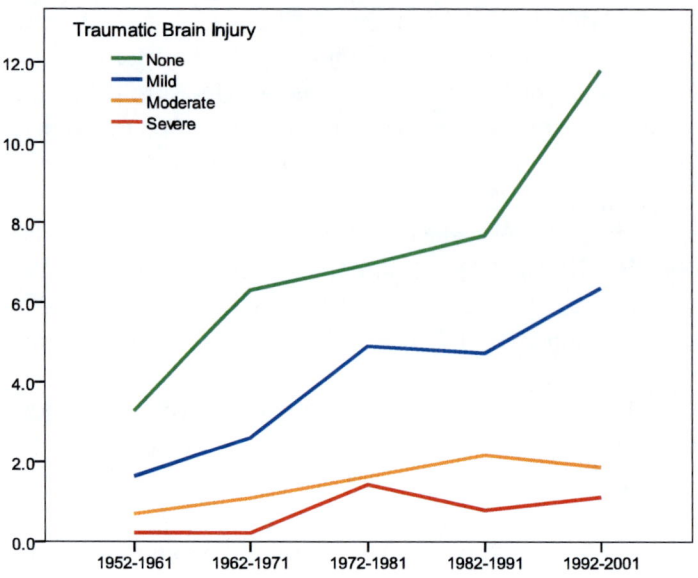

Figure 10. Incidence of TSCI and clinical concomitant TBI injury according classification of TBI and decade of injury, per million populations in Hordaland and Sogn og Fjordane counties (n = 336) [60].

**Table 8. Ordinal logistic regression analysis of severity of clinical TBI[a] on clinical variables and causes of injury in 336 patients with TSCI [60]**

| Variables | Odds ratio | 95 % CI[b] | p-value[c] |
|---|---|---|---|
| Age (years) | | | 0.439 |
| 0-29 | 1.36 | ( 0.71, 2.61) | |
| 30-59 | 0.95 | ( 0.53, 1.69) | |
| 60+ (ref[d]) | 1.00 | – | |
| Alcohol | | | < 0.001 |
| Yes | 3.62 | ( 2.10, 6.24) | |
| No (ref) | 1.00 | – | |
| Completeness of TSCI | | | 0.002 |
| Complete | 2.11 | ( 1.31, 3.42) | |
| Incomplete (ref) | 1.00 | – | |
| Level of TSCI | | | 0.032 |
| Cervical | 2.26 | ( 1.17, 4.39) | |
| Thoracic | 1.50 | ( 0.72, 3.12) | |
| Lumbosacral (ref) | 1.00 | – | |
| Causes of injury | | | < 0.001 |
| Car accidents | 1.89 | ( 0.83, 4.33) | |
| Motorcycle accidents | 3.95 | ( 1.31, 11.93) | |
| Bicycle accidents | 0.61 | ( 0.18, 2.10) | |
| Pedestrian accidents | 9.28 | ( 2.41, 35.68) | |
| Falls | 1.11 | ( 0.53, 2.32) | |
| Sport injuries | 0.86 | ( 0.31, 2.44) | |
| Other injuries (ref) | 1.00 | – | |

a) Classified into four levels corresponding to the International Head Injury Severity Scale.
1: No TBI, 2: Mild TBI, 3: Moderate TBI, 4: Severe TBI.
b) CI = confidence interval c) Likelihood ratio test d) ref = reference category.

In the multiple ordinal logistic regression models, all statistically significant variables were included. In addition, we included level of TSCI in the model. The analysis found a strong influence of alcohol, completeness of TSCI, cause of injury and level of TSCI on clinical TBI (Table 8). TBI is a leading cause of death and disability [62]. TSCI with a concomitant TBI has a significantly impact on TSCI rehabilitation outcome [58]. A TSCI will likely suppress the awareness of concomitant TBI unless the patient is unconscious on admission. Our results are most likely underestimates of the true incidence of TSCI with concomitant TBI [60]. The incidence of TSCI with concomitant TBI has increased during the last 50 years. Alcohol and completeness of injury are strong risk factors. Increased awareness of dual diagnoses is necessary [60].

## Work-Related TSCI

In western Norway, 22.9 % (77/336) of the patients had work-related TSCI [25]. Ninety six per cent of the cases with work-related TSCI were men in our population, similar to 95 % in the US and Australia [63,64].

**Table 9. Causes of work-related TSCI in Hordaland and Sogn og Fjordane counties, Norway 1952 – 2001 (n=336) [63]**

| Cause | Total number of TSCI | No. of work-related TSCI | Percentage of work-related TSCI |
|---|---|---|---|
| Fall | 153 | 37 | 24.2 |
| TA | 115 | 10 | 8.7 |
| Other | 39 | 30 | 76.9 |
| Sport | 29 | 0 | 0.0 |
| Total | 336 | 77 | 22.9 |

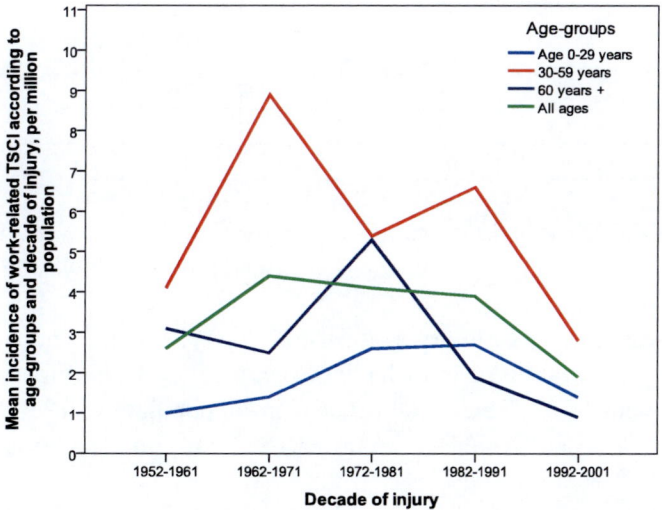

Figure 11. Mean incidence of work-related TSCI according to age-groups and decade of injury, in Hordaland and Sogn og Fjordane counties, Norway 1952 – 2001, per million populations [25].

The level of injury was cervical in 44.2 %. Fall was the main cause of work-related TSCI in our population (48.1 %), similar to the US and Australia [63,64]. The label "Other" in Table 9 denotes mainly patients hit by falling objects.

The incidence of work-related TSCI was highest among patients aged 30–59 years during all decades as shown in Figure 11. The incidence rate was highest in Australia among those age 25–34 years (4.9/mill) [63].

The total incidence in our region has decreased, probably due to legislation and penalty measurements regarding work-related injuries in Norway [65].

A decreasing trend was observed in Canada in the period 1947–1981, from 29.9 % in the period 1947–1973 to 1.8 % in the period 1996–2007 [66]. In the US, 13 % had a work-related TSCI in the period 1986–1991 [63,64]. A study from Australia found 13 % of TSCI to be work-related in the period 1986–1997, the percentages did however, not decline during the period [63].

## Alcohol-Related TSCI

In western Norway, 19 % of all TSCI-patients consumed alcohol prior to the accident, or were observed drunk on admittance to hospital. Of these, 87.5 % were men [25].

Fall was the most common cause of alcohol-related injuries in our population. In the group of patients aged 0–29 years at time of injury, both traffic accidents and falls occurred in 47.8 %. In the 30–59 and older than 60 year age groups, the cause was fall-related in 54.5 % and 84.2 % respectively [25].

**Table 10. Causes of alcohol-related TSCI in Hordaland and Sogn og Fjordane counties, Norway 1952–2001 (n=336) [25]**

| Cause | Total number of TSCI | No. of alcohol-related TSCI | Percentage of alcohol-related TSCI |
|-------|----------------------|-----------------------------|-------------------------------------|
| Fall  | 153                  | 39                          | 25.5 %                              |
| TA    | 115                  | 21                          | 18.3 %                              |
| Other | 39                   | 3                           | 7.7 %                               |
| Sport | 29                   | 1                           | 3.4 %                               |
| Total | 336                  | 64                          | 19.0 %                              |

A study from the US found that patients with cervical injuries were more likely to have used alcohol when injured (38 %) compared with patients with lower level injuries (23 %) [67].

Adjusting for age at time of injury and cause of injury, patients with cervical TSCI had a significantly increased relative odds of having used alcohol at the time of injury compared with participants with lower TSCIs (OR=2.06). In or population, 19.9 % of patients with cervical TSCI and 18.1 % of patients with lower TSCI had used alcohol at the time of injury [25].

Our data are based on medical records, and underreporting of alcohol-related injuries is probable. A study from Australia evaluated doctors recording of alcohol histories in patient records. The alcohol histories taken by doctors were judged to be adequate 74 % and 77 % of the time in 1992 and 1994 respectively [68].

Blood samples from 159 fatally injured drivers from 1989 and 1990, corresponding to 57 % of all fatally injured drivers in Norway during this period, were analysed for alcohol [69]. Alcohol was present in 28.3 % of the drivers, 27.0 % of those were above the legal limit of 0.0 5%. The Norwegian legal limit of blood alcohol concentration changed from 0.05 % to 0.02 % on January 1st 2001 [70].

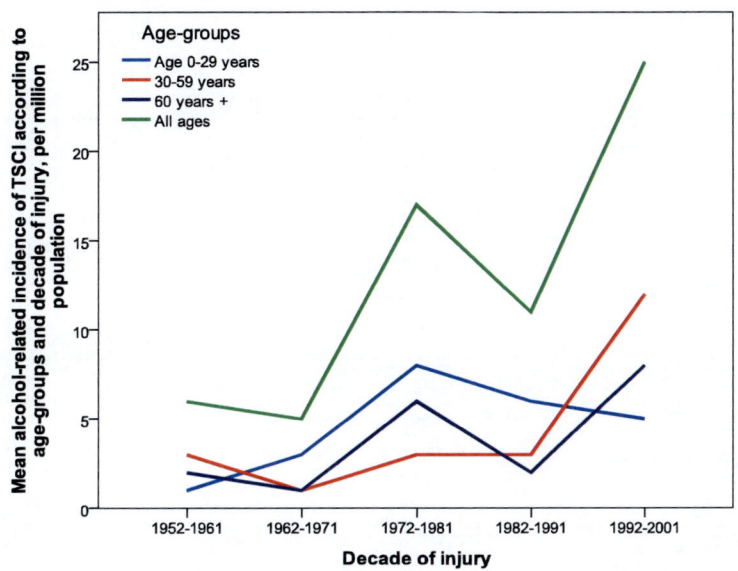

Figure 12. Mean incidence of alcohol-related TSCI according to age-groups and decade of injury, in Hordaland and Sogn og Fjordane counties, Norway 1952–2001, per million populations (n=336) [25].

## Survival and Mortality

TSCI causes dysfunction and complications in several organ systems, which may have an impact on survival. In 1927, Cushing described an 80 % mortality rate for World War I soldiers with TSCI in the first few weeks because of infections from bedsores and catheterization, with survival restricted to patients with incomplete lesions [71]. Internationally, the mortality of TSCI in the acute phase decreased from 30 % in the 1960s to 6 % in the 1980s [72]. Data from the United States show a reduction in mortality from the period 1973–1979 to the period 2000–2004 [73]. Despite this, patients with TSCI still have an increased risk of early death [74-77]. Studies from Denmark and Sweden reported a mortality rate of 1.3 % og 0 %, respectively during the first year after injury [78,79].

We compared the observed mortality with the expected mortality using a standardized mortality ratio (SMR) [80]. SMR is the ratio of the observed patient mortality and the mortality of the entire Norwegian population with the corresponding sex and year of birth.

There are two published studies from Norway. Lidal et al found an increased risk of death in patients with TSCI admitted to Sunnaas Rehabilitation Hospital; 1.8 for men and 4.9 for women, adjusted for age and gender [15].

**Table 11. Observed and expected number of deaths and SMRs by sex, periods of injury, level of injury, completeness, and age at injury in the Western Region of Norway [81]**

| Total mortality | N | Number of deaths | | SMR | (95 % CI) |
| --- | --- | --- | --- | --- | --- |
| | | Observed | Expected | | |
| *Gender* | | | | | |
| Male | 331 | 143 | 83.2 | 1.72 | (1.46, 2.03) |
| Female | 70 | 30 | 10.4 | 2.88 | (2.01, 4.12) |
| | | | | | |
| *Period* | | | | | |
| 1952-1961 | 32 | 28 | 14.2 | 1.97 | (1.36, 2.85) |
| 1962-1971 | 56 | 34 | 25.6 | 1.33 | (0.95, 1.86) |
| 1972-1981 | 82 | 42 | 20.4 | 2.06 | (1.52, 2.78) |
| 1982-1991 | 92 | 27 | 18.6 | 1.46 | (1.00, 2.12) |
| 1992-2001 | 139 | 42 | 14.8 | 2.84 | (2.10, 3.84) |
| | | | | | |
| *Level of injury* | | | | | |
| TLS | 188 | 59 | 30.4 | 1.94 | (1.51, 2.51) |
| Cervical | 213 | 114 | 63.2 | 1.80 | (1.50, 2.17) |
| | | | | | |
| *Completeness* | | | | | |
| Incomplete | 227 | 94 | 74.9 | 1.25 | (1.03, 1.54) |
| Complete | 174 | 79 | 18.7 | 4.23 | (3.39, 5.28) |
| | | | | | |
| *Level of injury and completeness* | | | | | |
| Incomplete TLS | 87 | 20 | 17.7 | 1.13 | (0.73, 1.76) |
| Incomplete Cervical | 140 | 74 | 57.3 | 1.29 | (1.03, 1.62) |
| Complete TLS | 101 | 39 | 12.7 | 3.07 | (2.24, 4.20) |
| Complete Cervical | 73 | 40 | 6.0 | 6.70 | (4.91, 9.13) |
| | | | | | |
| *Age* | | | | | |
| 0-20 years | 67 | 6 | 2.3 | 2.58 | (1.16, 5.75) |
| 21-30 years | 81 | 15 | 4.5 | 3.32 | (2.00, 5.51) |
| 31-40 years | 52 | 17 | 4.2 | 4.05 | (2.52, 6.52) |
| 41-50 years | 54 | 26 | 18.2 | 1.43 | (0.97, 2.09) |
| 51-60 years | 44 | 23 | 12.3 | 1.87 | (1.24, 2.81) |
| 61-70 years | 47 | 34 | 21.2 | 1.61 | (1.15, 2.25) |
| 71+ years | 56 | 52 | 30.8 | 1.69 | (1.28, 2.21) |
| *Total* | 401 | 173 | 93.6 | 1.85 | (1.59, 2.15) |
| *Cancer* | 401 | 19 | 22.6 | 0.84 | (0.54, 1.32) |
| *Cardiovascular* | 401 | 41 | 42.0 | 0.98 | (0.72, 1.33) |
| *Respiratory* | 401 | 17 | 8.7 | 1.96 | (1.22, 3.15) |
| *Genitourinary* | 401 | 3 | 1.5 | 1.99 | (0.64, 6.18) |
| *Accidental poisoning and suicide* | 401 | 10 | 1.7 | 5.79 | (3.11,10.75) |

A study from western Norway found that patients with TSCI had a nearly doubled risk of dying compared with others of the same gender and age with the SMR equal to 1.85 [81]. The risk was highest within the first 10 years after the injury. The risk did not change during the observation period. The group of patients with complete injury had a shorter average life expectancy relative to patients with incomplete injuries (SMR 4.23 vs. 1.25). Women had a reduced life expectancy compared to men (SMR 2.88 vs. 1.72). SMR was 6.70 for patients with complete cervical injuries and 3.07 for patients with complete lower level injuries. The average time from injury to death was 7.5 years, 6.9 years for patients with neck injury and 8.2 years for patients with lower level injuries (Table 11) [81].

In Norway, the mean life expectancy has increased for both genders from 1950 to 2008; 8 years for men and 10 years for women [82]. However, in our study the mean time from injury to death was shorter among women than among men, 7.4 years and 11.1 years respectively [81].

**Table 12. Unadjusted and adjusted relative mortality ratio (RMR) comparing the relative mortality (hazard) for the different categories for the included variables [81]**

| | | Unadjusted | | | Adjusted | |
|---|---|---|---|---|---|---|
| *Total mortality* | RMR | (95% CI) | p – value | RMR | (95% CI) | p – value |
| *Gender[a]* | | | | | | |
| Male | 1 | - | ref | 1 | - | ref |
| Female | 1.53 | (1.02, 2.29) | 0.038 | 1.96 | (1.29, 2.97) | 0.002 |
| | | | | | | |
| *Period[b]* | 0.40 | (0.11, 1.47) | 0.17 | 0.55 | (0.15, 2.04) | 0.38 |
| | | | | | | |
| *Level of injury and completeness[c]* | | | | | | |
| Incomplete TLS | 1 | - | ref | 1 | - | ref |
| Incomplete Cervical | 0.90 | (0.54, 1.50) | 0.69 | 1.35 | (0.79, 2.30) | 0.27 |
| Complete TLS | 2.40 | (1.39, 4.13) | 0.002 | 2.49 | (1.44, 4.30) | 0.001 |
| Complete Cervical | 4.18 | (2.41, 7.26) | <0.001 | 4.56 | (2.60, 8.00) | <0.001 |
| | | | | | | |
| *Age[b]* | 0.75 | (0.69, 0.82) | <0.001 | 0.81 | (0.74, 0.89) | <0.001 |

a) gender adjusted for level of injury, completeness, period of injury and age at injury.
b) per 10 year increase.
c) level and completeness of injury adjusted for gender, period of injury and age at injury.

Females had a significantly higher SMR than males; 2.88 vs. 1.72, after adjusting for age at time of injury, level, and completeness of injury and decade of injury. We compared the SMR for different covariates (age, sex, age at injury, period of injury, level of injury, completeness of injury) using a Cox model for time-dependent covariates [83]. The quantities estimated are referred to as relative mortality ratios (RMR). The RMR for women was 1.96 compared to men [81].

A higher female mortality relative to men has previously been reported in two other studies from Scandinavia. One study excluded patients requiring permanent respirator [78], and the other study excluded patients who died within one year post-injury [15]. Studies from UK and US however, have found a higher mortality rate for men relative to women [74,75,77].

The decreased survival was most significant in the group of patients with complete injuries. SMR was 6.70 times higher for the patients with complete cervical injuries, and 3.07 times higher for the patients with complete lower level injuries [81]. In the group of patients with incomplete injuries, there was an increased mortality in the first 10 years, but later the mortality did not differ from that of the Norwegian population in general [81].

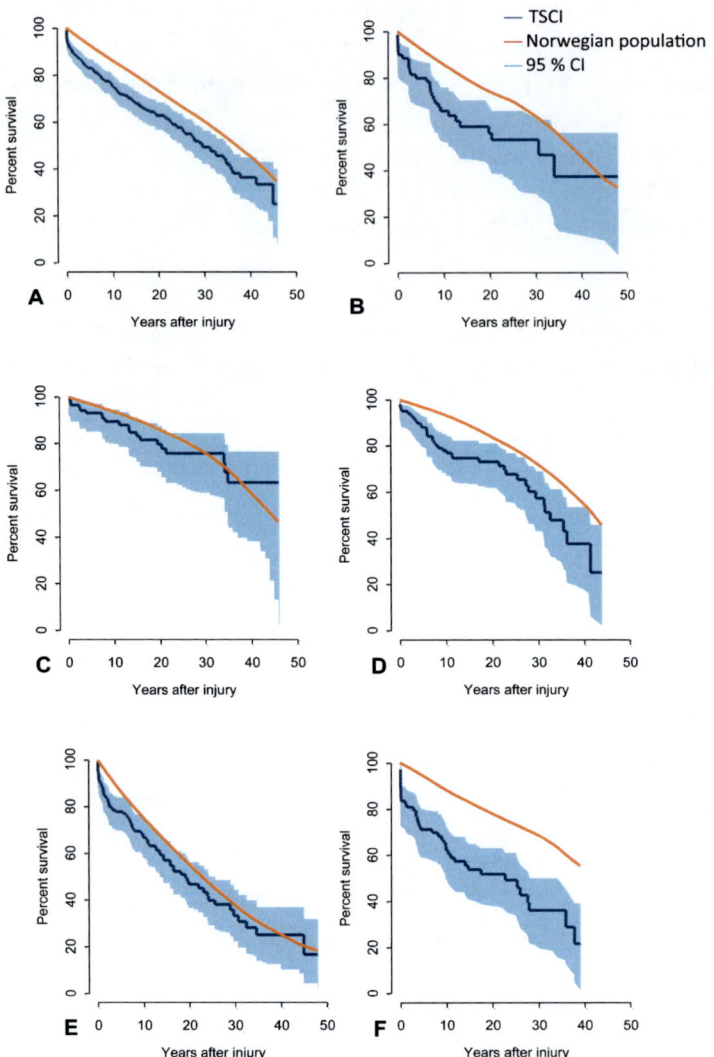

Figure 13. Survival probabilities of patients with TSCI injured 1952–2001, compared to the Norwegian population and with 95 % confidence interval. A: Men. B: Women. C: Incomplete TLS. D: Complete TLS. E: Incomplete cervical. F: Complete cervical [81].

## Time from Injury to Death

In the study from western Norway, the median survival time was 7.4 years; 6.7 years for women and 7.9 years for men; 6.8 years for cervical and 8.2 years for TLS injuries. During the entire period the mortality was 11.6 % within 30 days, 20.8 % with in one year, and 19.7 % during 1-5 years [81].

Generalized additive models (GAMs) represent a method of finding a smooth relationship between two or more variables through a scatter plot of data points. GAMs are useful where the relationship between the variables is expected to be complex, not easily fitted by standard linear or non-linear models [84,85]. GAMs are suitable for exploring the data set and visualizing the relationship between the dependent and independent variables.

The relation between 30 days mortality and year of injury is shown in Figure 14. The relation is clearly non-linear due to many factors both inside and outside hospital, as well as the patient population.

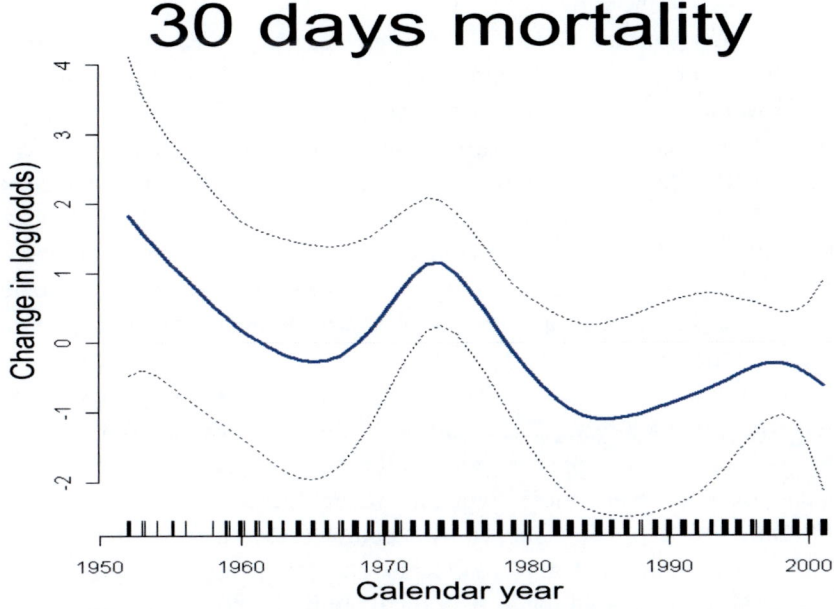

Figure 14. Generalized additive models for changes in log odds of death within 30 days after TSCI against calendar year of injury, with 95 % confidence intervals [25].

In the study from western Norway, 20.8 % of the patients died within one year [81]. This is lower than the 25 % reported from the US in 1967–1970 [86], and 48 % from Japan in 1953–1967 [87]. The American study included only patients who survived 72 hours post-injury [86] and the Japanese study included only those who were alive at admission to the hospital [87]. The first year mortality varied through the decades in our study: 10.8 %, 8.8 %, 33.3 %, 7.4 %, and 33.3 % (Figure 14) [81]. The increase in the last decade may partly be explained by an increasing number of elderly patients. These findings are in accordance with Furlan et al [88] who found that elderly individuals (older than 65 years) had significantly higher mortality than younger ones during the first year following TSCI.

## Causes of Death

In the last fifty years, the causes of late mortality in TSCI have changed significantly. Previously, urosepsis was the leading cause of death. Today significant advances in urologic management have led to dramatic changes in the leading causes of death. Pneumonia is now the leading cause of death among patients with cervical spinal cord injuries over the age of 55, while unintentional injury and suicide are frequent causes of death among patients with thoracic, lumbar and sacral injuries.

A study from Denmark found that the most common causes of death were respiratory diseases (especially pneumonia), suicide and ischemic heart disease [78]. A significant reduction in total mortality was observed from the first period 1953–1971 to the second period from 1972–1992.

Lidal found that the main causes of death were pneumonia/ influenza (16 %,) ischemic heart disease (13 %) and urogenital disease (13 %) in patients admitted to Sunnaas Rehabilitation Hospital in the period 1961–1982 [15].

In our study from western Norway, the cause-specific SMR was 1.96 for respiratory disease and 5.79 for suicide and accidental poisoning. Women had a significantly higher risk (SMR 37.59 for women, compared to 3.70 for men). The risk of dying from lung disease was highest in patients with neck injuries, while suicide and accidental poisoning occurred most frequently in patients with lower, incomplete injuries [81]. The most frequent causes of death during all decades were cardiovascular disease and respiratory disease (Figure 15) [81]. Deaths in TSCI individuals are often multi-factorial, and the precise cause of death in patients with multiple pathologies may be difficult to establish [89]. We included both underlying and contributing causes, because frequencies and descriptive information provide a more complete picture of the morbidity and the impact of particular causes of mortality [90].

Table 13 summarizes the underlying and contributing causes of death according to the level and completeness of injury [81]. Respiratory disease was the most frequent cause of death among patients with complete cervical injuries, while urogenital disease and suicide and accidental poisoning were most frequent among the patients with incomplete lower injuries [81]. Only 20 % of our patients with complete cervical TSCI had cardiovascular disease, which is surprising and may be due to underreporting. A study from Haukeland University Hospital found that although pulmonary emboli are the immediate cause of death in many cases, this clinical diagnosis is often missed [91]. Including both the underlying and the contributing causes of death gives better information regarding morbidity rather than examining only the underlying cause of death.

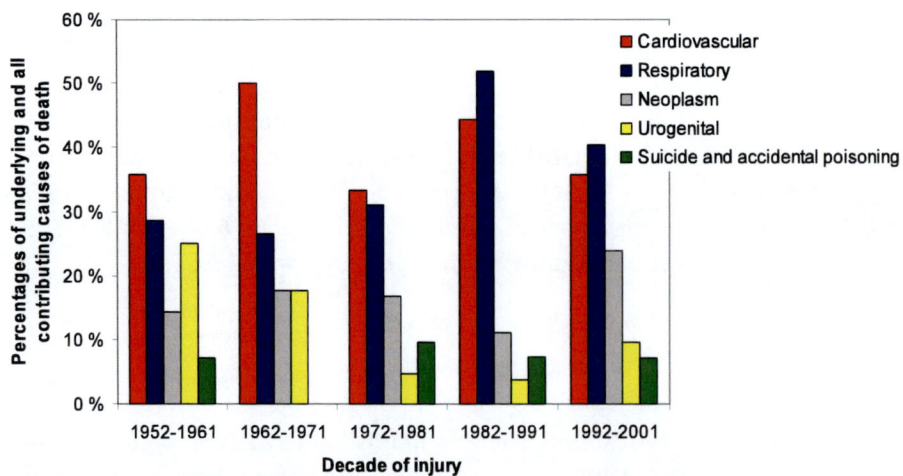

Figure 15. Percentages of five causes of death according to decade of injury, sum of the underlying cause and all contributing causes of death (n=173) [81].

**Table 13. Causes of death after TSCI during 1952–2001,
percentages given [81]**

| | All causes | | | | | |
|---|---|---|---|---|---|---|
| | Cervical | Cervical | TLS | TLS | | |
| | ASIA A | ASIA B-D | ASIA A | ASIA B-D | ALL | |
| | (Complete) | (Incomplete) | (Complete) | (Incomplete) | | |
| | (n=40) | (n=74) | (n=39) | (n=20) | (n=173) | p |
| | % | % | % | % | % | |
| Cardiovascular disease | 20 | 49 | 33 | 55 | 39 | 0.009 |
| Respiratory disease | 50 | 39 | 18 | 25 | 35 | 0.016 |
| | | | | | | |
| Neoplasm | 5 | 24 | 26 | 0 | 17 | 0.005 |
| Suicide and accidental poisoning | 5 | 3 | 8 | 20 | 6 | 0.044 |
| Nervous system disease | 20 | 15 | 23 | 5 | 17 | 0.312 |
| Digestive system disease | 3 | 4 | 10 | 5 | 5 | 0.424 |
| Musculoskeletal disease | 5 | 11 | 3 | 0 | 6 | 0.182 |
| Genitourinary disease | 15 | 9 | 15 | 5 | 12 | 0.538 |
| Mental disorder | 3 | 7 | 5 | 5 | 5 | 0.813 |
| Skin disease | 3 | 3 | 13 | 5 | 5 | 0.108 |
| Endocrine and metabolic disease | 3 | 5 | 3 | 0 | 3 | 0.627 |
| External causes | 70 | 31 | 33 | 10 | 38 | 0.000 |
| Other causes | 3 | 9 | 18 | 25 | 12 | 0.036 |

ICD codes converted to the European short-list for causes of death (EUROSTAT).

## Underlying Cause of Death

*Respiratory disease:* In our study the cause-specific SMR was 1.96 for respiratory disease [81]. A total of 9.8 % had respiratory disease as the main cause of death, lessr than reported by Lidal et al. (21.1 %) and Soden et al. (16.4 %) [15,92]. Respiratory disease was most frequent among our patients with cervical injuries, similar to the findings from Australia [92].

*Cardiovascular disease:* We found a SMR for cardiovascular disease of 0.98, which indicates that mortality due to cardiovascular disease among TSCI-patients is not increased compared to the general population [81]. This finding is similar to a hospital-based study from Sunnaas Rehabilitation Hospital, Norway in the period 1961–1982 and findings from Australia [15,92].

*Suicide:* In our study, the cause-specific SMR was 5.79 for suicide including accidental poisoning; 3.70 for men and 37.59 for women [81]. Soden et al. found a SMR of 4.4 for suicide in Australia [92]. We included accidental poisoning since suicide may be masked as such on the death certificate.

Suicide was a frequent cause of death among patients with incomplete TLS injuries (Table 13) [81]. A Danish study found a SMR for suicide of 4.6 for the period 1953–1990, highest for women and incomplete TSCI [93]. The suicide rate doubled from the period 1953–1971 to the period 1972–1990. Suicide was most frequent among patients with incomplete TLS injuries, nearly twice as high as the group of functionally complete tetraplegic patients [93]. The number of deaths from suicide and accidental poisoning in our population is small and the data should be interpreted with caution [81].

*Urogenital disease:* In our study the cause-specific SMR was 1.99 for urogenital disease [81]. Soden et al. found a SMR of 22.8 for diseases of the urinary system [92]. The main cause of death was urogenital diseases in 13 % for patients admitted to Sunnaas Rehabilitation Hospital, Norway in the period 1961–1982 [15]. The frequency of urogenital disease has decreased due to improved treatments of urinary tract infections [94,95].

*Cancer:* We found a SMR for cancer of 0.84 [81], comparable to the SMR of 1.0 for cancer in Australia [92].

A study has reported an increased risk of bladder malignancy in TSCI-patients with indwelling catheters [96]. Retrospective studies have suggested that the relative risk of a bladder neoplasm among TSCI is 16–28 times that of a normal population [97-99].

In our population only three patients (1.7 %) had neoplasm of bladder as either the underlying (two patients) or contributing cause of death (one patient) [81]. Kalisvaart et al. reviewed 1319 SCI-patients in the period 1983–2007, of these were 2.4 % (32/1319) diagnosed with bladder tumours [99].

Kalisvaart et al. found that 55 % of patients diagnosed with bladder cancer used an external catheter for a mean of 40 years with only 22.2 % having had an indwelling catheter, suggesting that the neurogenic bladder, not the indwelling catheter, may be the risk factor for bladder cancer [99].

# CONCLUSION

Studies from Norway have found an increasing incidence of TSCI during a 50-year period. The age-adjusted incidence of TSCI among adolescents has increased, whereas the age-adjusted incidence among children remained low during the 50 years.

TSCI was highly associated with car and pedestrian accidents among children. Among adolescence, TSCI was associated with car and motorcycle accidents. The most frequent cause of injury was falls, followed by traffic accidents. The frequency of TSCI due to traffic accidents has increased especially among men less than 30 years The frequency of TSCI due to falls and the frequency of incomplete cervical lesions have increased especially among men over 60 years at time of injury.

Falls and traffic accidents are potentially preventable mechanisms of injury. Awareness of these factors is important in prevention planning strategies.

The increasing proportion of older patients with cervical lesions poses a challenge to the health system. A high proportion of the elderly patients had cervical spinal stenosis and incomplete TSCI, and most of them regained good function.

The incidence of TSCI with concomitant TBI has also increased during the last 50 years. Alcohol and completeness of injury are strong risk factors. Increased awareness of dual diagnoses is necessary.

Patients with a TSCI, especially women, have an increased mortality despite modern treatment and care. Special attention should be paid to respiratory dysfunction, pulmonary infections, and suicide and accidental poisoning prevention strategies.

# REFERENCES

[1]     Ackery A, Tator C, Krassioukov A. A global perspective on spinal cord injury epidemiology. *J. Neurotrauma*, 2004;21(10):1355-70.

[2]     Chiu WT, Lin HC, Lam C, Chu SF, Chiang YH, Tsai SH. Review Paper: Epidemiology of Traumatic Spinal Cord Injury: Comparisons Between Developed and Developing Countries. *Asia Pac. J. Public Health*, 2010;22(1):9-18.

[3]     Cripps RA, Lee BB, Wing P, Weerts E, Mackay J, Brown D. A global map for traumatic spinal cord injury epidemiology: towards a living data repository for injury prevention. *Spinal Cord*, 2011;49(4):493-501.

[4]     van den Berg ME, Castellote JM, Mahillo-Fernandez I, de Pedro-Cuesta J. Incidence of spinal cord injury worldwide: a systematic review. *Neuroepidemiology*, 2010;34 (3):184-92.

[5]     Wyndaele M, Wyndaele JJ. Incidence, prevalence and epidemiology of spinal cord injury: what learns a worldwide literature survey? *Spinal Cord*, 2006;44(9):523-9.

[6]     Hagen EM, Rekand T, Gilhus NE, Gronning M. Diagnostic coding accuracy for traumatic spinal cord injuries. *Spinal Cord*, 2009;47(5):367-71.

[7]     Kurtzke JF. Epidemiology of spinal cord injury. *Neurol. Neurocir. Psiquiatr.*, 1977;18(2-3 Suppl):157-91.

[8]     Blumer CE, Quine S. Prevalence of spinal-cord injury - an international comparison. *Neuroepidemiology*, 1995;14(5):258-68.

[9]     Anon. Spinal cord injury facts and figures at a glance. *J. Spinal Cord Med.*, 2010;33(4):439-40.

[10]    Anon. Injury Prevention. Healthy Alaskans 2010 - Volume I: Targets for Improved Health. Alaska Department of Health Social Services, Division of Public Health; 2002.

[11]    Dryden DM, Saunders LD, Rowe BH, May LA, Yiannakoulias N, Svenson LW, et al. The epidemiology of traumatic spinal cord injury in Alberta, Canada. *Can. J. Neurol. Sci.*, 2003;30(2):113-21.

[12]    Martins F, Freitas F, Martins L, Dartigues JF, Barat M. Spinal cord injuries-- epidemiology in Portugal's central region. *Spinal Cord*, 1998;36(8):574-8.

[13]    Biering-Sorensen F, Pedersen V, Clausen S. Epidemiology of spinal-cord lesions in Denmark. *Paraplegia*, 1990;28(2):105-18.

[14]    Gjone R, Nordlie L. Incidence of traumatic paraplegia and tetraplegia in Norway: A statistical survey of the years 1974 and 1975. *Paraplegia*, 1978;16(1):88-93.

[15]    Lidal IB, Snekkevik H, Aamodt G, Hjeltnes N, Biering-Sorensen F, Stanghelle JK. Mortality after spinal cord injury in Norway. *J. Rehabil. Med.*, 2007;39(2):145-51.

[16]  Hagen EM, Eide GE, Rekand T, Gilhus NE, Gronning M. A 50-year follow-up of the incidence of traumatic spinal cord injuries in Western Norway. *Spinal Cord,* 2010;48(4):313-8.

[17]  Kraus JF, Franti CE, Riggins RS, Richards D, Borhani NO. Incidence of traumatic spinal cord lesions. *J. Chronic. Dis.*, 1975;28(9):471-92.

[18]  Maynard FM, Bracken MB, Creasey G, Ditunno JF, Donovan WH, Ducker TB, et al. International standards for neurological and functional classification of spinal cord injury. *Spinal Cord,* 1997;35(5):266-74.

[19]  Divanoglou A, Levi R. Incidence of traumatic spinal cord injury in Thessaloniki, Greece and Stockholm, Sweden: a prospective population-based study. *Spinal Cord,* 2009;47(11):796-801.

[20]  Ahoniemi E, Alaranta H, Hokkinen EM, Valtonen K, Kautiainen H. Incidence of traumatic spinal cord injuries in Finland over a 30-year period. *Spinal Cord,* 2008;46(12):781-4.

[21]  Razdan S, Kaul RL, Motta A, Kaul S, Bhatt RK. Prevalence and pattern of major neurological disorders in rural Kashmir (India) in 1986. *Neuroepidemiology,* 1994;13(3):113-9.

[22]  Rick Hansen Spinal Cord Injury Register. Spinal Cord Injury Facts and Statistics: Canada, 2010. http://rickhansenregistry.org/en/news-and-resources/sci-facts.html.

[23]  Dahlberg A, Kotila M, Leppanen P, Kautiainen H, Alaranta H. Prevalence of spinal cord injury in Helsinki. *Spinal Cord,* 2005;43(1):47-50.

[24]  Knutsdottir S. Spinal-cord injuries in Iceland 1973-1989. A follow-up-study. *Paraplegia,* 1993;31(1):68-72.

[25]  Hagen EM. Traumatic spinal cord injuries *A clinical and epidemiological study*. PhD Thesis. AIT AS, Oslo: The University of Bergen; 2010.

[26]  DeVivo MJ, Chen Y. Trends in New Injuries, Prevalent Cases, and Aging With Spinal Cord Injury. *Arch. Phys. Med. Rehabil.*, 2011;92(3):332-8.

[27]  Kannus P, Palvanen M, Niemi S, Parkkari J. Alarming rise in the number and incidence of fall-induced cervical spine injuries among older adults. *J. Gerontol. A Biol. Sci. Med. Sci.*, 2007;62(2):180-3.

[28]  Nobunaga AI, Go BK, Karunas RB. Recent demographic and injury trends in people served by the model spinal cord injury care systems. *Arch. Phys. Med. Rehabil.*, 1999;80(11):1372-82.

[29]  Pickett W, Simpson K, Walker J, Brison RJ. Traumatic spinal cord injury in Ontario, Canada. *J. Trauma,* 2003;55(6):1070-6.

[30]  Kannus P, Niemi S, Parkkari J, Palvanen M, Heinonen A, Sievanen H, et al. Why is the age-standardized incidence of low-trauma fractures rising in many elderly populations? *J Bone Miner Res* 2002;17(8):1363-7.

[31]  O'Connor PJ. Trends in spinal cord injury. *Accid. Anal. Prev.*, 2006;38(1):71-7.

[32]  Couris CM, Guilcher SJ, Munce SE, Fung K, Craven BC, Verrier M, et al. Characteristics of adults with incident traumatic spinal cord injury in Ontario, Canada. *Spinal Cord,* 2009;48(1):39-44.

[33]  Brolin K. Neck injuries among the elderly in Sweden. *Inj. Control Saf. Promot.*, 2003;10(3):155-64.

[34]  Jabbour P, Fehlings M, Vaccaro AR, Harrop JS. Traumatic spine injuries in the geriatric population. *Neurosurg. Focus*, 2008;25(5):E16.

[35] Krause JS, Kewman D, DeVivo MJ, Maynard F, Coker J, Roach MJ, et al. Employment after spinal cord injury: an analysis of cases from the Model Spinal Cord Injury Systems. *Arch. Phys. Med. Rehabil.*, 1999;80(11):1492-500.

[36] Falch JA, Kaastad TS, Bohler G, Espeland J, Sundsvold OJ. Secular Increase and Geographical Differences in Hip Fracture Incidence in Norway. *Bone*, 1993;14(4):643-5.

[37] Peden M. Global collaboration on road traffic injury prevention. *Int. J. Inj. Contr. Saf. Promot.*, 2005;12(2):85-91.

[38] Li J, Liu G, Zheng Y, Hao C, Zhang Y, Wei B, et al. The epidemiological survey of acute traumatic spinal cord injury (ATSCI) of 2002 in Beijing municipality. *Spinal Cord,* 2011;49(7):777-82.

[39] Dincer F, Oflazer A, Beyazova M, Celiker R, Basgoze O, Altioklar K. Traumatic spinal cord injuries in Turkey. *Paraplegia*, 1992;30(9):641-6.

[40] Pedersen V, Muller PG, Biering-Sorensen F. Traumatic spinal cord injuries in Greenland 1965-1986. *Paraplegia*, 1989;27(5):345-9.

[41] Knutsdottir S, Thórisdóttir H, Sigvaldason K, Jonsson H, Bjornsson A, Ingvarsson P. Epidemiology of traumatic spinal cord injuries in Iceland from 1975 to 2009. *Spinal Cord,* 2011,doi: 10.1038/sc.2011.105 [Epub ahead of print].

[42] Puisto V, Kaariainen S, Impinen A, Parkkila T, Vartiainen E, Jalanko T, et al. Incidence of Spinal and Spinal Cord Injuries and Their Surgical Treatment in Children and Adolescents A Population-Based Study. *Spine*, 2010;35(1):104-7.

[43] Augutis M, Malker H, Levi R. Pediatric spinal cord injury in Sweden; how to identify a cohort of rare events. *Spinal Cord,* 2003;41(6):337-46.

[44] Hagen EM, Eide GE, Elgen I. Traumatic spinal cord injury among children and adolescences during 50 years: a population-based study. *Spinal Cord,* 2011; 49 (9): 981-5.

[45] Statistics Norway. Statistical Yearbook of Norway 2009. Oslo, Norway: Statistics Norway; 2009.

[46] Vitale MG, Goss JM, Matsumoto H, Roye DP, Jr. Epidemiology of pediatric spinal cord injury in the United States: years 1997 and 2000. *J. Pediatr. Orthop.*, 2006;26(6):745-9.

[47] Augutis M, Levi R. Pediatric spinal cord injury in Sweden: incidence, etiology and outcome. *Spinal Cord,* 2003;41(6):328-36.

[48] DeVivo MJ, Vogel LC. Epidemiology of spinal cord injury in children and adolescents. *J. Spinal Cord Med.*, 2004;27 Suppl 1:S4-10.

[49] Apple DF, Anson CA, Hunter JD, Bell RB. Spinal-cord injury in youth. *Clinical Pediatrics*, 1995;34(2):90-5.

[50] Augutis M. Pediatric Spinal Cord Injury. PhD Thesis, Karolinska Institutet, Department of Neurobiology, Health Care Science and Society, Division of Neurorehabiliation, Stockholm, Sweden; 2007.

[51] Bilston LE, Brown J. Pediatric spinal injury type and severity are age and mechanism dependent. *Spine*, 2007;32(21):2339-47.

[52] Cifu DX, Seel RT, Kreutzer JS, Marwitz J, McKinley WO, Wisor D. Age, outcome, and rehabilitation costs after tetraplegia spinal cord injury. *NeuroRehabilitation*, 1999;12(3):177-85.

[53]  DeVivo MJ, Kartus PL, Rutt RD, Stover SL, Fine PR. The influence of age at time of spinal cord injury on rehabilitation outcome. *Arch. Neurol.*, 1990;47(6):687-91.

[54]  Cifu DX, Seel RT, Kreutzer JS, McKinley WO. A multicenter investigation of age-related differences in lengths of stay, hospitalization charges, and outcomes for a matched tetraplegia sample. *Arch. Phys. Med. Rehabil.*, 1999;80(7):733-40.

[55]  Go BK, DeVivo M, Richards J. The Epidemiology of Spinal Cord Injury. In: Stover SL, DeLisa JA, Whiteneck G, editors. Spinal Cord Injury Clinical Outcomes from the Model Systems. 1 ed. Gaithersburg, Maryland: *Aspen Publishers*; 1995. p. 21-55.

[56]  Hagen EM, Aarli JA, Gronning M. The clinical significance of spinal cord injuries in patients older than 60 years of age. *Acta. Neurol. Scand.*, 2005;112(1):42-7.

[57]  Sommer JL, Witkiewicz PM. The therapeutic challenges of dual diagnosis: TBI/SCI. *Brain Inj.*, 2004;18(12):1297-308.

[58]  Macciocchi SN, Bowman B, Coker J, Apple D, Leslie D. Effect of co-morbid traumatic brain injury on functional outcome of persons with spinal cord injuries. *Am. J. Phys. Med. Rehabil.*, 2004;83(1):22-6.

[59]  Tolonen A, Turkka J, Salonen O, Ahoniemi E, Alaranta H. Traumatic brain injury is under-diagnosed in patients with spinal cord injury. *J. Rehabil. Med.*, 2007;39(8):622-6.

[60]  Hagen EM, Eide GE, Rekand T, Gilhus NE, Gronning M. Traumatic spinal cord injury and concomitant brain injury; a cohort study. *Acta. Neurol. Scand.*, 2010;122(Suppl 190):51-7.

[61]  Teasdale G, Jennett B. Assessment of Coma and Impaired Consciousness - Practical. Scale. *Lancet*, 1974;2(7872):81-4.

[62]  Steyerberg EW, Mushkudiani N, Perel P, Butcher I, Lu J, McHugh GS, et al. Predicting Outcome after Traumatic Brain Injury: Development and International Validation of Prognostic Scores Based on Admission Characteristics. *PLoS Med.*, 2008;5(8):e165.

[63]  O'Connor P. Work related spinal cord injury, Australia 1986-97. *Inj. Prev.*, 2001;7(1):29-34.

[64]  Rosenberg NL. Occupational spinal cord injury: Demographic and etiologic differences from non-occupational injuries. *Neurology*, 1993;43(7):1385-8.

[65]  The Working Environment Act, LOV 1977-02-04 nr 04, Ministry of Labour and Social Inclusion, (1977).

[66]  Tator CH, Duncan EG, Edmonds VE, Lapczak LI, Andrews DF. Changes in epidemiology of acute spinal-cord injury from 1947 to 1981. *Surg. Neurol.*, 1993;40(3):207-15.

[67]  Garrison A, Clifford K, Gleason SF, Tun CG, Brown R, Garshick E. Alcohol use associated with cervical spinal cord injury. *J. Spinal Cord Med.*, 2004;27(2):111-5.

[68]  Burns L, Adams M. Alcohol-history taking by nurses and doctors--how accurate are they really? *J. Adv. Nurs.*, 1997;25(3):509-13.

[69]  Gjerde H, Beylich KM, Morland J. Incidence of Alcohol and Drugs in Fatally Injured Car Drivers in Norway. *Accid. Anal. Prev.*, 1993;25(4):479-83.

[70]  Road Traffic Act, Ministry of Transport and Communications, (1965).

[71]  Cushing H. Organization and activities of the neurological service American expeditionary forces. In: Ireland MW, editor. The medical department of the United States Army in the world war. Volume XI Surgery, Part One General surgery, Orthopedic surgery, Neurosurgery.Washington, D.C.: Government Printing Office, Washington, *D.C.*, USA; 1927. p. 749-58.

[72] Ducker TB. Treatment of spinal-cord injury. *N. Engl. J. Med.*, 1990;322(20):1459-61.

[73] Strauss DJ, DeVivo MJ, Paculdo DR, Shavelle RM. Trends in life expectancy after spinal cord injury. *Arch. Phys. Med. Rehabil.*, 2006;87(8):1079-85.

[74] DeVivo MJ, Krause JS, Lammertse DP. Recent trends in mortality and causes of death among persons with spinal cord injury. *Arch. Phys. Med. Rehabil.*, 1999;80(11):1411-9.

[75] Frankel HL, Coll JR, Charlifue SW, Whiteneck GG, Gardner BP, Jamous MA, et al. Long-term survival in spinal cord injury: a fifty year investigation. *Spinal Cord,* 1998;36(4):266-74.

[76] Garshick E, Kelley A, Cohen SA, Garrison A, Tun CG, Gagnon D, et al. A prospective assessment of mortality in chronic spinal cord injury. *Spinal Cord,* 2005;43(7):408-16.

[77] Saunders LL, Selassie AW, Hill EG, Nicholas JS, Varma AK, Lackland DT, et al. Traumatic spinal cord injury mortality, 1981-1998. *J. Trauma,* 2009;66(1):184-90.

[78] Hartkopp A, Bronnum-Hansen H, Seidenschnur AM, Biering-Sorensen F. Survival and cause of death after traumatic spinal cord injury. A long-term epidemiological survey from Denmark. *Spinal Cord,* 1997;35(2):76-85.

[79] Divanoglou A, Westgren N, Seiger A, Hulting C, Levi R. Late mortality during the first year after acute traumatic spinal cord injury: a prospective, population-based study. *J. Spinal Cord Med.,* 2010;33(2):117-27.

[80] Andersen PK, Vaeth M. Simple parametric and nonparametric models for excess and relative mortality. *Biometrics,* 1989;45(2):523-35.

[81] Hagen EM, Lie SA, Rekand T, Gilhus NE, Gronning M. Mortality after traumatic spinal cord injury: 50 years of follow-up. *J. Neurol. Neurosurg. Psychiatry,* 2010;81(4):368-73.

[82] Statistics Norway. Causes of Death 1995-2006. Oslo, Norway: Statistics Norway; 2009.

[83] Andersen PK, Borch-Johnsen K, Deckert T, Green A, Hougaard P, Keiding N, et al. A Cox regression model for the relative mortality and its application to diabetes mellitus survival data. *Biometrics,* 1985;41(4):921-32.

[84] Hewson PJ. Cycle helmets and road casualties in the UK. *Traffic Inj. Prev.,* 2005;6(2):127-34.

[85] Hastie TJ, Tibshirani R. Generalized additive models. 1990.

[86] Rish BL, Dilustro JF, Salazar AM, Schwab KA, Brown HR. Spinal cord injury: a 25-year morbidity and mortality study. *Mil. Med.,* 1997;162(2):141-8.

[87] Nakajima A, Honda S, Yoshimura S, Ono Y, Kawamura J, Moriai N. The disease pattern and causes of death of spinal cord injured patients in Japan. *Paraplegia,* 1989;27(3):163-71.

[88] Furlan JC, Bracken MB, Fehlings MG. Is age a key determinant of mortality and neurological outcome after acute traumatic spinal cord injury? *Neurobiol. Aging.,* 2010;31(3):434-46.

[89] Goldacre MJ. Cause-specific mortality: understanding uncertain tips of the disease iceberg. *J. Epidemiol. Community Health,* 1993;47(6):491-6.

[90] DeVivo M, Stover SL. Long-Term Survival and Causes of Death. In: Stover SL, Demetriades D, Whiteneck G, editors. Spinal Cord Injury Clinical Outcomes from the Model Systems. 1 ed. Gaithersburg, Maryland: *Aspen Publishers*; 1995. p. 289-316.

[91] Karwinski B, Svendsen E. Comparison of clinical and postmortem diagnosis of pulmonary embolism. *J. Clin. Pathol.,* 1989;42(2):135-9.

[92] Soden RJ, Walsh J, Middleton JW, Craven ML, Rutkowski SB, Yeo JD. Causes of death after spinal cord injury. *Spinal Cord,* 2000;38(10):604-10.

[93] Hartkopp A, Bronnum-Hansen H, Seidenschnur AM, Biering-Sorensen F. Suicide in a spinal cord injured population: its relation to functional status. *Arch. Phys. Med. Rehabil.,* 1998;79(11):1356-61.

[94] Bakke A, Digranes A, Hoisaeter PA. Physical predictors of infection in patients treated with clean intermittent catheterization: A prospective 7-year study. *Br. J. Urol.,* 1997;79(1):85-90.

[95] Bakke A, Vollset SE. Risk-Factors for Bacteriuria and Clinical Urinary-Tract Infection in Patients Treated with Clean Intermittent Catheterization. *J. Urol.,* 1993;149(3):527-31.

[96] West DA, Cummings JM, Longo WE, Virgo KS, Johnson FE, Parra RO. Role of chronic catheterization in the development of bladder cancer in patients with spinal cord injury. *Urology,* 1999;53(2):292-7.

[97] Groah SL, Weitzenkamp DA, Lammertse DP, Whiteneck GG, Lezotte DC, Hamman RF. Excess risk of bladder cancer in spinal cord injury: evidence for an association between indwelling catheter use and bladder cancer. *Arch. Phys. Med. Rehabil.,* 2002;83(3):346-51.

[98] Subramonian K, Cartwright RA, Harnden P, Harrison SCW. Bladder cancer in patients with spinal cord injuries. *BJU Int.,* 2004;93(6):739-43.

[99] Kalisvaart JF, Katsumi HK, Ronningen LD, Hovey RM. Bladder cancer in spinal cord injury patients. *Spinal Cord,* 2010;48(3):257-61.

In: Epidemiology of Spinal Cord Injuries
Editors: V. Rahimi-Movaghar, S. B. Jazayeri et al.

ISBN: 978-1-61942-894-2
©2012 Nova Science Publishers, Inc.

*Chapter 9*

# TRAUMATIC SPINAL CORD INJURY IN SWEDEN

## *Richard Levi [1], Anestis Divanoglou [1] and Marika Augutis [2]*
[1]Division of Rehabilitation Medicine, Umeå University, Sweden
[2]Dept. of Research and Development, Sundsvall Hospital, Sweden

## 1. USE OF REGISTRIES IN SCI EPIDEMIOLOGY IN SWEDEN

The country of Sweden has an unusually long tradition of population registration, dating back to 1749 when a specific governmental institution, *"Tabellverket"* [1] was founded for this specific purpose. Since then, several nationwide population-based disease or effect registers have been developed [2]. The drop-out rates are typically very low, usually under 5%. The registers are frequently utilized for research, evaluation, planning and other purposes by a variety of users [3].

Furthermore, there is a unique system of individual so-called personal registration numbers (PRN) for the identification of every Swedish resident [3].

This, together with availability of modern computer-based techniques, provides facilities for easy linkage of exposure and outcome data down to the level of individual patients [2].

Population-based administrative registers are practical and cost-effective when utilized for epidemiological purposes [4]. However, there are caveats when using such databases for scientific research [5]. Since the primary purpose of many such registers is administrative rather than scientific, this may reflect negatively on data quality [2].

In the literature there are many cautions about the use of surveys based on register studies, pointing to biases in the reporting methods, data collection systems and classification patterns [6]. The use of discharge diagnoses for identification of cases, for example, may be problematic due to variations in coding procedures, coding errors, incomplete coding, lack of specificity in available codes and clinical errors in diagnosis [4].

Data collection of rare events (such as Traumatic Spinal Cord Injury) from population-based registers poses particular problems due to the large amount of data that has to be screened in order to obtain a study population large enough on which to base conclusions. The implication is that verification of every single case must be made very carefully to avoid misclassifications and/or differences in classification.

In our studies we found that registries can be an expedient way to identify a Traumatic Spinal Cord Injury (TSCI) population but that the initial, registry-described case identification needs subsequent refinement and quality control in order to be useful for a specific study. Such quality control is time-consuming but necessary, since the validity of incidence estimates obviously is dependent on how well true cases are recognized, identified and verified [7-10].

In many countries population based registers do not exist, and estimates of diseases or injuries then have to be based on either retrospective data from individual hospitals or prospective estimates attempting to capture all cases within a geographic area.

Yet another way to collect information on the epidemiology of TSCI is through Quality registers. The Swedish SCI Council, with delegates from the six university hospitals, has formed a national consensus regarding fundamental indicators of quality of care, as well as documentation of treatment and results. From 1997 until 2011, the so-called Nordic Spinal Cord Injury Registry (NSCIR) collected data from spinal units in several Nordic countries, Sweden among them. The registry was used as a source for specific research and development projects, facilitated international collaboration as well as enhanced preventive efforts [11, 12]. In 2011, the NSCIR was ceased and replaced by the more general "WebRehab" register for rehabilitation medicine. It is at this time not possible to predict whether this will affect the possibility for monitoring SCI in Sweden.

## 2. PEDIATRIC SCI IN SWEDEN

The incidence of TSCI among children under the age of 16 was known to be low in Sweden, although actual studies had not been performed. Due to lack of centralization of pediatric TSCI (pedTSCI) care and also due to the fact that the extant quality register used by spinal units in Sweden rarely covers the pediatric group (as such patients are generally not treated at these units), the only way to determine TSCI incidence in children was to use population based registers.Our principal aim of this study, performed in 1999, was to assess etiology and early outcome of TSCI in children (0-15 years) in Sweden during 1985-1996, a period of time chosen to obtain enough cases given the low incidence of SCI.

### 2.1. Method

Identification of persons with TSCI aged 0-15 years at time of injury was performed in several steps through population-based registries, local registries and by supplementary informal sources as shown in figure 1. As an initial step, the study population was operationally defined and criteria for inclusion and exclusion were set (Table 1). The pedTSCI population was assessed according to the following descriptors: a. gender, b. age at injury, c. cause of injury [13, 14] and d. cause of death [15, 16].

*Gross neurological and functional outcome* was assessed among survivors by review of medical records and/or additional clinical observations.

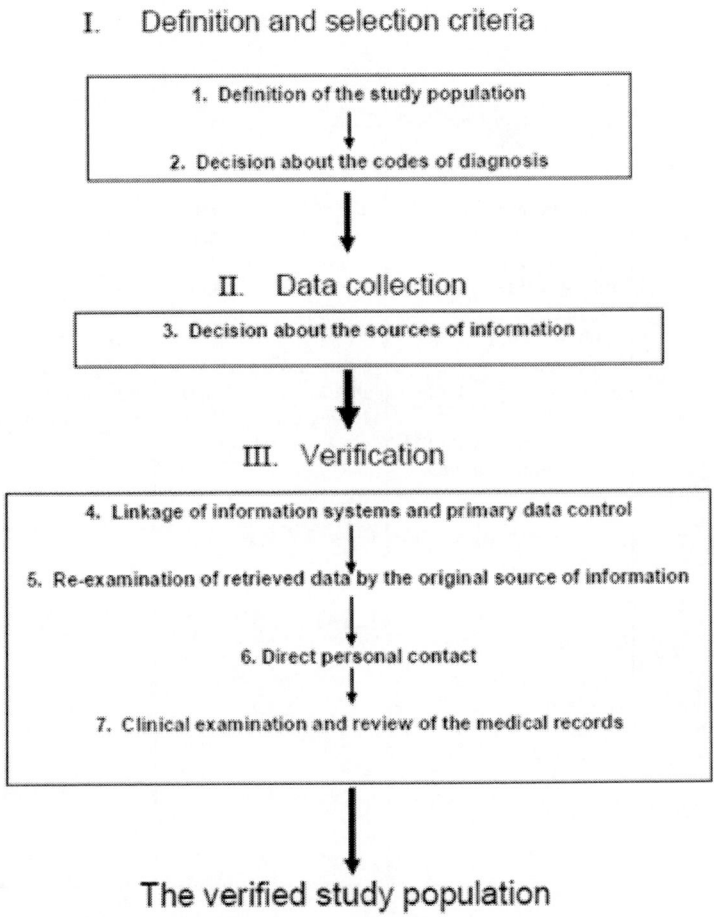

I.   Definition and selection criteria

1. Definition of the study population

2. Decision about the codes of diagnosis

II.   Data collection

3. Decision about the sources of information

III.   Verification

4. Linkage of information systems and primary data control

5. Re-examination of retrieved data by the original source of information

6. Direct personal contact

7. Clinical examination and review of the medical records

The verified study population

Figure 1. Process chart of finding a verified population of pedTSCI.

*Mortality* directly related to the TSCI was operationally defined as all deaths which had occurred within one year post-injury. Subjects that died later than one year post-injury were allocated to the survivor group.

*Etiological classification:* Through the interviews, ten cases initially classified as fall accidents, and two cases initially classified as traffic accidents, were re-classified as sports injuries. *Care providers:* Patients were treated at county hospitals, and/or university clinics with or without specialized SCI units. The data sources utilized were the Hospital Discharge Register (HDR) [3], medical records and patients themselves. If a patient had been treated in two or more hospitals, the hospital where the patient had been treated the longest period was indicated. Thereafter a decision was made regarding what sources of information should be used. Verification was made in four steps (Figure 1): 1. Linkage of retrieved data from different data sources were performed, in order to avoid duplicates, as well as to identify and eliminate obvious errors. 2. Retrieved data were sent back to the original source, with a request for validation of the recorded diagnosis. 3. Personal contact was undertaken in order to corroborate data from the medical records. 4. If ambiguity with regard to diagnosis and/ or outcome remained, a clinical examination and/or additional review of medical records were performed.

**Table 1. Criteria on operational definitions used in the study**

| Definition | Exclusion criteria | Inclusion criteria | Requested classification codes from the Swedish National Board of Health and Welfare | |
|---|---|---|---|---|
| Impairment resulting from traumatic lesions of the cauda equina or the spinal cord proper. Lesions with complete sensory-motor restitution were also included, as defined by American Spinal Injury Association (ASIA), impairment Scale grade E, but with documented evidence of previous symptoms and signs of SCI for at least two weeks after the injury [60]. When the incidence was estimated, mortality directly related to the traumatic event was operationally defined as death occurring within one year post injury [61] | Children with isolated root lesions or no injury to the intraspinal neural elements. Children with congenital malformations of the spinal cord. Children with acquired SCI of non-traumatic etiology. | The injury must have occurred in Sweden between the years 1-1-1985 until 31-12-1996. At the time of the injury the child should be between 0-15 years of age. | The Swedish version of the 9th edition of the International Classification of Disease (rev. ICD 9 used in the period 1987-1995 and their equivalents in the 8th edition of this classification) [14, 62]. | |
| | | | 806 A-X | *Fracture of the spine with a SCI* |
| | | | 952 A-X | *SCI without any signs of damage to the spinal vertebrae* |
| | | | 767E | *Birth injuries, injuries to the spine and the spinal cord* |
| | | | 344 A-X | *Other paralyses* |

### 2.1.1. Calculation of Estimated Incidence

The incidence estimates of pedTSCI were calculated based on data from population registers and County Habilitation centers for the years 1-1-1985 to 31-12-1996.

The cumulative total population of Swedish children below 16 years of age during the 12 year period was 20.171.823 children, with an average population growth of 1.680.000 children/year (max/min: 1.767.000/1.613.000) [16].

Instead of using the cumulative total population as a basis for incidence, information from each year was used. The annual incidence can be treated as a random variable over the 12-year study period. The expected value and confidence interval was then based on the annual incidences.

## 2.2. Results

Initial register screening identified 384 cases, which by subsequent analysis were found to include a large number of false positives (i.e. incorrect diagnostic coding). Ultimately, 35 living cases could be fully verified and 14 deceased cases could be pragmatically verified (Figure 2).

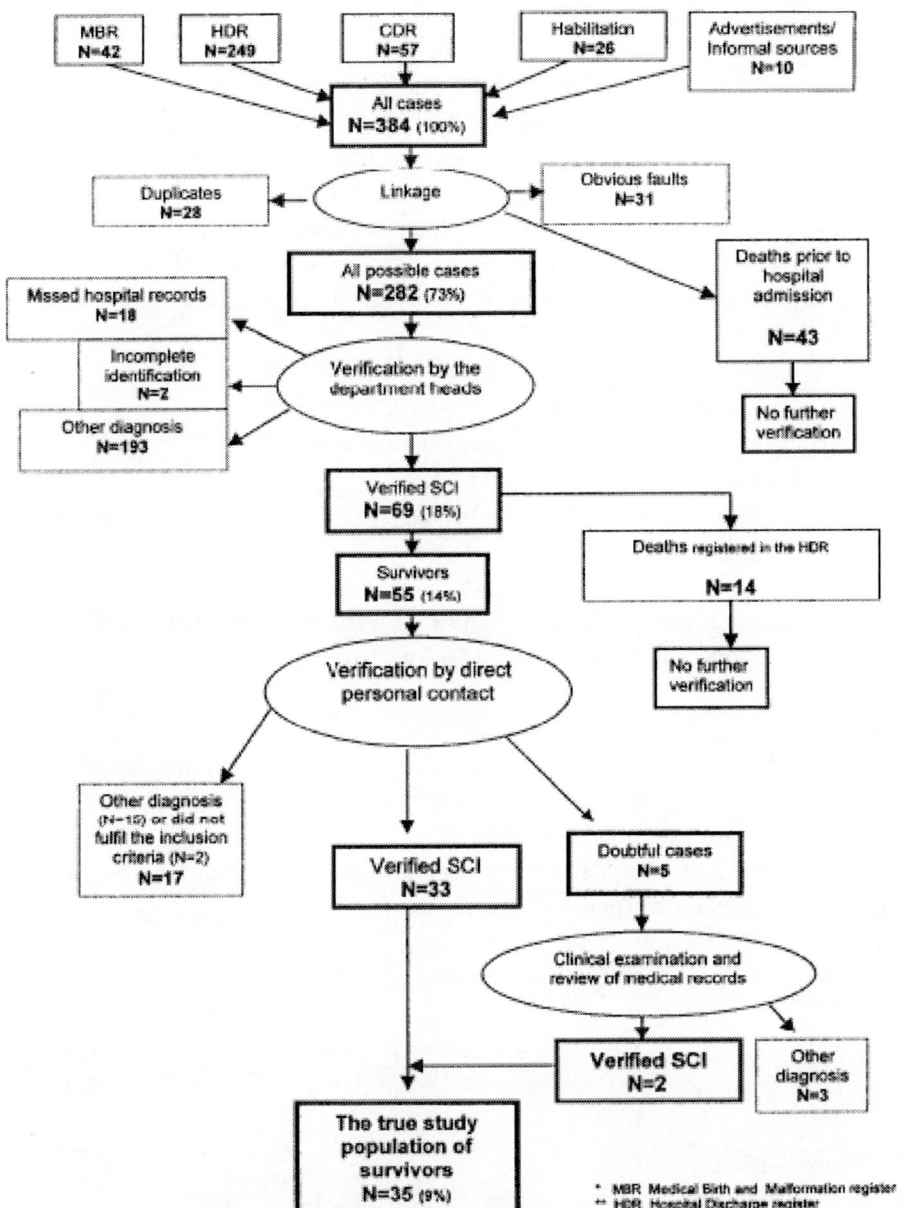

Figure 2. Flow-chart of the process of finding children and adolescents (0-15 years) with pedSCI in Sweden, 1985-1996.

The study population included three groups of children and adolescents:

1. For cases identified as dead prior to hospital admission (N=43), data from the Cause of Death register [15, 17] were used as verification. Autopsy protocols were not reviewed.

2. For cases identified as dead within one year post-injury (N=12), the head of the department at the treating hospital verified the diagnosis by retrospectively reviewing

the medical records. The information originated from the Hospital Discharge register [18] and the Cause of Death register [15, 17].

3.  For survivors (n=37), retrieved data were checked against the medical records by a senior staff physician at the treating hospital. Subjects were then directly contacted for further verification of diagnosis, after which the remaining putatively true cases were interviewed and in some cases also examined for final verification and additional data retrieval. The information originated from the Hospital Discharge register (N=34) [18], Habilitation Centers (N=2) and informal contacts (N=1). (Two cases died three years and nine years post injury, respectively, and information was retrieved from medical records).

### 2.2.1. Incidence for Ages 0-15 Years

The incidence was 4.6 /million children/year (95% CI 3.6-5.5). When excluding pre-hospital fatalities, the incidence was 2.4 (95% CI 1.8-3.1).

Twenty-one children (23%) of the total group (N=92) were aged 15 years at the time of the injury.

Out of survivors (N=37), 12 children were 15 years of age (32%). Out of the children dead prior of hospital admission (N=43), 7 children were aged 15 years (16%). Two children out of the group who died within one year post-injury were aged 15 years.

### 2.2.2. Mortality

Fifty-five children (60%) of the total group (N=92) died within one year after the SCI.

### 2.2.2.1. Deaths Prior to Hospital Admission

Forty-two of the 43 children dead at the scene of the accident or who died on the way to the hospital were injured in traffic accidents (figure 3).

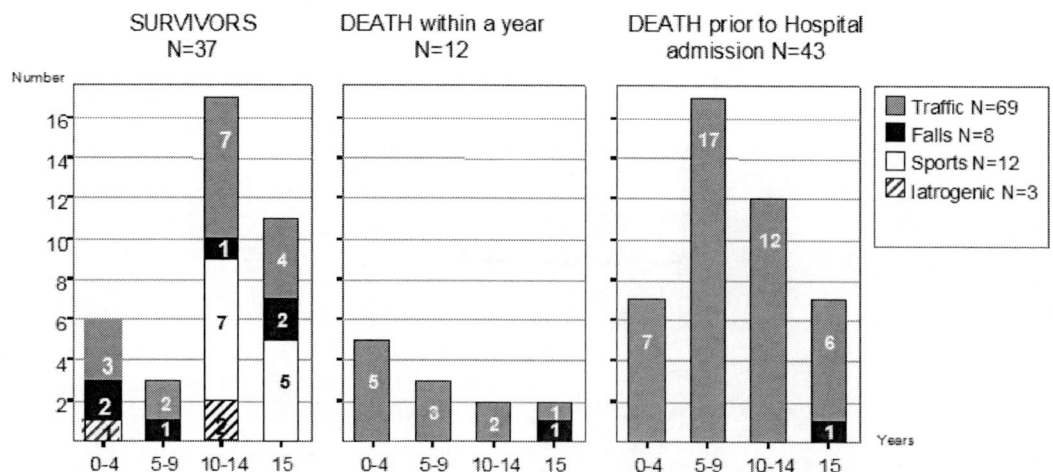

Figure 3. Causes of injury by age group and outcome, N=92.

As a principle diagnosis, three had SCIWORA, (ICD 952) and the others were registered as SCI (ICD 806.00). Average age at injury was 9 years (SD=4; range 2-15 years), 19 were girls and 23 were boys. The retrieved register information gave no information about the level of injury.

### 2.2.2.2. Deaths within One Year Post-Injury

Twelve children died during initial hospitalization; all within three months post-injury. All but one child were injured by traffic accidents *(figure.3)*.

The average age at injury for this group was 7.3 years (SD=5.3; range 0-15 years), including 10 girls and 2 boys. All patients had cervical injuries except one child that suffered a thoracic injury, with an additional brain injury.

### 2.2.2.3. The Survivors

Children surviving at least the first year post-injury (N=37) had an average age at injury of 11.9 years (SD 4.4; range 2-15 years).

### *2.2.3. Associated Injuries*

Of the total group (N=92), 38 children (41%) had associated injuries such as extremity fractures, thoracic injuries, abdominal injuries or head injuries. All head injuries but one were caused by traffic accidents.

### *2.2.4. Causes of Injury*

### Traffic Accidents

Among fatalities, traffic accidents dominated (figure 4). None of the bicyclists survived. The mean age was 9.2 years (SD 3.6; range 4-15).

The distribution of traffic accidents by age groups is shown in Table 2. The pedestrians had a mean age of 8.9 years (SD 2.8; range 5-14). Among survivors (10-15 years), sports related injuries (43%) were as common a cause of injury as traffic accidents (39%) (Figure 3).

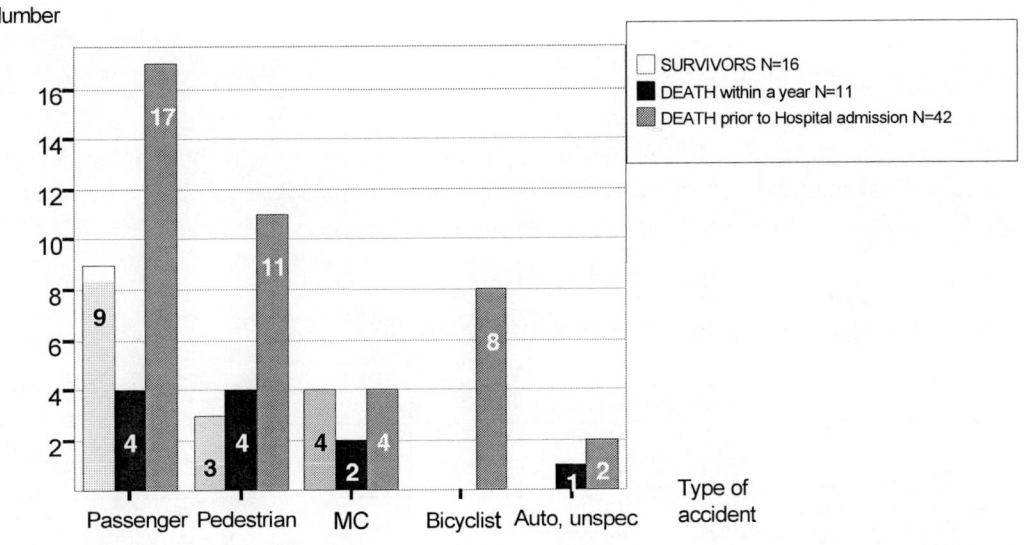

Figure 4. Distribution of traffic accidents by outcome, N=69.

**Table 2. Distribution of traffic accidents by age groups, N=69**

| Type of traffic accident | Age groups | | | | |
|---|---|---|---|---|---|
| | 0-4 years | 5-9 years | 10-14 years | 15 years | Total |
| Passengers | 13 | 6 | 8 | 3 | 30 |
| Pedestrians | 0 | 11 | 7 | 0 | 18 |
| Bicycle | 1 | 4 | 2 | 1 | 8 |
| Moped/MC | 0 | 0 | 3 | 7 | 10 |
| Unspecified | 1 | 1 | 0 | 1 | 3 |
| Total | 15 | 22 | 20 | 12 | 69 |

## Falls

Out of six fall-related injures among the survivors, four children were injured by falling from heights. Only one girl was injured in a falling accident (Figure 3), the remained were boys.

## Iatrogenic Injury

Three children, two girls and one boy, sustained a TSCI related to surgery for spinal deformity (Figure 3).

### 2.2.5. SCIWORA

Of the total group (N=92), five children were registered as Spinal Cord without radiological abnormality (SCIWORA). Among the fully verified survivors, three children had sustained a SCIWORA (aged 3, 4, 9 years).

### 2.2.6. Gender

There were 47 males and 45 females. The distribution of males increased by age among the survivors.

### 2.2.7. Types of Lesions

Distribution of level of lesions is shown in Table 3. Cervical injuries among the survivors were as common as thoracic lesions (N=16). The average age for children with cervical lesions was 12.2 years (SD 4.2; range 3-15 years), for children with thoracic lesions 11.1 years (SD 4.8; range 2-15 years) and for children with lumbar lesions 13.2 years (SD 1.3; range 11-15 years). Almost half (N=17) of the group of survivors had a complete SCI (ASIA grade A).

**Table 3. Distribution of injury level and care provider among the survivors, N=37**

| Level of injury | Level of care and rehabilitation | | | |
|---|---|---|---|---|
| | University | County Hospital | SCI-unit | Total |
| Cervical | 2 | 4 | 10 | 16 |
| Thoracic | 1 | 7 | 8 | 16 |
| Lumbar | 0 | 1 | 4 | 5 |
| Total | 3 | 12 | 22 | 37 |

### 2.2.8. Care Provider

The survivors (N=37) were treated in 18 different hospitals. Distribution of care provider and level of lesion is shown in Table 3.

The average age of cases treated at a SCI unit was 14 years (SD 1.3; range 9-15 years), whereas cases treated elsewhere had a lower average age, 8 and 8.9 years, respectively.

## 2.3. Discussion

We were able to verify the prevalent belief that pedTSCI is rare in Sweden. We found that the method of using the population based registers was very time-consuming. The frequency of false positive diagnoses (over 70%) found in the HDR made direct analysis useless without additional quality control.

It is our opinion that the identification of spinal cord lesions of *non-traumatic* etiology in the HDR would have been next to impossible.

One possible solution to these problems is the development of specific "quality registers" for rare diagnoses such as SCI. Several such registers have in fact been developed by the National Board of Health and Welfare in Sweden. The SCI Council in Sweden has produced a consensus document on basic quality indicators of SCI care, as well as a set of descriptors of treatments and outcomes.

A national database which collects data from all major SCI units was launched in 1997. This database is a potentially useful source for research projects and may facilitate collaborative projects [11, 12]. Internationally, the development of a so-called core data set has further standardized and improved the data collection and reporting pertaining to SCI [19, 20]. It is obviously of importance to also determine the reliability of these standards for pedSCI [21].

Despite these efforts, there remains the problem of cases missed by the available registers. The care of pedTSCI in Sweden remains severely scattered and is not systematically monitored as it would be at the designated SCI centers. In particular, the youngest children are treated in pediatric settings which lack contact with adult SCI centers and which are unaware of the national SCI database and lack familiarity with the SCI core data set.

## 2.4. Conclusion

Traffic accidents are the main cause of pedTSCI in Sweden.

The incidence of pediatric trauma in Sweden is among the lowest in the world. This is likely a result of vigorous preventative work performed over the last 50 years. Laws and regulations have made the environment for children safer, as have systematic information and education efforts aimed at parents [22, 23].

Still, accidents remain the most common causes of death among children and adolescents aged 1-14 years in Sweden [22, 23]. Children are vulnerable in traffic accidents due to the complex situations that frequently arise and which exceed their cognitive, developmental, behavioural, physical and sensory abilities to avoid injury. Children are impulsive and have difficulties in judging speed, spatial relations and distances.

Additionally, adolescents in particular tend to be risk-prone and easily influenced by emotions, stress, and peer pressure [24]. They frequently act in the adult environment, but they lack the experience and mature behaviour of an adult.

Sport is another leading cause of pedTSCI in Sweden, especially so among adolescents. This is in accordance with reports from other countries [25-29]. Preventative measures, e.g. strict rules and adequate equipment, should be ensured in sports which carry a risk for SCI.

SCI prevention should be tailored according to the specific risk profile of each age group. As Sweden until now has focused most prevention strategies on younger children [30], there is now a need for national coordination and methodological development of preventative efforts towards adolescents.

# 3. SCI AMONG ADULTS IN SWEDEN

Data presented below are part of the Stockholm Thessaloniki Acute Traumatic Spinal Cord Injury Study (STATSCIS). In summary, STATSCIS evaluated the demographic and injury characteristics [9], clinical characteristics on admission [31], early treatment [31], clinical process [31, 32], first year mortality [33], and other key outcomes at one year post-trauma [32] of the incident Traumatic Spinal Cord Injury (TSCI) populations in a Northern (Stockholm, Sweden) and in a Southern (Thessaloniki, Greece) European Union Region.

The two regions followed different approaches of care for managing acute TSCI; Stockholm followed a systems approach with a centralized and predefined clinical process that includes a Spinal Injury Unit (SIU), whereas Thessaloniki appeared with a generic "non-system" approach scattered over dozens of wards.

## 3.1. Method

### 3.1.1. Setting

The following data refer to Greater Stockholm region in Sweden (hereafter: Stockholm). In accordance with the Nomenclature of Territorial Units for Statistics (NUTS) adopted by the European Commission, what in the present text is referred to as the the "greater Stockholm region" consists of Stockholm County and Gotland County, Sweden. As of early 2003, Sweden had a population of almost 8.9 million. In 2007, Stockholm's population over 15 years of age was just over 1.6 million. Within Stockholm, there is a comprehensive SCI system of care, consisting of one hospital based SIU, two inpatient rehabilitation centres and one outpatient clinic for lifelong follow-up.

### 3.1.2. Inclusion Criteria

All of the following criteria had to be satisfied for inclusion:

1. acute traumatic spinal cord or cauda equina lesion;
2. age ≥16 years at the time of injury;
3. inpatient care at a hospital of Stockholm at any time between September 2006 and October 2007;

4. survival for at least 7 days post trauma;
5. Swedish residency

For data referring to mortality, only the Incidence Cohort was considered, i.e. that of injury occurring during the first 12 months of the study period (September 2006 to September 2007).

### 3.1.3. Identification of Cases

Identification of acute TSCI cases was obtained through a surveillance system with both passive and active components. In Stockholm, there is a comprehensive system of care, consisting of one hospital based SIU, two inpatient rehabilitation centres, and one outpatient clinic for life-long follow-up.

All parts of the system share a battery of registration forms, the so-called Nordic Spinal Cord Injury Registry (NSCIR).

The NSCIR was the passive component of case-identification, and it was coordinated by the principal investigator (A.D.) both in order to avoid inclusion of false positive cases (e.g. non-traumatic or chronic SCI) and also to ensure inclusion of outliers (e.g. cases not treated in the system). An additional active surveillance component was added by contacting all Intensive Care Units (ICUs) in the region, which were not typical locations for treatment of TSCI.

This design was chosen since, although the regional SCI system of care is highly centralized, it may occasionally be the case that severe multi-trauma cases with TSCI receive acute treatment in other hospitals. Thus, a letter of inquiry was sent to all seven ICUs in the region, asking if during the study period the unit had hospitalised any potential case with acute TSCI who had died.

### 3.1.4. Cohorts

STATSCIS included two types of cohorts: the incidence (II) and the inception (IV) cohorts (Figure 5). The incidence cohorts (II) consisted of cases injured after the start of registration (middle of September 2006) and during the 12 following months.

The inception cohorts (IV) consisted of the incidence cohorts, and additionally included two more subgroups; the first comprising cases hospitalized at the initiation of STATSCIS on September 2006; and the second comprising cases injured after the first 12 months of registration but before end of October 2007. This method was chosen in order to increase the sample size and assure inclusion of all incident cases. More specifically, the period between middle of September 2007 and end of October 2007 served as a trajectory period.

In that way, we ensured the inclusion of cases that were injured during the first 12 months of the study, but which were identified at a later stage (e.g. early hospitalisation in a smaller hospital, injury occurring abroad, delayed final diagnosis).

STATSCIS, importantly, did not include cases that died during the first week post-trauma. This methodological choice was made due to the following reasons:

(1) Deaths that occur early after trauma are often difficult to assess accurately.
(2) Lack of systematic data in early fatal trauma cases.
(3) The contribution of TSCI, its consequences and complications to death are difficult to assess in early trauma deaths.

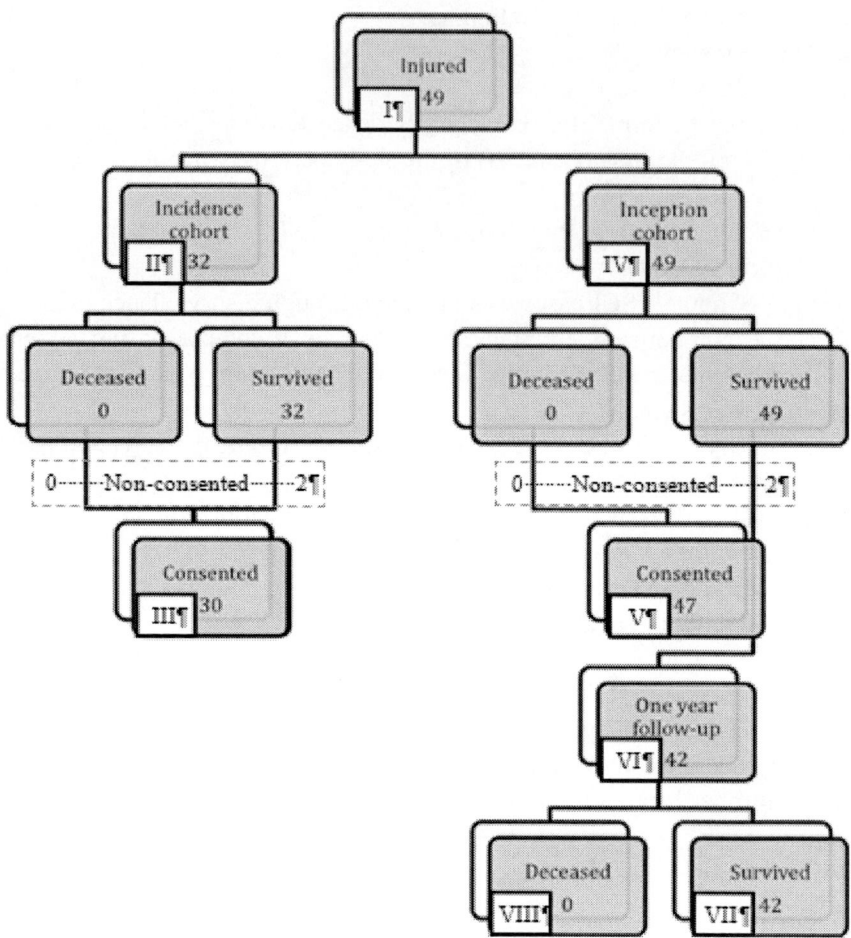

Figure 5. Cohort in Stockholm.

(4) Pre-hospital trauma deaths are categorized generally, and not based on a specific diagnosis.

(5) Many early trauma deaths occur irrespectively of the given treatment due to the severity of injuries. Our goal was to isolate cases where management could play a significant role in survival.

PedTSCI was not included due to its rare nature, and the different type of management that is usually required.

### 3.1.5. Data Collection

Each case was individually followed-up during the first year post-trauma. All data collection was carried out according to a subset of the NSCIR (www.nscic.se). The subset consisted of the Acute Form, the Neurological Assessment Form, the Pain Form, the Urological Function Form, the Bowel Function Form, the Spasticity Form, the Respiratory Function Form, the Pressure Ulcer Form, the ADL Form and the Circulatory Function Form.

The NSCIR forms were used on admission, at discharge and at one year post-trauma. Data were obtained by physical examination, including the International Standards for

Neurological classification for SCI; medical records review, including EMS notes and death certificate; personal communication with the attending physicians and staff; and communication with each case and a first degree relative. Use of multiple sources of information was necessary since a single complete source was not available.

Clinical neurological examination including assessment according to the International Standards was performed in all cases. All such examinations, which provided data for the present study, were performed by physicians and physiotherapists specialized in SCI. Clinical diagnosis of TSCI was confirmed by neuro-imaging studies.

Data were gathered according to the routine process of the NSCIR. One of the authors (AD) carefully coordinated all data collection throughout the study period. Furthermore, after obtaining an approval by the Nordic SCI Council, A.D. performed a large part of data entry in the system of NSCIR, thus being able to control for missing and mismatched data.

Quality assurance was performed by cross-checking data in the registry forms with medical records, in order to maximise validity and minimise missing data. All retrieved data were re-evaluated in detail by the authors jointly for purposes of medical accuracy and uniform interpretation, e.g. as regards extra-spinal injuries and any secondary morbidity.

The web-based registration forms of the NSCIR were used to store data in Stockholm. An additional computer-based module was developed that allowed for registration of the patient's clinical course, including inter-facility transfers and Length of Stay (LOS).

## 3.2. Results and Discussion

### 3.2.1. Incidence

The annual incidence of TSCI (for individuals older than 15 years of age who survived for at least 7 days post-trauma) was 19.4/million for Stockholm. Recent studies from other EU countries report annual survival incidences of TSCI per million inhabitants of 10.4 in the Netherlands [34] (survived first hospitalization), 33.6 in Greece [9] (survived first week after injury), 13.1 in Ireland (35) (survived acute care), 25.4 in Portugal (36) (survived 30 days after injury), 19.4 in France [37] (older than 15 years who survived acute care).

Our figure for annual incidence rate of TSCI in Stockholm is nearly double that presented previously [38]. This might be due to the fact that previous estimates were purely based on raw registry data from a single component of the system, and without systematically performing quality assurance procedures. Although direct comparison of incidence rates between studies is hampered by methodological differences, it may nonetheless be concluded that Stockholm has a relatively low incidence of TSCI.

### 3.2.2. Demographics and Injury Characteristics

Overall, 49 individuals in Stockholm sustained a TSCI during the study period. Demographic and injury characteristics are provided in Table 4. Out of 47 individuals who consented to STATSCIS, 36 were males (77%) and 11 females (23%), with a mean age of 47 years (SD=+18, Median=46). Just 23% of the individuals in Stockholm group belonged to the 16-30 age-group, nearly as many as to the 31-45 age-group, 19% belonged to the 46-60 age group, 28% to the 61-75 age-group, and only 4% to the >75 years age-group.

One out of seven individuals (15%) was a foreigner living in Sweden, one out of ten (11%) acquired their injury during work, and six (13%) while travelling abroad. The peak months for occurrence of TSCI were August and September and the peak day was Saturday.

Falls were the leading cause of injury as they occurred in 22 individuals (47%). Transportation accidents occurred in 11 (23%), sports-related injuries (including diving) in 8 (17%), iatrogenic in 2 (4%), assault in 1 (2%) and other causes in 3 (6%). Within the category of falls, 4 were intentional and 18 unintentional; 10 occurred on the same level or from less than 1 meter height, 4 from 1-3 meter, 3 from more than 3 meters and 1 unknown. Regarding individuals injured in transportation accidents, 2 were car occupants, 5 motorcycle riders, 1 pedestrian and 3 other/unknown.

While falls affected all age-groups, transportation accidents occurred in only three out of five age-groups; 16-30, 31-45 and 61-75 with a peak in the middle one.

Regarding the youngest age-group, sports-related injuries (including diving) affected more individuals as compared to transportation accidents (Figure 6).

In Sweden, the leading cause of injury has shifted during the last decade from transportation to fall accidents. As in Australia, such a trend could probably be attributed to the success of public health measures directed at transport-related injury, as well as to the increasing need for prevention programs directed at fall-related injuries [39].

## Table 4. Demographic and injury characteristics

|  | Stockholm |
|---|---|
| Consented cases | 47 |
| Gender (Male:Female) *Males* *Females* | 3:1 36 (77%) 11 (23%) |
| Age (Mean, Median, Stand. Dev.) *16-30* *31-45* *46-60* *61-75* *>75* | 47, 46, ±18 11 (23%) 12 (26%) 9 (19%) 13 (28%) 2 (4%) |
| Foreign background | 7 (15%) |
| Level of education *Basic* *Further* *Advanced* | 14 (30%) 18 (38%) 15 (32%) |
| Aetiology *Sports-related including diving* *Fall* *Assault* *Iatrogenic* *Transportation* *Other* | 8 (17%) 22 (47%) 1 (2%) 2 (4%) 11 (23%) 3 (6%) |
| Work-related | 5 (11%) |

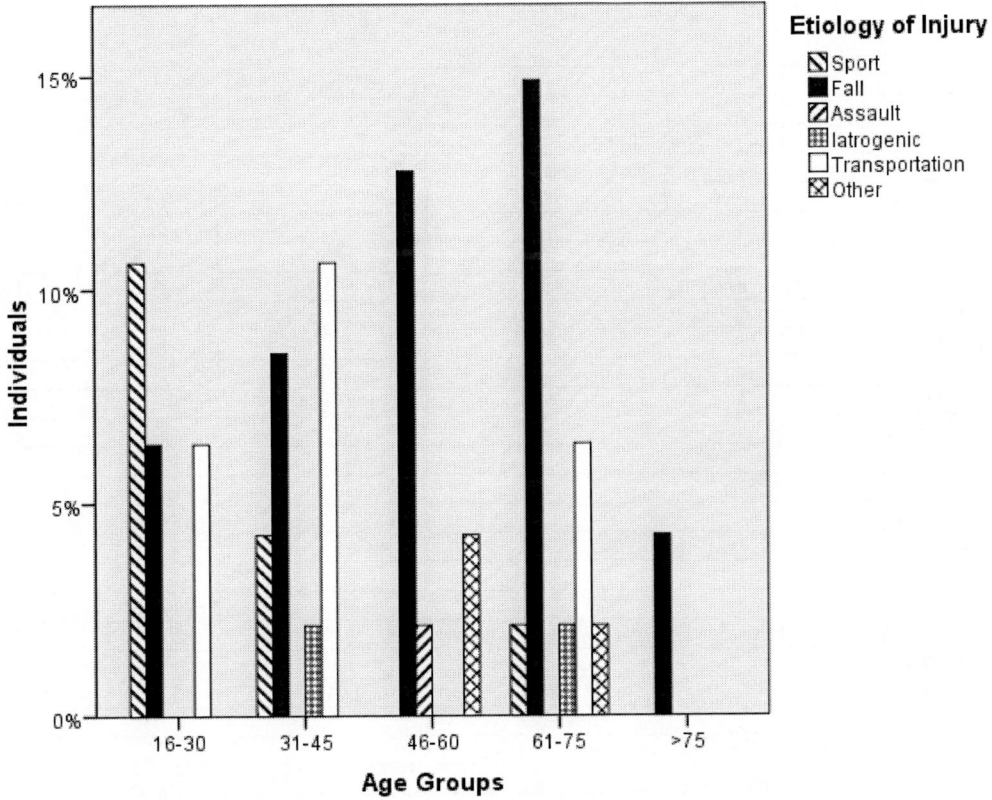

Figure 6. Etiology of injury.

### 3.2.3. Core Clinical Characteristics on Admission

With regard to neurological status of cases on admission, about 30% of TSCI cases had a high cervical neurological lesion (C1-C4), about 10% had a low cervical lesion (C5-C8), about 45% a thoracic lesion (T1-T12) and about 10% had a lumbo-sacral lesion. Approximately 35% of lesions were classified as ASIA Impairment Scale (AIS) grade A, 5% as AIS grade B, 20% as AIS grade C, and 30% as AIS grade D. (Figure 7).

Seven out of ten cases had normal level of consciousness (LOC). Upper extremities and thorax injuries were the most common extra-spinal injuries. One out of ten cases had a life-threatening extra-spinal injury. (Table 5).

### 3.2.4. Acute Key Therapeutic Interventions

Transfers from the scene of trauma to a tertiary level hospital were carried out mainly by road ambulance and in a few cases by air transport. The vast majority of cases (83%) were transferred directly to a tertiary level hospital, whereas the rest were first transferred to a lower level hospital. Overall, nearly all cases were transferred from the scene of trauma to a tertiary level hospital within the same day of injury.

Overall, the goal seems to be to transfer the case as soon as possible to a tertiary hospital, and then to provide treatment within the designated system.

### Table 5. Core clinical characteristics on admission

|  | Stockholm (n=47) | |
| --- | --- | --- |
|  | *n* | *(%)* |
| Consciousness on first hospital admission |  |  |
| *Normal* | *30* | *(64)* |
| *Impaired* | *9* | *(19)* |
| *Unconscious* | *2* | *(4)* |
| *Missing* | *6* | *(13)* |
| Extra spinal injuries - Present | 23 | (49) |
| Extra spinal injuries – Severity |  |  |
| *Mild* | *11* | *(23)* |
| *Serious* | *8* | *(17)* |
| *Life-threatening* | *4* | *(9)* |
| Extra Spinal Injuries – Topography |  |  |
| *Skull* | *6* | *(13)* |
| *Upper extremities* | *10* | *(21)* |
| *Thorax* | *11* | *(23)* |
| *Abdomen* | *1* | *(2)* |
| *Pelvis* | *3* | *(6)* |
| *Lower extremities* | *5* | *(11)* |
| Co-morbid Spinal Disorder – Present | 12 | (26) |
| *Rheumatoid arthritis* | *0* | *(0)* |
| *Spinal stenosis* | *7* | *(15)* |
| *Mb Bechterew* | *2* | *(4)* |
| *Degenerative spinal disease* | *2* | *(4)* |
| Pre-morbid non-spinal disorder |  |  |
| *Diabetes Mellitus* | *1* | *(2)* |
| *Arteriosclerotic Cardio/ Cerebrovascular Disease* | *6* | *(13)* |
| *Parkinson Disease* | *0* | *(0)* |
| *Major Psychiatric Disorder* | *3* | *(6)* |
| *Abuse* | *5* | *(11)* |

### Table 6. Acute key therapeutic interventions

|  | Stockholm (n=47) | |
| --- | --- | --- |
|  | *n* | *(%)* |
| Spinal Surgery | 46 | (98) |
| Additional spinal surgery | 4 | (9) |
| Mechanical ventilation | 10 | (21) |
| *Acute* | *9* | *(19)* |
| *Post-acute* | *1* | *(2)* |
| Tracheostomy | 7 | (15) |
| *Early* | *4* | *(9)* |
| *Late* | *3* | *(6)* |
| Initiation of Corticosteroids | 31 | (66) |
| Anti-coagulant treatment | 45 | (96) |

Nearly 20% received mechanical ventilation and seven out of ten patients who received ventilation also underwent a tracheostomy (Table 6). Spinal surgery was performed in nearly all cases (98%) after an average of 3 days (Median=1, SD=4).

Despite the absence of conclusive data on optimal timing for performing spinal surgery, it has been recommended that surgical decompression and stabilization should be performed early after acute TSCI, especially in the presence of progressive neurological deterioration [40, 41].

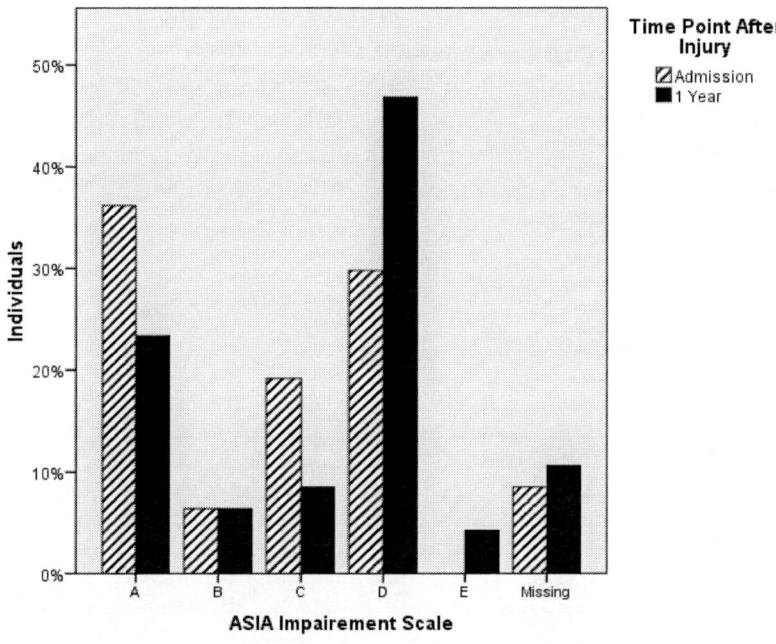

Figure 7. ASIA Impairment scale on admission and at 1 year post injury.

### 3.2.5. Mortality

The annual case mortality rate was 0%, as none of the 32 cases of the incidence cohort died during the first year post-trauma. This figure refers to the cases who had already survived the first week post-trauma.

The purpose of STATSCIS was to evaluate the impact of the presence of a system of care on outcomes after a TSCI. Therefore, it was beyond the scope of this study to investigate first week post-trauma mortality.

As has been shown previously [42], pre- and early in-hospital deaths (occurring during the first week after trauma) were significantly associated with more severe injuries, compared with late in-hospital deaths. Furthermore, as reported by the Liverpool Hospital Trauma Death Peer Review Committee [43] a greater proportion of potentially avoidable trauma deaths occurred after and not during the first week of admission. Considering our inclusion criteria, and especially the 7 days survival cut-off, we could assume that the most severely injured who died were excluded from this study. Precise comparisons with other studies are hampered by methodological differences that greatly affect the estimated mortality rates. In the population-based study from Portugal, 26% of those with acute TSCI who had survived the first week after trauma died during the following months [36]. Other studies reported in-hospital mortality rates after acute TSCI to be 5.7% to 8% in Canada [44-46], 8.6% in Germany [47], and 11.9% in Teresina/ Brazil [48]. The 1-year TSCI mortality rate was reported to be 18.8% in Greece [33], 5.8% in Australia [49] and 3.6% in US Model Spinal

Cord Injury System [50]. A more recent study from the US Model Spinal Cord Injury System revealed a 40% decline in mortality during the first two years after trauma since 1970s [51].

### 3.2.6. Associated Conditions and Complications

Clean intermittent catheterization (four out of ten cases) and suprapubic catheter (two out of ten) were the two methods for bladder management for those who could not initiate voiding normally. No case had an indwelling urethral catheter in place at one year post trauma. Long-term use of an indwelling urethral catheter is known to be responsible for higher morbidity [52-54].

No case was on a ventilatory support or had a tracheostomy in place at one year follow-up. Data on associated conditions and their management are provided in Table 7 and medical complications are provided in Table 8.

### Table 7. Associated conditions and their management

|                              | Stockholm (n=42) | |
| --- | --- | --- |
|                              | *n* | *(%)* |
| BLADDER                      |     |       |
| Awareness of bladder filling |     |       |
| *Yes*                        | 25  | *(60)* |
| *No*                         | 17  | *(40)* |
| Bladder management method    |     |       |
| *Normally initiated*         | 17  | *(40)* |
| *Intermittent catheterization* | 16 | (38) |
| *Indwelling catheter*        | 0   | (0)   |
| *Suprapubic catheter*        | 9   | (21)  |
| *Other*                      | 0   | (0)   |
| BOWEL                        |     |       |
| Awareness of bowel filling   |     |       |
| *Yes, directly*              | 18  | *(43)* |
| *Yes, indirectly*            | 8   | *(19)* |
| *No*                         | 16  | *(38)* |
| Colostomy                    | 0   |       |
| CIRCULATION                  |     |       |
| *Orthostatism*               | 2   | *(5)* |
| Autonomic Dysreflexia        | 4   | *(17)** |
| RESPIRATORY                  |     |       |
| *Tracheostomy*               | 0   | *(0)* |
| *Ventilator*                 | 0   | *(0)* |
| PAIN                         |     |       |
| *Above NL of lesion*         | 7   | *(17)* |
| *At NL of lesion*            | 18  | *(43)* |
| *Below NL of lesion*         | 15  | *(36)* |
| SPASTICITY                   |     |       |
| *No*                         | 15  | *(36)* |
| *Mild*                       | 12  | *(29)* |
| *Moderate*                   | 11  | *(26)* |
| *Severe*                     | 4   | *(10)* |

Abbreviations: NL, Neurological level.

\* percent counted considering only the cases being at a risk to develop Autonomic Dysreflexia; 31 cases in Thessaloniki and 23 cases in Stockholm.

**Table 8. Medical complications**

| | Stockholm (n=42) | |
|---|---|---|
| | *n* | *(%)* |
| RENAL | | |
| Urinary Tract Infection | | |
| *None* | *11* | *(26)* |
| *1-2* | *20* | *(48)* |
| *> 3* | *11* | *(26)* |
| Pyelonephritis | *3* | *(7)* |
| Orchitis | *0* | *(0)* |
| Other | *4* | *(10)* |
| PRESSURE ULCERS | | |
| During the last year | | |
| *None* | *24* | *(57)* |
| *One* | *8* | *(19)* |
| *Two – Four* | *10* | *(24)* |
| *Five or more* | *0* | *(0)* |
| On 1 year follow-up | | |
| *Yes* | *7* | *(17)* |
| *No* | *35* | *(83)* |
| PULMONARY | | |
| *Pneumonia* | *8* | *(19)* |
| *Tracheal stenosis* | *0* | *(0)* |
| *Other* | *2* | *(5)* |
| MUSCULOSCELETAL | | |
| *Heterotopic ossification* | *2* | *(5)* |
| *Decreased spinal mobility* | *0* | *(0)* |
| *Others* | *2* | *(5)* |
| CIRCULATION | | |
| *Sepsis/ bacteraemia* | *1* | *(2)* |
| *Cardiac arrhythmias* | *0* | *(0)* |
| *DVT* | *0* | *(0)* |
| *Compartment syndrome* | *1* | *(2)* |
| *Pulmonary embolism* | *1* | *(2)* |

Urinary tract infection (UTI) was the most common complication during the first year post-trauma, as half of the cases had experienced one or two incidents. One out of four cases had multiple UTIs ($\geq$3). Acquiring a pressure ulcer of any degree still remains the second most common complication, as two out of five cases acquired at least one ulcer during the first year post trauma. Nearly every fifth case went through the first year follow-up having a pressure ulcer. DVT and PE were rare, probably due to routine administration of anticoagulant prophylaxis early after injury. It might be that acquiring one low grade pressure ulcer in the acute stage is more or less inevitable. The lack of data on ulcer grading and location do not allow for further analysis of this issue in the present study.

Data from other settings report rates of pressure ulcers on the first annual follow-up year post-trauma to range between 12-36% [55-58]. In some of these studies, pressure ulcers were the most frequent medical complication, with an increasing rate in later follow-ups [57]. Cases transferred early to a SCI-system were reported to suffer a statistically significant fewer ulcers as compared to those admitted later [59].

### 3.2.7. Length of Stay

For assessment of LOS (Table 9), cases were divided in two groups, depending on their motor completeness on admission – AIS grades A and B formed the 'initially motor complete' group (IMC), whereas AIS grades C and D formed the 'initially motor incomplete' group (IMIC). Sixteen IMC cases (84%) and 8 IMIC cases (42%) were hospitalized in an Intensive Care Unit (ICU) for a similar median period (8 days and 7 days respectively). All cases were hospitalized in the Spinal Injury Unit (SIU), the IMC for a median period of 53 days and the IMIC for a median period of 35 days. Similarly, nearly all cases were subsequent treated at an in-patient rehabilitation facility; IMC for a median period of 51 days and IMIC for a median period of 38 days. Total in-patient LOS for IMC was 119 days and for IMIC was 76 days.

As becomes evident when considering data on process and LOS, long stays in ICU were avoided, and cases were concentrated in the SIU and in the two designated post-acute in-patient rehabilitation centres. The clinical process seems very straight forward for the vast majority of the cases. A precise comparison with other studies is not possible, mainly due to methodological differences, especially on defining accurately each component of care.

Motor completeness on admission seemed to play some role in hospitalisation in an ICU, as IMC cases were more likely to receive treatment in such a facility.

### Table 9. Length of Stay[1]

|  | Initially Motor Complete mean (s.d.) median IQR N (%) | Initially Motor Incomplete mean (s.d.) median IQR N (%) |
|---|---|---|
| Intensive Care Unit | 11 (11) 8 [1-22] 16 (84) | 7 (6) 7 [1-12] 8 (42) |
| General Hospital Ward | 9 (8) 5 [4-13] 13 (68) | 10 (9) 8 [4-14] 16 (84) |
| Spinal Injury Unit | 62 (36) 53 [41-78] 19 (100) | 34 (14) 35 [21-47] 19 (100) |
| In-patient Rehabilitation Center | 55 (23) 51 [40-74] 18 (95) | 33 (16) 38 [19-41] 18 (95) |
| Total In-patient | 121 (37) 119 [90-156] 19 (100) | 74 (30) 76 [45-97] 19 (100) |

[1]Four cases in Stockholm were not considered as information on initial motor completeness was missing.

The clinical course in Stockholm is determined almost entirely by the co-ordinated system, which is based on functional outcomes. It should be remembered, however, that the system of care extant in Stockholm is by no means typical or representative of the situation at large in Sweden. As a rule, most acute TSCI patients receive early treatment at one of the six University hospitals with a SIU. Thereafter, particularly but not exclusively in the northern half of the country, patients are transferred to local hospitals for post-acute in-patient rehabilitation. Despite decades of discussions, a fully centralized system of care has as of yet not been implemented. To the contrary, the trend in later years has unfortunately been one of increasing decentralization and dispersion of patients.

The standardised process in Stockholm and generally in Sweden allows for a successful identification of both incident and prevalent TSCI cases, with a possibility of life-long follow-up and continuous quality assurance. Nonetheless, we believe that the new registry in Sweden, should have clearly defined information needs and purposes, right level of compliance with the International Core Data Set, and continuous connection it with other registries.

## 3.3. Conclusion

- Incidence rate for TSCI in Stockholm, Sweden is 19.4/ million/ year, which is a relatively low figure as compared to other countries.
- The leading cause of injury was falls that peaked in the 61-75 age group. The peak months for occurrence of TSCI were August and September and the peak day was Saturday.
- Mortality during the first year post injury is 0% for those who survive the first week post injury.
- Clinical course is highly centralized in the greater Stockholm area. Nearly all cases undergo spinal surgery for decompression and/ or spinal stabilization very soon after injury.
- Urinary tract infections and pressure ulcers remain the most common complications during the first year post-injury.
- Total in-patient LOS reaches approximately 4 months for IMC and two and half months of IMIC.

## REFERENCES

[1] Sköld P. Kunskap och kontroll. Den svenska befolkningsstatistikens historia. Umeå: *Almqvist and Wiksell International,* 2001.

[2] Malker H. Register- Epidemiology in the Identification of Cancer Risks. Arbete och Hälsa - vetenskaplig skriftserie. Solna: *National Board of Occupational Safety and Health,* 1988. p. 1-50.

[3] Welfare tNBoHa. In English - the National Patient Register. Stockholm: Socialstyrelsen; 2011 [updated 2011; cited 2011 2011-03-11]; Available from: http://www.socialstyrelsen.se/register/halsodataregister/patientregistret/inenglish.

[4] Steinberg EP, Whittle J, Anderson GF. Impact of claims data research on clinical practice. *Int. J. Tech. Asess. Health Care,* 1990;6(2):282-7.

[5] Flood A. Peaks and pits of using large data bases to measure quality of care. *Int. J. Tech. Assess. Health Care,* 1990;6(2):253-62.

[6] Dickman CA, Rekate HL, Sonntag VKH, Zambramski JM. Pediatric Spinal Trauma: Vertebral Column and Spinal Cord Injuries in Children. *Pediatr. Neurosci.,* 1989;15(5):237-56.

[7] Augutis M, Levi R. Pediatric spinal cord injury in Sweden: incidence, etiology and outcome. *Spinal Cord,* 2003 Jun;41(6):328-36.

[8] Augutis M, Malker H, Levi R. Pediatric spinal cord injury in Sweden; how to identify a cohort of rare events. *Spinal Cord,* 2003;41(6):337-46.

[9]   Divanoglou A, Levi R. Incidence of traumatic spinal cord injury in Thessaloniki, Greece and Stockholm, Sweden: a prospective population-based study. *Spinal Cord,* 2009 Nov;47(11):796-801.

[10]  Levi R. The Stockholm Spinal Cord Injury Study: Medical, Economical and Psycho-social Outcomes in a Prevalence Population [Doctoral Dissertation]. Stockholm: Karolinska Institute; 1996.

[11]  Ingvarsson PE. Årsrapport från Nationella Ryggmärgsskaderådet (NRR): Ryggmärgsskaderegistret i Sverige (RYSS) 1997: Stiftelsen Nationella Ryggmärgsskaderådet; 1998 Contract No.: Document Number|.

[12]  Levi R, Ertzgaard P. Quality Indicators in Spinal Cord Injury Care: A Swedish Collaborative Project. *Scand. J. of Rehabil. Med. Suppl.,* 1998;38(Supplement,):1-80.

[13]  Socialstyrelsen. Klassifikation av sjukdomar 1968: tillrättalagd för sjukhusbruk = International statistical classification of diseases, injuries and causes ofdeath, 1965 revision adapted for indexing of hospital records and morbidity statistics.

[14]  Systematisk förteckning = Systematic list. 4. uppl. ed. Stockholm: Utg.; 1968.

[15]  Socialstyrelsen. Klassifikation av sjukdomar 1987. Stockholm: Socialstyr.; 1986.

[16]  Statistics NBo. Causes of death 1995. Stockholm: Statistics Sweden; 1995.

[17]  SCB. Population Statistics. Part III, Distribution by sex, age marital status and citizenship by municipality etc.: Statistics Sweden; 1985-1996.

[18]  Statistics. NCBo. Cause of Death 1983. Stockholm; 1985.

[19]  Statistics. NCBo. In-patient statistics 1981 in somatic hospitals. Stockholm: Statistics Sweden; 1984.

[20]  Biering-Sorensen F, Charlifue S, DeVivo M, Noonan V, Post M, Stripling T, et al. International Spinal Cord Injury Data Sets. *Spinal Cord,* 2006 Sep;44(9):530-4.

[21]  DeVivo M, Biering-Sorensen F, Charlifue S, Noonan V, Post M, Stripling T, et al. International Spinal Cord Injury Core Data Set. *Spinal Cord,* 2006 Sep;44(9):535-40.

[22]  Mulcahey MJ, Gaughan J, Betz RR, Johansen KJ. The International Standards for Neurological Classification of Spinal Cord Injury: reliability of data when applied to children and youths. *Spinal Cord,* 2006 Oct 3.

[23]  Berfenstam R. Barnolycksfall. Stockholm: The Swedish Council on Technology Assessment in Health Care; 1997. Report No.: 132 Contract No.: Document Number|.

[24]  Janson S. Så skadar sig barn. Stockholm: Gothia; 2005.Administration UDoTNHTS. Traffic Safety Facts 1999. NHTSAwww.nhtsa.dot.gov; 1999.

[25]  Apple D, Anson C, Hunter J, Bell R. Spinal cord injury in youth. *Clin. Pediatr.,* 1995;34:90-5.

[26]  DeVivo M, Kartus P, Rutt R, Stover S, Fine R. The Influence of Age at Time of Spinal Cord Injury on Rehabilitation Outcome. *Arch. Neurol.,* 1990;47:687-91.

[27]  Hamilton M. pediatric spinal injury: review of 174 hospital admissions. *J. Neurosurg.,* 1992;77:700-4.

[28]  Kewalramani LS, MSOrth., Tori J. Spinal Trauma in Children. *Spine,* 1980;5(1):11-8.

[29]  Stover S. Review of forty years of Rehabilitation Issues in Spinal Cord Injury. *The Journal of Spinal Cord Medicine,* 1995;8(3):175-81.

[30]  SOU. Från barnolycksfall till barns rätt till säkerhet och utveckling. Slutbetänkande från Barnsäkerhetsdelegationen. (In Swedish with English summery). In: SOU, editor. Stockholm: Edita Norstedts Tryckeri AB; 2003. p. 127.

[31] Divanoglou A, Seiger A, Levi R. Acute management of traumatic spinal cord injury in a Greek and a Swedish region: a prospective, population-based study. *Spinal Cord,* Jun;48(6):477-82.

[32] Divanoglou A, Westgren N, Bjelak S, Levi R. Medical conditions and outcomes at 1 year after acute traumatic spinal cord injury in a Greek and a Swedish region: a prospective, population-based study. *Spinal Cord,* Jun;48(6):470-6.

[33] Divanoglou A, Westgren N, Seiger A, Hulting C, Levi R. Late mortality during the first year after acute traumatic spinal cord injury: a prospective, population-based study. *J. Spinal Cord Med.,* 33(2):117-27.

[34] Van Asbeck FWA, Post MWM, Pangalila RF. An epidemiological description of spinal cord injuries in The Netherlands in 1994. *Spinal Cord,* 2000 Jul;38(7):420-4.

[35] O'Connor RJ, Murray PC. Review of spinal cord injuries in Ireland. *Spinal Cord,* 2006 Jul;44(7):445-8.

[36] Martins F, Freitas F, Martins L, Dartigues JF, Barat M. Spinal cord injuries - Epidemiology in Portugal's central region. *Spinal Cord,* 1998 Aug;36(8):574-8.

[37] Albert T, Ravaud JF. Rehabilitation of spinal cord injury in France: a nationwide multicentre study of incidence and regional disparities. *Spinal Cord,* 2005 Jun;43(6):357-65.

[38] Norrbrink Budh C. Pain following spinal cord injury. Stockholm: Karolinska institutet; 2004.

[39] O'Connor PJ. Trends in spinal cord injury. *Accid. Anal. Prev.,* [Article]. 2006 Jan;38(1):71-7.

[40] Consortium for Spinal Cord Medicine. Early acute management in adults with spinal cord injury: a clinical practice guideline for health-care professionals. *J. Spinal Cord Med.,* [Review]. 2008;31(4):403-79.

[41] Fehlings MG, Perrin RG. The timing of surgical intervention in the treatment of spinal cord injury: a systematic review of recent clinical evidence. *Spine,* [Review]. 2006 May;31(11):S28-S35.

[42] Soreide K, Kruger AJ, Vardal AL, Ellingsen CL, Soreide E, Lossius HM. Epidemiology and contemporary patterns of trauma deaths: Changing place, similar pace, older face. *World J. Surg.,* [Article]. 2007 Nov;31(11):2092-103.

[43] Sugrue M, Caldwell E, D'Amours S, Crozier J, Wyllie P, Flabouris A, et al. Time for a change in injury and trauma care delivery: A trauma death review analysis. *Anz. Journal of Surgery,* [Article]. 2008 Nov;78(11):949-54.

[44] Pickett GE, Campos-Benitez M, Keller JL, Duggal N. Epidemiology of traumatic spinal cord injury in Canada. *Spine,* [Article]. 2006 Apr;31(7):799-805.

[45] Tator CH, Duncan EG, Edmonds VE, Lapczak LI, Andrews DF. Neurological recovery, mortality and length of stay after acute spinal cord injury associated with changes in management. *Paraplegia,* [Article]. 1995 May;33(5):254-62.

[46] Furlan JC, Kattail D, Fehlings MG. The Impact of Co-Morbidities on Age-Related Differences in Mortality after Acute Traumatic Spinal Cord Injury. *J. Neurotrauma.,* [Article]. 2009 Aug;26(8):1361-7.

[47] Botel U, Glaser E, Niedeggen A. The surgical treatment of acute spinal paralysed patients. *Spinal Cord,* [Article]. 1997 Jul;35(7):420-8.

[48] Leal MB, Borges G, de Almeida BR, Aguiar ADX, Vieira M, Dantas KD, et al. Spinal cord injury: Epidemiologycal study of 386 cases with emphasis on those patients

admitted more than four hours after the trauma. *Arq. Neuropsiquiatr.,* [Article]. 2008 Jun;66(2B):365-8.

[49] O'Connor PJ. Survival after spinal cord injury in Australia. *Arch. Phys. Med. Rehabil.,* [Article]. 2005 Jan;86(1):37-47.

[50] DeVivo MJ, Black KJ, Stover SL. Causes of death during the 1st 12 years after spinal-cord injury. *Arch. Phys. Med. Rehabil.,* [Article]. 1993 Mar;74(3):248-54.

[51] Strauss DJ, DeVivo MJ, Paculdo DR, Shavelle RM. Trends in life expectancy after spinal cord injury. *Arch. Phys. Med. Rehabil.,* [Article]. 2006 Aug;87(8):1079-85.

[52] Consortium for Spinal Cord Medicine. Bladder management for adults with spinal cord injury: a clinical practice guideline for health-care providers. *J. Spinal Cord Med.,* [Review]. 2006;29(5):527-73.

[53] Weld KJ, Dmochowski RR. Effect of bladder management on urological complications in spinal cord injured patients. *J. Urol.,* [Article]. 2000 Mar;163(3):768-72.

[54] Burns AS, Rivas DA, Ditunno JF. The management of neurogenic bladder and sexual dysfunction after spinal cord injury. *Spine,* [Article]. 2001 Dec;26(24):S129-S36.

[55] Chen D, Apple DF, Hudson LM, Bode R. Medical complications during acute rehabilitation following spinal cord injury—current experience of the Model Systems. *Arch. Phys. Med. Rehabil.,* [Article]. 1999 Nov;80(11):1397-401.

[56] Haisma JA, van der Woude LH, Stam HJ, Bergen MP, Sluis TA, Post MW, et al. Complications following spinal cord injury: Occurrence and risk factors in a longitudinal study during and after inpatient rehabilitation. *J. Rehabil. Med.,* [Article]. 2007 May;39(5):393-8.

[57] Johnson RL, Gerhart KA, McCray J, Menconi JC, Whiteneck GG. Secondary conditions following spinal cord injury in a population-based sample. *Spinal Cord,* [Article]. 1998 Jan;36(1):45-50.

[58] Pagliacci MC, Celani MG, Spizzichino L, Zampolini M, Aito S, Citterio A, et al. Spinal cord lesion management in Italy: a 2-year survey. *Spinal Cord,* 2003 Nov;41(11):620-8.

[59] Domingo M. Organisation of an autonomous Spinal Injuries Unit. *Paraplegia,* [Article]. 1967 Nov;5(3):170-6.

[60] Johnson R, Gabella G, Gerhart K, McCray J, Menconi J, Whiteneck G. Evaluating sources of traumatic spinal cord injury surveillance data in Colorado. *Am. J. Epidemiol.,* 1997;146:266-72.

[61] Augutis M, Malker H, Levi R. Pediatric spinal cord injury in Sweden; how to identify a cohort of rare events. *Spinal Cord,* 2003 Jun;41(6):337-46.

[62] Welfare. TSNBoHa. Klassifikation av sjukdomar mm systematisk förteckning. 4:e ed. Stockholm: Socialstyrelsen, 1968.

In: Epidemiology of Spinal Cord Injuries
Editors: V. Rahimi-Movaghar, S. B. Jazayeri et al.

ISBN: 978-1-61942-894-2
©2012 Nova Science Publishers, Inc.

*Chapter 10*

# SPINAL CORD INJURY IN TURKEY

## *Kemal Nas*

Department of Physical Medicine and Rehabilitation, Faculty of Medicine,
University of Dicle, Diyarbakır, Turkey

## ABSTRACT

Traumatic spinal cord injury (SCI) often results in profound and long-term disability, which is life changing for the injured individual and his or her family. These injuries also have tremendous social costs associated with expensive health care treatment, rehabilitation, and lost productivity. The estimated annual incidence of traumatic SCI is 12.7 per million inhabitants in Turkey. The mortality rate of SCI is estimated to be 12%-15% in Turkey. SCI patients became either tetraplegic (32.18%) and paraplegic (67.82%) after injury. The most common level of injury was C5 among tetraplegics, T12 and L1 for paraplegics. The most prevalent associated injury was head trauma followed by extremity fractures. Regarding the etiology, traffic accident is the most common cause of spinal cord injury, the second most-common cause is falls from height and the third is gunshot injury. The incidences of gunshot wounds and injuries from falls are higher in Turkey than other countries, which can be explained by special socio-economic and cultural differences. The high incidence of gunshot wounds is the result of the violence experienced mainly in south-eastern of Turkey. Moreover, the higher frequency of falls from height can be associated with the fact that most falls occurred in the summer when it is very hot in this region and people are forced to sleep on the top of their houses, which do not have barriers along the roof perimeter. Traumatic SCI is more frequent among males than females and among those between the ages of 15 and 39 years. Considering that traffic accidents, falls from height and gunshot wounds are the leading cause of traumatic SCI, it can be concluded that the prevention measures should be focused mainly on these types of traumas in order to reduce the frequency of SCI in Turkey.

## INTRODUCTION

Neurological deficits often produce long-term effects that persist throughout life and are associated with severe disability and handicap. Since SCI causes extensive lifelong consequences, epidemiological data are of fundamental importance in tracing its occurrence, deciding upon preventive strategies, and planning clinical resources and social services [1]. Therefore, epidemiologic studies provide local estimates of incidence and prevalence, identify high-risk groups, and, thus, provide insight into priorities for resource allocation, etiologic research, and prevention efforts. They also provide a baseline from which to gauge the effectiveness of interventions [1,2].Reported traumatic SCI annual incidence rate have ranged from 6 [3] to 56.1 [4] cases per million, with traffic accident, falls, violence and sports activities identified as leading causes of injury. A descriptive review [5] of the incidence of traumatic SCI showed that these rates have remained more or less stable over the last 3 decades. However, this review only reported crude incidence rates and did not take into account differences in age distribution and population size across geographical areas [1]. Over the past 2 decades, many countries have made great effort to complete traumatic SCI research to establish useful epidemiological guidelines, to provide information regarding the magnitude of the traumatic SCI problem and to help identify the risk factors for traumatic SCI [6]. Recent studies have demonstrated certain differences between the causes of SCI in developing and in developed countries [7-11]. Common causes of SCI throughout the world are traffic accidents, gunshot wounds, knife wounds, falls from height and landslide accidents [7,12-16] whereas, the main causes of SCI in Turkey appear to be road accidents, falls from flat-roofed houses and gunshot wounds injuries [16]. In Turkey, five epidemiological studies related to SCI were conducted in Istanbul [15], Ankara [17], the south-eastern part of Turkey [7,16] and nation-wide [18].It is believed that the characteristics of SCI may exhibit certain differences in certain time periods even in the same population. There may also be differences between developing and developed countries in terms of SCI characteristics [7]. In this chapter we aimed to review the incidence, gender distribution, etiological factors, injury levels, mortality rate, seasonality, associated disability, and associated traumas of SCI in Turkey.

## Incidence

SCI incidences have been reported between 6 and 56.1/million in previous studies from different countries throughout the world [10,13-16,19-21]. There may be differences in SCI incidence in different regions of the same country. This is the case also in Turkey, where the reported incidences were 21.1/million in Istanbul [15] , 11.9-16.9 /million in south-eastern Anatolia [7,16] and 12.7/million in Turkey as a whole [18]. From a socio-economic standpoint, the most developed and crowded city in Turkey is Istanbul. Motor vehicle usage is very common in this city. Public health services are widely distributed and health workers are more qualified in Istanbul compared with the other parts of the country. South-eastern Anatolia is an underdeveloped rural region where agriculture is the most important source of income. Public health services are insufficient. Different rates were reported from these two distinct regions of Turkey [7,15,16,18]. Socio-economic, cultural and political factors may play a role in the differences between SCI incidences reported in two studies by Karamehmetoğlu and colleagues [15,16]. The incidence rates of traumatic SCI varied widely between developed countries and developing countries. Developing countries [6,18,22] had lower incidence rates compared with those of developed ones [6,23,24]. The risk of death was increased in traumatic SCI cases in the acute post-injury period due to insufficient health facilities in the developing countries. This situation may explain the low SCI incidence in developing countries as fewer individuals survive the initial injury to be counted as a SCI patient. Among developed countries, the incidence rates of traumatic SCI dropped from 52.2 to 13.1 per million people [6,25,26]. Among developing countries, the incidence rates range between 12.7 and 29.7 per million people [6,18,27].

## Age and Gender

Although there were almost equal numbers of males and females in the population, SCI was approximately three times more common in males than females. As reported in other studies, men have a greater risk of SCI [10,12-16,19]. In a developing country such as Turkey, men are the breadwinners and they often work in jobs with high risk of injury. On the other hand, women are usually at home as housewives and as a consequence they are protected from many outside dangers. Therefore, the variations may due to different socio-economic and cultural backgrounds and the higher ratio of incidence in males can be explained by examination of the etiological factors [7]. Studies carried out in Turkey have reported gender ratios between 2.5-5.8:1 [7,16,18].Karamehmetoğlu and colleagues found male/female ratio to be 3.1:1 in 115 male and 37 female patients with SCI. The mean age of the study population was 33 years, 34 for male patients and 31 for females. SCI was most prevalent between 20 and 29 years of age inclusive with only one peak in this age group [15]. In another study, there were 64 males and 11 females with SCI, yielding a male:female ratio was 5.8:1. SCI was most prevalent between 20-29 years inclusive with only one peak in this age group [16].

In their study Karacan et al. have found a ratio of 2.5:1 males to females in their study group composed of 415 males and 166 females. The most prevalent age groups were 20-29 followed by 30-39 [18]. Gur et al. found that there were 416 male and 123 female patients with SCI; the male:female ratio was 3.38:1. The high percentage of patients in the 15-44 years age group is striking as 409 (77.73%) of the patients fall into this group. The 15-29 year age group with 261 (48.42%) patients is the highest risk age sub-group [7]. Dinçer et al. reported the male:female ratio to be 3.1:1 in a study of 1694 patients, including 1282 (75.68%) males and 412 (24.32%) females [17]. Patient characteristics of epidemiologic studies for SCI in Turkey are presented in Table 1.

The most common cause of SCI in Turkey is motor vehicle accidents. Statistical reports from the General Directorate of Security revealed the fact that 3.92% of men and 5.31% of women involved in the accidents died and 97.07% of men and 95.21% of women were injured as the result of these accidents.

According to these reports male or female gender cannot be considered as a risk factor for death or injury. These results may be interpreted to suggest that men are more prone to motor vehicle accidents than women in Turkey [18]. Reported data from the National Statistics Institute revealed that 35.9% of the working population are female in Turkey [18,28]. In fact, the rate of falls and traffic accidents are almost equal between men and women. However due to different rates of working outside the home, women are less prone to traffic accidents and falls and hence to SCI [18].

**Table 1. Patient characteristics of epidemiologic studies for SCI in Turkey**

| Reference | Period (year) | Place | Sample size | Age (Mean ±SD) | M(Mean ±SD) | F(Mean ±SD) | M/F |
|---|---|---|---|---|---|---|---|
| Dinçer | 1974-1985 | Ankara | 1694 | 26.8±? | ? | ? | 3.11/1 |
| Karamehmetoğlu | 1992 | Istanbul | 152 | 33±? | 34±? | 31±? | 3/1 |
| Karamehmetoğlu | 1994 | South-eastern | 75 | 31.3±12.8 | 31.2±13 | 31.4±11.7 | 5.8/1 |
| Karacan | 1992 | nation-wide (Turkey) | 581 | 35.5±15.1 | 35.4±14.8 | 35.9±16 | 2.5/1 |
| Gur | 1990-1999 | South-eastern | 539 | 30.62±13.21 | ? | ? | 3.38/1 |

## Cause of SCI

Traffic accidents have been found to be the most common cause of spinal cord trauma in the literature. However, the incidences of gunshot wounds and injuries from falls are also higher in Turkey than other countries, which can be explained by socio-economical and cultural differences. The high incidence of gunshot wounds is attributed to violence which was prevalent in the south-eastern part of Turkey before 1995. Moreover, the higher frequency of falls from a height may be explained by the fact that most falls occurred in the summer. When the weather in this region is very hot most people sleep on the top of their houses, which are flat-roofed. There have been previous reports about injuries secondary to falls from height [7,29-31]. But there is only one report, which was carried out in south-eastern region of Turkey [7,32], about falls from flat-roofed houses. In this region, children and older people have the highest risk of accidental falls from flat-roofed houses accidentally. The simple houses common in this region have no barriers around their roofs and falls from them cause serious morbidity and mortality. The main aspect of prevention for this source of injury should focus on creating a safe environment, for example, though the compulsory construction of pitch-roofed buildings or of a barrier around the perimeter of the room of flat-roofed buildings [7]. The third highest cause of SCI in south-eastern region, gunshot wounds, is a specific problem to this part of Turkey which contains active areas of armed conflict. There are no available data about SCI due to conflict in this region so the actual incidence of SCI is difficult to accurately characterize but may be higher than that found in previous few studies [7,15-17]. Improved quality of life, social dynamics of the community and better access to education, sports facilities and community centers for young people would decrease deaths related to political violence in this region [7]. Causes of SCI reported for epidemiologic studies in Turkey are presented in Figure 1. Kurtaran et al. reported that the most common cause of injury was car accidents (45.3%) followed by falls (34.4%) and gunshot injuries (9.4%)[33]. In another study, it was found that the most common cause of injury was car accidents (51%) followed by falls (24%) and gunshot injuries (11%)[34]. Müslümanoğlu et al. found that living in suburban areas rather than urban areas may account for the fact that falls cause a higher percentage of SCI than motor vehicle accidents in some studies of the etiological factors for SCI [35]. Cosar et al. found that the cause of injury in traumatic SCI patients was car accidents in 55.1%, falls in 33.9% and gunshot wounds for 7.9% of patients with SCI [36]. Study characteristics of epidemiologic surveys of SCI in Turkey are presented in Table 2.

## Table 2. Study Characteristics of epidemiologic survey in Turkey

| Reference | Incidence | Study Population (Specific) | Study Location | Simple Size | Study Design | Causes of Injury |
|---|---|---|---|---|---|---|
| Dinçer 1992 | ? | Traumatic SCI | Ankara Rehabilitation center | 1694 | Retrospective cohort | Car accidents (35.41%)<br>Falls (29.51%),<br>Gunshot wound (29.51%)<br>Stab wounds (0.49%) |
| Karamehmetoğlu 1995 | 21 | Traumatic SCI | I.U. Cerrahpaşa PMR<br>Istanbul rehabilitation center<br>Neurosurgery Okmeydanı Hospital<br>Neurosurgery Haydarpaşa Hospital<br>Neurosurgery Şişli Eftal Hospital<br>PMR Kartal Insurans hospital<br>Neurosurgery Kartal Hospital<br>PMR Kartal State Hospital | 152 | Retrospective cohort | Falls (43%)<br>Car accidents (41%)<br>Gunshot wound (5%)<br>Stab wounds (2%) |
| Karamehmetoğlu 1997 | 16.9 | Traumatic SCI | Dicle University hospital PMR | 75 | Retrospective cohort | Falls (37.3%)<br>Gunshot wound (29.3%)<br>Car accidents (25.3%)<br>Stab wounds (1.3%) |
| Karacan 2000 | 12.7 | Traumatic SCI | I.U. Cerrahpaşa University PMR<br>Dokuz Eylül University PMR<br>Akdeniz University PMR<br>Erciyes University Hospital PMR<br>Ankara Military Hospital PMR<br>Kastomonu Rehabilitation center<br>Trakya University Hospital PMR<br>Ankara rehabilitation center<br>100. Yıl University Hospital PMR<br>Dicle University Hospital PMR<br>Bakırköy State Hospital PMR<br>Afyon State Hospital PMR | 581 | Retrospective cohort | Car accidents (48.8%)<br>Falls (36.5%)<br>Stab wounds (3.3%)<br>Gunshot wound (1.9%) |
| Gur 2004 | 11.9 | Traumatic SCI | Dicle University Hospital PMR<br>Diyarbakır State Hospital<br>Diyarbakır Military Hospital<br>Diyarbakır Insurance Hospital | 539 | Retrospective cohort | Car accidents (37.12%)<br>Falls (31.90)<br>Gunshot wound (21.34%)<br>Stab wounds (3.79%) |

I.U: Itanbul University, PMR: Physical Medicine and Rehabilitation

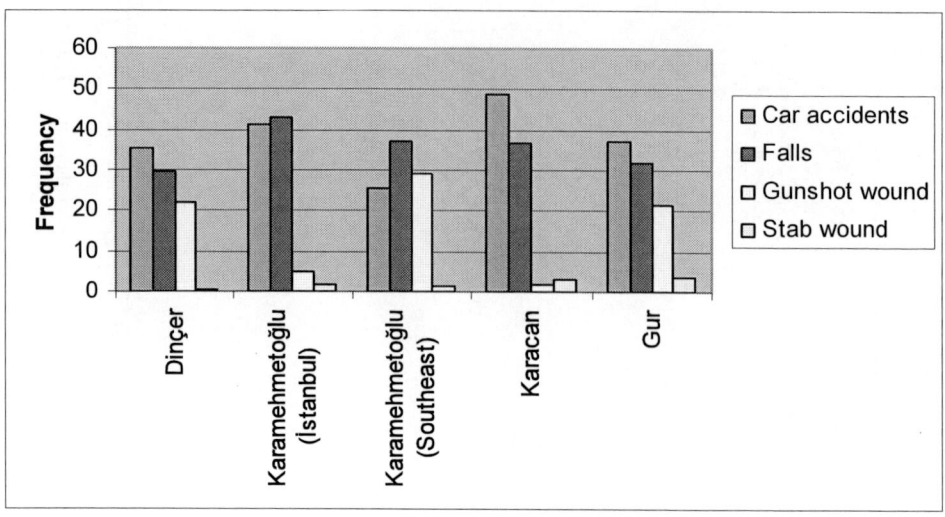

Figure 1. Frequency of SCI causes in epidemiologic studies published from Turkey.

## SCI Level

According to current literature, the most common levels of injury were C5 and C6 among tetraplegics and T12 and L1 among paraplegics. Cases with paraplegia are twice as common as those with tetraplegia. This may be the result of high mortality rates among tetraplegics during critical care and transportation in the early post-injury period, leading to underreporting of these cases [18].

Karacan et al. showed that eighty-seven patients (32.18%) were tetraplegic and 394 patients (67.6%) were paraplegic. The most common level of injury was C5 (57.4%) among tetraplegics and T12 (17.7%) among paraplegics [18]. Karamehmetoğlu et al. found that 31 patients (41.3%) were tetraplegic and 44 (58.7%) patients were paraplegic. In tetraplegic patients the commonest level was C5 whereas, it was L1 in paraplegic patients [16]. In another study, 50 patients (33%) were found to be tetraplegic and 102 (67%) patients paraplegic. In the tetraplegic patients, the commonest level was C5, compared to L1 in paraplegic patients [15]. In their study, Gur et al. reported 30 ( 5.56%) persons with upper-cervical tetraplegia (C1-4) and 118 (21.89%) persons with lower-cervical tetraplegia (C5-T1) or paresis in their 10-years study period,. Among the paraplegic or paretic patients, 47 (8.72%) had a high thoracic level of SCI (T2-6), 140 (25.97%) had a low thoracic level of SCI ( T7-L2) and 204 ( 37.84%) had a lumbosacral level of SCI [7].Kurtaran et al. reported that paraplegic patients were less likely to have incomplete (28.1%) than complete lesions (54.7%), and tetraplegic patients were similarly less likely to have had complete (6.8%) than incomplete lesions (10.4%)[33]. In another study, most of the patients were paraplegic or had incomplete injuries. Paraplegic patients were more likely to have incomplete (53%) than complete lesions (24%), similar to tetraplegic patients who were more likely to have incomplete (15%) compared to complete (8%) lesions [34].

## Seasonal Distribution

In a study conducted in Turkey, SCI was most frequently observed during the summer (32%) and spring (27.6%) seasons. During all seasons, traffic accidents were found to be the leading cause of SCI, but were most common in summer (37.3%) [18]. In another study, the seasonal distribution of SCI showed highest rates during the spring with falls as the most common cause. In summer, traffic accidents were the main cause [16]. Dinçer et al. observed that rates of traffic accidents and falls peaked in summer months of June, July, and August followed by May and September. This pattern may be due to increased tourism during these months [17].

Karacan et al also suggested that seasonal distribution of SCI showed increased rates during summer. Although SCI cases due to car accidents were more common during summer, the General Directorate of Security reported that motor vehicle accidents were more common in winter and autumn. These seemingly contradictory results can be best explained by other reported data from General Directorate of Security indicating that the number of accidents resulting in death and injury is greater in summer compared to winter and autumn [18].

## Mortality

Karacan et al. reported that it was estimated that 12% to 15% of deaths at the time of admission to hospital are associated with SCI [18]. In another study, this rate was estimated at 12-25%. The most common associated injury was head trauma. Severe head trauma as a common cause of death might obscure the actual incidence of SCI [15].

## Associated Trauma

There was no associated trauma in more than 77% of patients with SCI. The most common associated trauma was head trauma, followed by extremity fractures, burns, pneumothorax and others [15]. In another study, the most prevalent associated injuries was head trauma (9.8%) followed by extremity fractures (7.9%), hemothorax (2.2%), burns (1%) and pneumothorax (0.5%) [18]. Thirty eight percent of the patients had an associated trauma, the commonest being head injury, followed by extremity fractures, pneumothorax, hemothorax, and burns (şafak 1997). In another study, a total of 123 (24.49%) patients had associated traumas, the most frequent type being extremity fractures (11.69%), followed by head injury (4.08%), pneumothorax (3.71%), hemothorax (2.2%), burn (0.3%) and others (2.41%) [7].

## The Distribution of Patients According to Profession

SCI is an important condition that leads to serious social and economical consequences both for the life of affected individual and his/her family. One of the objectives of rehabilitation is to facilitate returning to work, thus easing the burden on patients' lives. The majority of patients with SCI are young; thus, they should be evaluated on the basis of not only their condition but also on rehabilitation approaches that will facilitate social and occupational reintegration [33,37]. Working is considered to be an essential part of social integration after a major trauma because it increases the self-confidence of an individual, and contributes to self-expression, and the first step toward returning to work after an injury is dependent on successful post-injury rehabilitation [38]. Occupational production is the most important for participation of adults to the economical and social life [39]. After SCI, the most prominent factors determining the ability to return to work include: younger age, younger age at injury onset and higher education. Having a less-severe injury, race/ethnicity and gender were also associated with employment outcomes [33,40]. One of the important factors that contributes to socialization of SCI patients is return to work. In various studies evaluating employment status after SCI, the rate of returning to work was found to be 11.5-74% [39]. A recent study from Turkey has reported a rate of 36% for return to work after injury, and the same study has acknowledged that in developing countries, even those individuals without any disability have difficulty in finding profitable jobs. Although employers in Turkey are obliged to employ enough disabled individuals to make up 5% of their employee population, they prefer to employ those with lesser degrees of disability than patients with SCI [41]. In another study, most of those who worked before injury in occupations requiring physical activity, such as farming, driving, construction work and automotive repair do not return to work; rather, they retired for reasons of disability or remained unemployed. Most patients in rural areas for social reasons do not obey even their routine outpatient visits. Therefore, these patients do not show great ambition to return to work. The rate of returning to work was found to be 14.6% [33].

Kurtaran et al. reported that before injury, 138 patients were employed in gainful occupations, 26 were housewives, 10 were retired, 7 were students and 11 patients were unemployed. Only 15 patients (7.8%) returned to their original occupation after injury. Thirteen patients (6.8%) were currently working in another job, 1 patient (0.5%) was a student, 10 (5.2%) were retired both before and after injury, 40 (20.8%) were retired because of disability, 26 (13.5%) were housewives, and 87 patients (45.3%) were currently unemployed. Only 28 patients (14.6%) returned to work after injury [33].

Gur et al. reported that the occupations of the sample, at the time of SCI, included civil servants (22.63%), housewives (20.22%), and soldiers (15.03%). Most of the housewives were from agricultural regions, and were unpaid but contributed to farm work [7]. With respect to the frequency of SCI according to profession, it was highest in civil servants, followed by housewives and soldiers [7].

Karamehmetoğlu et al. reported that individuals were at high risk of SCI if the performed outside work in high-risk environments such as on high buildings or in environments with few safety precautions and if they drove an automobile. On the other hand, women are usually at home as housewives where they are protected from many risks for SCI [15].

# CONCLUSION

SCI may vary according to country and the region within that country. Specifically in Turkey, SCI from falls off flat-roofed houses and gunshots are more frequent causes compared to SCI etiology in other countries. Accordingly, patients with SCI in Turkey are younger and predominantly male in gender. On the other hand, the leading etiology for SCI may change in summer as traffic accidents and falls from height are the leading causes in this season.

# REFERENCES

[1] van den Berg MEL, Castellote JM, Mahillo-Fernandez I, de Pedro-Cuesta J. Incidence cord injury of spinal worldwide: a systematic review. *Neuroepidemiology*, 2010; 34: 184-192.

[2] van den Berg MEL, Castellote JM, Mahillo-Fernandez I, de Pedro-Cuesta J, Mahillo-Fernandez I. Survival after spinal cord injury: a systematic review. *J. Neurotrauma.*, 2010; 27: 1517-1528.

[3] van Asbeck FWA, Post MWM, Pangalila RF. An epidemiological description of spinal cord injuries in The Netherlands in 1994. *Spinal Cord*, 2000; 38: 420-424.

[4] Martins F, Freitas F, Martins L, Dartigues JF, Barat M. Spinal cord injuries-epidemiology in Portugal's central region. *Spinal Cord*, 1998;36:574-578.

[5] Wyndaele M, Wyndele JJ. Incidence, prevalence and epidemiology of spinal cord injury: what learns a worldwide literature survey?. *Spinal Cord*, 2000; 44: 523-529.

[6] Chiu WT, Lin HC, Lam C, Chu SF, Chiang YH, Tsai SH. Epidemiology of traumatic spinal cord injury: Comparisons between developed and developing countries. *Asia Pacific J. Public Health*, 2010; 22(1): 9-18.

[7] Gur A, Kemaloglu S, Cevik R, Sarac AJ, Nas K, Kapukaya A, Sahin H, Guloglu C, Bakır A .Characteristics of traumatic spinal cord injuries in south-eastern Anatolia, Turkey: a comparative approach to 10 years' experience. *Int. J. Rehabil. Res.*, 2005; 28(1): 57-62.

[8] Dixon GS, Danesh JN, Caradoc-Davi JH. Epidemiology of spinal cord injury in New Zealand. *Neuroepidemiology*, 1993; 312: 88-95.

[9] Price C, Makintubee S, Hendon W, Istre GR. Epidemiology of traumatic spinal cord injury and acute hospitalization and rehabilitation charges for spinal cord injuries in Oklahoma 1988-1990. *American Journal of Epidemiology*, 1994; 139: 37-47.

[10] Shingu H, Ikata T, Katoh S, Akatsu T. Spinal cord injury patients in Japan: a nationwide epidemiological survey in 1990. *Paraplegia*, 1994; 32: 3-8.

[11] da Paz AC, Beraldo PS, Almeida MC, Neves EG, Alves CM, Khan P. Traumatic injury to the spinal cord. Prevalence in Brazilian hospitals. *Paraplegia*, 1992; 30: 636-640.

[12] Chen CF, Lien IN. Spinal cord injuries in Taipei, Taiwan: 1978-1981. *Paraplegia*, 1985; 23: 364-370.

[13] Biering Sporensen F, Pederson V, Clausen S. Epidemiology of spinal cord lesions in Denmark. *Paraplegia*, 1990; 28: 105-118.

[14] Garcia-Renses J, Herruzo Cabrera R, Martinez-Moreno M. Epidemiological study of spinal cord injury in Spain 1984-1985. *Paraplegia*, 1991; 28: 180-190.

[15] Karamehmetoglu ŞS, Ünal Ş, Karacan I, Yilmaz H, Tagay HS, Ertekin M. Traumatic spinal cord injuries in Istanbul, Turkey. An epidemiological study. *Paraplegia*, 1995; 33: 469-471.

[16] Karamehmetoglu ŞS, Nas K, Karacan I, Sarac AJ, Koyuncu H, Ataoglu S, Erdoğan F. Traumatic spinal cord injuries in southeast Turkey. An epidemiological study. *Spinal Cord*, 1997; 35: 531-533.

[17] Konig W, Fowein RA. Incidence of spinal cord injuries in the Federal Republic of Germany. *Neurosurgery Review*, 1989; 12: 562-566.

[18] Knutsdottir S. Spinal cord injuries in Iceland: 1973-1989. A follow-up study. *Paraplegia*, 1993; 31: 68-72.

[19] Lan C, Lai JS, Chang KH, Jean YC, Lien IN. Traumatic spinal cord injuries in the rural region of Taiwan: an epidemiological study in Hualien Country. 1986-1990. *Paraplegia*, 1993; 31: 398-403.

[20] Karacan I, Koyuncu H, Pekel O, Sumbuloglu G, Kırnap M, Dursun H, et al. Traumatic spinal cord injuries in Turkey: a nationwide epidemiological study. *Spinal Cord*, 2000; 38: 697: 701.

[21] Hoque MF, Grangeon C, Reed K. Spinal cord lesions in Bangladesh: an epidemiological study 1994-1995. *Spinal Cord*, 1999; 37: 858-861.

[22] Burke DA, Linden BD, Zhang YP, Maiste AC, Shields CB. Incidence rates and populations at risk for spinal cord injury: a regional study. *Spinal Cord*, 2001; 39: 274-278.

[23] Pickett GE. Campos-Benitez M, Keller JL, Dug dal N. Epidemiology of traumatic spinal cord injuries in Canada. *Spine*, 2006; 31: 799-805.

[24] Dryden DM, Saunders LD, Rowe BH, et al. The epidemiology of traumatic spinal cord injury in Albert, Canada. *Can. J. Neurol. Sci.*, 2003; 30: 113-121.

[25] O'Connor BJ, Murray PC. Review of spinal cord injuries in Ireland. *Spinal Cord*, 2006; 44: 445-448.

[26] Silberstein B, Rabinovich S. Epidemiology of spinal cord injuries in Novosibirsk, Russia. *Paraplegia*, 1995; 33: 322-325.

[27] Dinçer F, Oflazer A, Beyazova M, Çeliker R, Basgöze O, Altioklar K. traumatic spinal cord injuries in Turkey. *Paraplegia*, 1992; 30: 641-646.

[28] State Institute of Statistics Prime Ministry, Republic of Turkey. *Statistical year-book of Turkey,* 1992.

[29] Mathis RD, Levine SH, Phifer S. An analysis of accidental free falls from a height: the 'spring break' syndrome. *Journal of Trauma1*,993; 34: 123-126.

[30] Risser D, Bönsch A, Schneider B, Bauer G. Risk of dying after a free fall from height. *Forensic Science International*, 1996; 78: 187-191.

[31] Weisskopf M, Hoffmann R, Südkamp NP, Haas NP. Dens fracture and multiple fracture of the thoracic spine after fall from great height. Diagnostic standard. *Unfahirurllchirurg*, 1996; 99: 520-524.

[32] Yagmur Y, Kiraz M, Kara IH. Looking at trauma and deaths. Diyarbakır city in Turkey. *Injury*, 1999; 30: 111-114.

[33] Kurtaran A, Akbal A, Ersöz M, Selçuk B, Yalçın E, Akyüz M. Occupation in spinal cord injury patients in *Turkey Spinal Cord*, 2009; 47: 709-712.

[34] Demiral G, Yılmaz H, Gençosmanoğlu B, Kesiktaş N. Pain following spinal cord injury. *Spinal Cord*, 1998; 36: 25-28.

[35] Müslanoğlu L, Aki S, Öztürk Y, Soy D, Filiz M, Karan A, Berker E. Motor, sensory and functional recovery in patients with spinal cord lesions. *Spinal Cord*, 1997; 35: 368-389.

[36]  Cosar SNS, Yemisci OU, Oztop P, Cetin N, Sarifakioğlu B, Yalbuzdağ SA, Ustaomer K, Karataş M. Demographic characteristic after traumatic and non-traumatic spinal cord injury: a retrospective comparison study. *Spinal Cord*, 2010; 48: 862-866.

[37]  Scönherr MC. Vocational perspectives after spinal cord injury. *Clin. Rehabil.*, 2005; 19: 200-208.

[38]  Oppermann JD. Interpreting the meaning individuals ascribe to returning to work after traumatic brain injury: a qualitative approach. *Brain Inj.*, 2004; 18: 941-955.

[39]  Lidal IB, Huynh TK, Biering-Sorensen F. Return to work following spinal cord injury: a review. *Disabil. Rehabil.*, 2007; 29: 1341-1375.

[40]  Krause JS. Years to employment after spinal cord injury. *Arch. Phys. Med. Rehabil.*, 2003; 84: 1282-1289.

[41]  Yavuer G, Ergin S. Productivity of patients with spinal cord injury in Turkey. *Int. J. Rehabil. Res.*, 2002; 25: 153-155.

In: Epidemiology of Spinal Cord Injuries
Editors: V. Rahimi-Movaghar, S. B. Jazayeri et al.

ISBN: 978-1-61942-894-2
©2012 Nova Science Publishers, Inc.

*Chapter 11*

# EPIDEMIOLOGY OF TRAUMATIC SPINAL CORD INJURY IN UNITED KINGDOM, FRANCE, ITALY, GERMANY AND THE NETHERLANDS

*Amirali Sayadipour[1], Mohammad Reza Rasouli[2] and D. Greg Anderson[2]*
[1]Drexel University College of Medicine, PA, US
[2]Thomas Jefferson University, PA, US

## ABSTRACT

The incidence of SCI is widely variable, from 9 to 53 cases per million population inhabitants per year in the international literature. The life expectancy of patients with spinal cord injury (SCI) has been improved over the years through enhancements in emergency care, acute medical and surgical stabilization and rehabilitation. In the past, the main focus of researchers has been the prevention and treatment of complications such as urinary tract infection and skin break down. However recently, the focus of research has been expanded to include methods of mobility restoration and optimization of an affected individual's quality of life. This report will attempt to summarize the available data on SCI care in certain large medical systems in Europe.

## UNITED KINGDOM

The United Kingdom has a nationalized system of medical care, divided into four regions covering England, Scotland, Wales and Northern Ireland. The National Health Service (NHS) is charged with providing comprehensive healthcare services to UK citizens and in certain situations to non-citizens. Spinal care has evolved since the end of the second World War into a regionalized entity providing care in designated centers. Although exact figures regarding spinal cord injured patients are not available country-wide for the 20th and 21st century time frame, published studies are available which shed light on the incidence and management of SCI in the United Kingdom (UK).

One study, published in 1976, from Lodge Moor Hospital in Sheffield UK described the center as serving a population of about 5 million people. As a regional center, SCI cases were transferred to this Hospital within 24-48 hours of the injury. Between 1955 and 1974, there were 900 cases of traumatic SCI, with 99 (11%) in patients over 60 years old. When the data was broken down by five-year intervals, an increasing incidence of SCI was found with about a 3-fold increase between 1955 and 1974. The most common injury mechanisms involved a fall at home (54%), traffic accident (28%) or accident at work (15%). Only 2 cases SCI were related to sporting activities. Cervical injuries were most common, comprising 84%. The incidence for males and females was almost equally distributed (53% vs. 47% respectively), despite the fact that 80% of the overall hospital population was male. Mortality in the acute phase (1st six weeks) was 80% for quadriplegics with complete lesions, versus 23% for quadriplegics with incomplete injuries. For patients dying within the acute phase, the leading causes of death were respiratory failure, pulmonary embolism and heart failure. The death rate for paraplegics was lower at 13% in the same timeframe. For patients discharged to home, about half achieved longer term survival of up to 13 years. However, 19 patients (20%) were transferred to long-term hospital facilities and had survival time of less than five years. [1]

The National Spinal Injuries Centre in Stoke Mandeville Hospital was founded in 1944 as one of the world's first dedicated SCI centers. Between 1944 and 1977, 150 patients (142 males and 8 females) were admitted because of a SCI following diving accidents. Most of the patients were between 15 and 29 years of age. The patient make up was predominantly British, however, many of the injuries occurred outside the UK as a result of military members serving abroad. This injury pattern spiked in the mid-1960s as a result of the high number of British service members serving abroad at that time. Injuries involved the cervical spine in 142 patients, with 107 patients having injuries within the C5-7 region. At the time of hospital discharge, 79 patients had complete lesions and 71 had incomplete lesions. [2]

Spinal cord injuries from rugby were evaluated in another report. During six seasons between 1977 and 1983, five SCI's were reported among 2500 players, an incidence of 1 per 3000 player per season. Treatment consisted of early reduction with skull traction, with/without anterior fusion. The outcome demonstrated full recovery in two patients; persistent quadriplegic in one patient and residual weakness or altered sensation in two patients. Most rugby injuries were noted to occur within the first few matches of the season, suggesting that a lack of match fitness may have been a causative factor. [3]

A records review from that Midland Centre at the Robert Jones and Agnes Hunt Orthopedic Hospital was conducted between 1960 and 1986. During this interval, there were a total of 935 cases of acute SCI treated at the center. Overall, 7.6% (91 cases) had multiple level injuries and 71 cases had a non-contiguous injury. Non-contiguous injuries most commonly affected the lower cervical spine or cervicothoracic junction. About half (55%) of the patients had an incomplete neurologic deficit. In the setting of a multilevel non-contiguous injury, 70% of patients were observed to have complete quadriplegia. [4]

The Spinal Injuries Association (SIA) was founded in 1974 in London. The SIA is the largest organization representing spinal cord injured individuals in the UK. At the time of writing of the manuscript, the SIA had a staff of 30 full and part-time researchers and 6000 members. The SIA is involved in the design of spinal units and has input on the triage system for SCI in the UK. The SIA also deals with practical issues for SCI patients such as the design of toilets for the disabled. The organization also works on behalf of SCI patients for independent living rights including driver's licenses and access to businesses and public venues. The SIA publishes research papers and books such as *So You're Paralyzed* and *World Wheelchair Traveler*. [5]

A retrospective study of SCI survivors in the UK over a period of 48 years (1943-1991) aimed to identify risk factors for mortality following SCI. The study consisted of 3179 patients (81% males and 19% females), with an age distribution of 57% under 30; 22% 31-45 and the 21% over 45 years of age. The most common cause of death was pneumonia (23%) followed by urinary tract infection (19%) and heart disease (18%). This data was noted to be a departure from the major cause of death (UTI) seen in the early years of data collection within the UK. The report also highlighted the increased rate of suicide in the later years of the study. [6]

Another retrospective study involved 221 episodes of readmission to the hospital following SCI from January 1994 to December 1995 at a Regional Spinal Injuries Center in Southport, UK. The investigators collected data on the causes of readmission to the hospital, the duration of hospitalization and the mortality rate. Urinary tract disorders were the most common reason of readmission (43%) with an average length of stay was 3 days. Cardio-respiratory diseases were the second most common cause of readmission with average hospital stay of 6 days. The mortality rate for the patients readmitted to the hospital was 2.7%. The authors recommend liberal use of visiting nurses and telephone advise for tetraplegic patients, especially during the early stage post-injury phase.[7]

A retrospective study of 432 patients with spinal injuries over a period of 5-year (1998-2003) was conducted to look at the effects of delayed admission to the Spinal Center. This report included 108 complete and 115 incomplete injuries. Although the average time between the injury and referral was 10.7 days, admission of the patient to the Spinal Center was delayed in 26% of cases for a variety of logistical reasons. The authors found that a delay between injury and the referral to the Spinal Center did not influence on the length of hospital stay, however a delay between referral and admission caused a significant increase in the length of hospitalization.[8]

Another report involved 19,538 injured children from the Trauma Audit and Research Network (TARN) Database which includes about 50% of the trauma receiving hospitals in England and Wales from 1989 to 2000. Although uncommon, the authors noted that SCI in younger children (≤ 8 years of age) posed unique challenges. In this population, automobile accidents were the leading cause of injury (49.8% of all spinal injuries and 66% of injuries with a SCI). Multilevel fractures and associated non-spinal injuries were common with this population, particularly closed head injuries. For this reason, whole spine radiography was recommended by the authors. [9]

## REFERENCES

[1]    Watson N. Pattern of spinal cord injury in the elderly. *Paraplegia*, 1976 May;14(1):36-40].

[2]    Frankel HL, Montero FA, Penny PT. Spinal cord injuries due to diving. *Paraplegia*, 1980 Apr;18(2):118-22.

[3]    McCoy GF, Piggot J, Macafee AL, Adair IV. Injuries of the cervical spine in schoolboy rugby football. *J. Bone Joint. Surg. Br.,* 1984 Aug;66(4):500-3.

[4]    Gupta A, el Masri WS. Multilevel spinal injuries. Incidence, distribution and neurological patterns. *J. Bone Joint. Surg. Br.,* 1989 Aug;71(4):692-5.

[5]    Hart J. Spinal injury associations: a British perspective. *Paraplegia,* 1992 Jan;30(1):37-8.

[6]    Frankel   HL, Coll   JR, Charlifue   SW, Whiteneck   GG, Gardner   BP, Jamous MA, Krishnan KR, Nuseibeh I, Savic G, Sett P. Long-term survival in spinal cord injury: a fifty year investigation. *Spinal Cord,* 1998 Apr; 36(4):266-74.

[7]    Vaidyanathan S, Soni BM, Gopalan L, Sett P, Watt JW, Singh G, Bingley J, Mansour P, Krishnan KR, Oo T. A review of the readmissions of patients with tetraplegia to the Regional Spinal Injuries Centre, Southport, United Kingdom, between January 1994 and December 1995. *Spinal Cord,* 1998 Dec; 36(12):838-46.

[8]    Amin A, Bernard J, Nadarajah R, Davies N, Gow F, Tucker S. Spinal injuries admitted to a specialist centre over a 5-year period: a study to evaluate delayed admission. *Spinal Cord,* 2005 Jul; 43(7):434-7.

[9]    Martin   BW, Dykes   E, Lecky   FE.    Patterns and risks in spinal trauma.    *Arch.   Dis. Child,* 2004 Sep; 89(9):860-5.

# FRANCE

There are almost 1,000 new cases of SCI annually in France, giving an annual incidence of approximately 1 per 100,000 populations. About half of new SCI cases are due to road traffic accidents.

A retrospective study of 351 cases of traumatic SCI was reported from the Rhone-Alpes region at Henry Gabrielle Hospital during 6 years from 1970 to 1975. The incidence and prevalence of traumatic SCI were 1.27 per100, 000 and 25 per 100,000 population respectively in the Rhone-Alpes region.

The mean age of patients with a traumatic spinal cord injury was 39 years old. The male/female ratio was 3.68 (78.63% in males versus 21.37% in females). The most common injury mechanisms involved a motor vehicle accident in 31.8%, a fall in 24.25% and a motorcycles or bicycles accident in 15.4%. The incidence of tetraplegia was highest in motor vehicle accidents, while thoracolumbar lesions were more common in falls and suicide attempts. [1]

A nationwide survey was conducted to define the annual incidence of SCI in France among 380 medical centers. For individuals over the age of 15, there were 19.4 per million population or 934 new cases per year in 2000. This finding represented a substantial increase compared to the rate of SCI reported in 1970s by Minaire et al. [2]

In one retrospective study of the 10-year period from 1997–2006, there were noted to be 21,623 cases of spinal trauma, including 1523 cases of major spinal trauma. Cervical injuries with SCI were the most common (58%), with a peak incidence in the age range of 20–30 years old. Males suffered a significantly higher rate of SCI compared to females. [3]

In a recent French observational study, data from the Rhône Road Trauma Registry was evaluated. Two 6-year observation periods with a gap interval between them was analyzed

(1996-2001 and 2003-2008). Interestingly, in spite of a significant drop in road trauma and injury rates, there was no change in the incidence or mortality of SCI. One reason for the lack of improvement in the mortality and incidence of SCI was suggested to be a greater underestimate of SCI rates in earlier studies due to the lack of inclusion of patients that died prior to reaching the hospital or within the first 24 hours of the injury. [4]

# REFERENCES

[1]    Minaire P, Castanier M, Girard R, Berard E, Deidier C, Bourret J. Epidemiology of spinal cord injury in the Rhonealpes region, France, 1970-75. *Paraplegia*, 16 (1978-79) 76-87.

[2]    Albert T, Ravaud JF; Tetrafigap group. Rehabilitation of spinal cord injury in France: a nationwide multicentre study of incidence and regional disparities. *Spinal Cord*, 2005 Jun; 43(6):357-65.

[3]    Lieutaud T, Ndiaye A, Frost F, Chiron M; Registry Group. A 10-year population survey of spinal trauma and spinal cord injuries after road accidents in the Rhône area. *J. Neurotrauma*, 2010 Jun; 27(6):1101-7.

[4]    Lieutaud T, Ndiaye A, Laumon B, Chiron M._Spinal cord injuries sustained in road crashes are not on the decrease in France: A study based on epidemiological trends. *J Neurotrauma*, 2011 Sep 6 [Epub ahead of print].

# ITALY

The incidence of SCI in Italy has been estimated from 18 to 20 per million. [1]

A prospective, multi-centered observational study was conducted to estimate the survival, complications, re-admissions rates and maintenance of neurologic status with traumatic SCI. A total of 511 patients with SCI were administered a standardized questionnaire via telephone between 1997 and 1999. Of this group, 79% completed the interview. Fifty three percent of patients with SCI had complications in the first 6 months of injury. The most common complications were urological (53.7%), pain, spasticity and pressure sores. More than half of patients (56.8%) had re-admissions to the hospital after the initial injury period. Reasons for re-admission included the need for additional rehabilitation (31.7%), urological complications (24.2%), medical assessment (19.8%), removal of spinal instrumentation (12.3%), management of pressure sores (7.9%) and osteoarticular complications (11%). Bowel autonomy and bladder continence were reported in 70.5% and 85% of patients, respectively. The re-admission rate was higher in male subjects (p<0.05). Mortality was positively correlated with older age (p<0.001), female gender (p<0.05), tetraplegia (p<0.001), lack of bladder/ bowel autonomy (p<0.001), shorter length of stay in rehabilitation (p<0.05) and pressure sores (p<0.001) on discharge. [2]

Another study evaluated a cohort of patients receiving emergency care, acute intervention and rehabilitation for traumatic SCI. The male to female ratio for this study was 4:1 and the mean age of the patients was 38.5 years. Overall, 53.8% of patients had motor vehicle accidents, followed by falls (22.6%). Surgery was performed in 80% of patients. Of those, almost 50% of surgical procedures were done within the first 24 hours. During acute care, pressure ulcer was the most frequent complication. [1]

Another multicenter retrospective study of patients with SCI was conducted, looking at factors influencing the length of stay between 1989 and 1994. During this period, 859 patients were enrolled in the study from seven rehabilitation centers in central and northern Italy. The male to female ratio was 4:1 and the mean age was 38 years. Overall, 75% of SCIs were traumatic in origin. Pressure ulcers accounted for 25% of the total cost of care. The prevalence of pressure ulcer was 34% in traumatic SCI series. Neurologic recovery was seen in 74%. The mean LOS was 143 ± 89 days for traumatic SCI patients.[3]

## REFERENCES

[1]    Pagliacci MC, Celani MG, Zampolini M, Spizzichino L, Franceschini M, Baratta S, Finali G, Gatta G, Perdon L; Gruppo Italiano Studio Epidemiologico Mielolesioni. An Italian survey of traumatic spinal cord injury. The Gruppo Italiano Studio Epidemiologico Mielolesioni study. *Arch. Phys. Med. Rehabil.*, 2003 Sep;84(9):1266-75.

[2]    Pagliacci MC, Franceschini M, Di Clemente B, Agosti M, Spizzichino L; GISEM. A multicentre follow-up of clinical aspects of traumatic spinal cord injury. *Spinal Cord*, 2007 Jun; 45(6):404-10.

[3]    Celani MG, Spizzichino L, Ricci S, Zampolini M, Franceschini M; for the Retrospective Study Group on SCI. Spinal cord injury in Italy: A multicenter retrospective study. *Arch. Phys. Med. Rehabil.*, 2001 May;82(5):589-96.

## GERMANY

A retrospective German study was conducted to define the demographics of spinal trauma. There were 562 traumatic spine fractures, evaluating the rate the correlations and effects of age, gender and cause of accident on the type of vertebral fracture and fracture distribution, the likelihood to sustain an associated injury or neurological deficit from 1996 to 2000. The study consisted of 61% male and 39% female with the overall male to female ratio of 1.6:1.

They divided the study group based on a fracture mechanism into three subgroups: compression, distraction, rotation. Compression and distraction fractures were similar in male and female, however rotation fracture was significantly higher in male patients (m: f=2.8:1). The mean age was 43.8 years. Fall (39%) was the most common cause of mechanism of injury followed by traffic accidents (26.5%).

There was a correlation between the accident mechanism and type of the fracture. Simple fall predominantly caused a compression fracture and evenly distributed over the whole spine. While traffic accidents induced significantly more fractures of the cervical and thoracic spine and caused a distraction fracture. Fall from great height also caused a distraction type of fracture. Patients with cervical spine fracture had the highest risk (65%) of suffering from an associated injury compare to thoracic (50.6%) and lumbar (52.3%) per spinal region. The highest incidence of associated injuries was seen in patients with multilevel fractures (96.5%).In terms of neurological deficit, 75.3% exhibited no deficit, 11.2% showed a complete motor and sensory deficit and 13.5% had an incomplete neurological deficit. Patients with cervical spine fractures tend to have the highest number of complete motor and sensory neurological deficits (19.7%). [1]

Another study investigated all spinal cord injuries of 21 special centers in Germany from 1976 to 1996 about 20 years. 1500 cases were treated per annum. 75% of those injuries were traumatic versus 25% of non-traumatic. Male had the highest SCI ranged from 73% to 71% compared to female from 29% to 27%. The average was very stable in both genders. 62% of patients with SCI were paraplegic, 38% were tetraplegic. Of 22,212 recent cases with SCI, 35% had traffic accident injury, 14% work injury, 4% sports and diving, 5% suicide and 1% killing attempts. The most common reason of readmission was disorders of soft tissues (23%) followed by urinary tract disorder (21%).

Their investigation data demonstrate very stable trends within 20 years period. The special centers carried out treatment and consultation in about 22,000 recent cases, 45,000 readmissions and 80,000 out- patients. [2]

Others studied the incidence of SCI in the Germany as well. They used three sources which included the data of the central office for paraplegic patients, The German workmen's compensation and the hospital discharge data. They reported the overall incidence of SCI about 36 per million inhabitants for new cases and 72 per million inhabitants for the existing cases. [3]

## REFERENCES

[1]    Leucht P, Fischer K, Muhr G, Mueller EJ. Epidemiology of traumatic spine fractures. *Injury*, 2009 Feb; 40(2):166-72.

[2]    Exner G, Meinecke FW. Trends in the treatment of patients with spinal cord lesions seen within a period of 20 years in German centers. *Spinal Cord*, 1997 Jul; 35(7):415-9.

[3]    Köning W, Frowein RA. Incidence of spinal cord injury in the Federal Republic of Germany.

[4]    *Neurosurg. Rev.*, 1989; 12 Suppl 1:562-6.

## THE NETHERLANDS

The incidence of SCI varies between 9 and 16 /million/annum in the Europe. In The Netherlands, acute spinal cord injured patients are first admitted to trauma, orthopedic, neurological and neurosurgical departments of university and general hospitals. Then patients are transferred to a rehabilitation institution. [2, 4]

A multicenter, prospective study sought to document the Dutch experience with SCI. In this study, 205 individuals were enrolled and compared to the international experience for SCI management.

The study setting was 8 Dutch rehabilitation centers, specializing in SCI between August 2000 and July 2003. All subjects ranged in age from 18–65 years. During the 3-year period, 68% of the enrolled patients were noted to have complete lesions. Fifty nine percent were classified as having paraplegia. The most common causes of the SCI trauma included traffic accidents (42%), followed by falls (23%) and sports accidents (15%). Male gender was predominant (74%).

The length of clinical rehabilitation varied between 2 months to more than a year, depending on the level and severity of the neurologic injury and the presence of co-morbidities. The investigators concluded that the length of stay in rehabilitation centers in The Netherlands was longer (212–387 days) compared to Denmark (149–2 85 days), Australia (43–206 days) and the USA (78-45 days).[1]

A retrospective study was conducted on 479 patients with SCI to ascertain the incidence of SCI in The Netherlands in 1994. The investigators found an incidence of a traumatic neurologic injury to the spinal cord of about 10.4 per million inhabitants per year in the Netherlands. An injury was characterized as a SCI if there traumatic loss of motor, sensory, and/or bladder and bowel function below the level of the lesion which lasted for more than 2 weeks. Overall, 48.7% of cases had complete injuries. Seventy percent were admitted to a rehabilitation center with a mean acute care hospital stay of 31 days. [2]

In another multi-centered prospective study, 919 patients with traumatic and non-traumatic SCI were admitted to 11 rehabilitation centers in the Netherlands and Flanders between 2002 and 2007. In this report, the majority of patients had non-traumatic lesions (54.7%).

The male/female ratio was 2.8:1 in the traumatic group. The mean age of the patients was 43.4 years. The mean length of stay at a rehabilitation center was 183.3 days. The longest stays were required by patients with traumatic, motor complete, cervical lesions. Compared to the USA, Australian and Italian patients , the Dutch/Flemish SCI population showed a more even gender distribution, older age, and less severe SCI lesions on average.[3]

An older retrospective study was conducted on 293 patients with SCI between 1982 and 1993 to describe the Dutch SCI care system during those years. At that point, the mean length of stay in a rehabilitation center was 154 days. There were found to be sixteen new SCI patients per million population per year. The male to female ratio was 2.2: 1 and the mean age was 45.1 years. [4]

# REFERENCES

[1]    de Groot S, Dallmeijer AJ, Post MW, van Asbeck FW, Nene AV, Angenot EL, van der Woude LH. Demographics of the Dutch multicenter prospective cohort study 'Restoration of mobility in spinal cord injury rehabilitation'. *Spinal Cord*, 2006 Nov; 44(11):668-75.

[2]    van Asbeck FW, Post MW, Pangalila RF. An epidemiological description of spinal cord injuries in The Netherlands in 1994. *Spinal Cord*, 2000 Jul;38(7):420-4.

[3]    Osterthun R, Post MW, van Asbeck FW; Dutch-Flemish Spinal Cord Society.

[4]    Characteristics, length of stay and functional outcome of patients with spinal cord injury in Dutch and Flemish rehabilitation centres. *Spinal Cord*, 2009 Apr;47(4):339-44.

[5]    Schönherr MC, Groothoff JW, Mulder GA, Eisma WH. Rehabilitation of patients with spinal cord lesions in The Netherlands: an epidemiological study. *Spinal Cord*, 1996 Nov; 34(11):679-83.

# SECTION III: EPIDEMIOLOGY OF SPINAL CORD INJURIES IN ASIA

In: Epidemiology of Spinal Cord Injuries
Editors: V. Rahimi-Movaghar, S. B. Jazayeri et al.
ISBN: 978-1-61942-894-2
©2012 Nova Science Publishers, Inc.

*Chapter 12*

# SPINAL CORD INJURY IN INDIA: DEMOGRAPHICS, MORBIDITY AND EMPLOYMENT

### *Nalina Gupta*

MPT (Neurosciences)
Head, Department of Physiotherapy,
College of Applied Education and Health Sciences, Meerut, India

## ABSTRACT

In India, approximately 1.5 million people live with deficits caused by spinal cord injury. Every year, 10,000 new cases are added to this group. The majority of SCIs occur in males in the 16-30 age group. However, this is only an estimate since there is no reliable national database. There is a decline in the male to female SCI ratio which reflects the changing social norms as females in India become more active and outgoing. There is a gradual trend towards an increased incidence of road traffic accidents indicating a gradual urbanization of society and an increase in the number of vehicles on the roads in India. In earlier studies, pressure sores and urinary tract infections were the most prevalent morbidities in individuals with spinal cord injury. In more recent studies, on the other hand, pain and spasticity were found to be more prevalent. Psychiatric morbidity in individuals with spinal cord injury is given more attention than in the past. There is scant literature on quality of life, re-integration into the community and employment of patients with spinal cord injury in India. Major barriers for community reintegration are architectural and environmental obstacles, poor socio-economic status and associated co-morbidities. Most studies from India are hospital based and there is still no existing national database. Thus, there is a need to have a multi-centric effort in India to establish a reliable national database.

## INTRODUCTION

Spinal Cord Injury (SCI) was described by the Edwin Smith Papyrus as "an ailment not to be treated" over 5000 years ago.[1] More than eighty percent of the world's population lives in more than 100 developing countries where little is known about the epidemiology of

SCI. Constraints on resources and research funding, the priority of curable diseases over SCI lesions, and a lack of general interest by the medical community to address a prolonged and often permanent disability contribute to this relative ignorance.[2]

There is no reliable national SCI database in most developing countries, mainly because of poorly managed medical record systems.[3] Studies regarding the demographics, morbidity and employment status of SCI patients have been undertaken at many centers in India – these studies will be reviewed in this chapter.

In India, approximately [1.5] million people live with spinal cord injury. Every year, an estimated 10,000 new cases are added to this group but this number is difficult to confirm because of the lack of a national database.[4] The majority of SCI patients are males in the 16-30 year age group. In this chapter, we will discuss three aspects of spinal cord injury in India: demographics, morbidity and employment.

# DEMOGRAPHICS

In 1986, Chacko et al evaluated the problems encountered in a general hospital in rural India. Two hundred and eighteen individuals with spinal cord injury admitted in the hospital were analyzed. One hundred and twenty five of these individuals had a neurological deficit. They found the male to female ratio to be 13.5:1. More than 60% of injuries occurred within the 3rd and 4th decade of life and the most common cause for spinal cord injury were falls from height followed secondly by traffic accidents.[5]

Chacko et al emphasized that the rescue and retrieval systems in India were inadequate as was knowledge regarding precautions necessary when transporting a SCI patient. The study highlighted the necessity of appropriate preventive measures, and also reemphasized the short-comings of spinal cord injury treatment in general hospitals.[5]

Shanmugasundaram was the principal investigator and Project Director of the PL.480 Paraplegia project, Madras and the ICMR Paraplegia Project (1979-1987).[6] He found in his 1987 study that falls from heights or into wells (66%) were the most common mode of spinal cord injury in India[7] followed by road traffic accidents (14%). The male to female ratio was 8.98:18 and patients with SCI at Madras were mostly males in their second to fourth decades of life.[7] Singh R et al. found the male to female ratio to be 3.7:1 and falls from height as the major cause of spinal cord insult followed by road traffic accidents.[8]

Singh et al conducted a study between January 2000 and December 2001 in Haryana, India. All the patients with traumatic spinal injuries reporting to the Accident and Emergency Department and all outpatients and inpatients of the orthopedic department were included in the study. Patients who died before reaching hospital were not taken into account. A detailed history was asked regarding their demographic characteristics such as age, gender, occupation, socio-economic status, and mode of trauma. Other questions regarding their pre-hospital care, mode of transfer, time since injury etc. were also queried. Total subjects reported were 483. [8]

Singh et al found the male to female ratio to be 2.96:1. The average age at injury was 35.4 and the most prevalent age group was 20-29 followed by 30-39. The most common cause of injury was fall from height (roof, trees, electricity pole (44.5%) followed by motor vehicle accidents (34.7%)). Falls were more prominent in the second and third decades and roadside accidents in the third and fourth decade. The first lumbar vertebrae was the most common level of injury followed by the twelfth thoracic vertebra; the cervical spine was the next most common site of injury (C5 and C6 were most common injured levels).[8]

A hospital based study performed by Agrawal et al in Karnataka also reported predominance of male victims with a ratio of men to women of 3.6:1.The largest number of patients were in the 20-39 year age range. Mechanisms of injury recorded were fall from height (58.9%), fall of weight (7.2%), Motor Vehicle Accident (21.3%) and non-traumatic causes (12.6%).[9]

Pandey et al enrolled sixty patients with spinal cord injury admitted to their hospital (ISIC, Delhi) between August 2005 and May 2006 for analysis. Eighty five percent of individuals were males with a mean age at injury of 34 years. There was an average delay of 45 days prior to admission to a spinal unit. This delay may be due to a lack of awareness on the part of patients/doctors regarding specialized spinal centers. In 62.5% of cases, patients transported themselves to the facility without spinal precautions because of this lack of awareness regarding proper precautions against secondary injury.[10]

Since most of the studies mentioned above were hospital based, we (Gupta et al) attempted to collect data regarding the demographic characteristics and morbidity trends for SCI patients from hospitals all over India between August 2004 to May 2006. This postal survey had a response rate of 46% and identified 276 individuals with paraplegia. Individuals age 18 or older with paraplegia and evidence of a complete spinal cord lesion from any cause were included in the study. Subjects could be either community dwelling or institutionalized. The most common age groups at the time of injury were 18-25 years and 40-50 years and we found a male to female ratio of 5.42:1. A fall from height was the leading cause for spinal cord insult (25%), followed by road traffic accidents (17.4%). Fall from a height was the commonest cause for the spinal cord insult in all age groups (especially in the 40-50 age group) and road traffic accidents were the leading cause in the 18-25 years age group. The most common level of injury in individuals with paraplegia was lumbar (60.1%).[11]

Manjeet et al conducted a study from January 2006 to July 2008 in the Jammu division. All subjects with traumatic spinal cord injury with or without neurological deficit who were admitted to the emergency wing of Government Medical College in Jammu were included in the study. A total of four hundred and three (n=403) cases were analyzed. They found the male to female ratio to be 2.98:1 and the most prevalent age group was 20-30 years followed by 30-40 years. Falls from a height including roof, trees, electricity pole and Hill tops (50%, n = 201) were the commonest cause of spinal cord injury followed by motor vehicle accidents (30.3% n = 122). Falls were more prominent in the second and third decades whereas road traffic accidents were more common in third and fourth decade. This study likely reflects the trend in most of the hilly states in India.[12]

An epidemiological study was performed in 2010 by the Indian Spinal Injuries Centre (ISIC), Delhi to determine the demographic profile of those treated at the facility over the previous 12 years. The study analyzed 1,138 patients treated in ISIC from both rural and urban areas. Road traffic accidents (43.5%) were the most common cause of SCIs and disability. Another important cause was fall from height (38.04%). The male to female ratio was found to be 5.6:1.[13]

Clinical and radiological features of SCI were analyzed for 212 patients treated between 2006 and 2010 at Acharya Vinoba Bhave Rural Hospital, Maharashtra India, a tertiary hospital in a rural setting. 80.6% of these individuals were males and a fall from a height was the commonest mode of spinal injury (54.8%), followed by road traffic accident (28.38%). Mean time between injury and arrival at the hospital was 74.4 hours.[14] If we closely analyze the trends in the literature (Table 1), we see that there has been a decline in the male to female ratio compared to studies from 20 or 25 years ago.

### Table 1. Demographic trend of individuals with spinal Cord Injury in India

| Author/Centre | Year | Place | Type of study | Male: Female | Prevalent age/decade at injury | Etiology Fall | RTA |
|---|---|---|---|---|---|---|---|
| Chacko et al [5] | 1986 | Karnataka, South India | Hospital based | 13.5:1 | 3$^{rd}$ -4$^{th}$ decade of life | 55.2% | --- |
| Shanmuga Sundaram [6,7] | 1987 | Madras, South India | Madras Project | 8.9:1 | 2$^{nd}$ -4$^{th}$ decade of life | 66% | 14% |
| Singh R et al [8] | 1994 | India | --- | 3.7:1 | --- | --- | --- |
| Singh R et al [8] | 2003 | Haryana, North India | Hospital based | 2.9:1 | Average age at injury 35.4 years | 44.5% | 34.7% |
| Agrawal P et al[9] | 2006 | Karnataka, South India | Hospital based | 3.6:1 | --- | 58.9% | 21.3% |
| Pandey VK et al[10] | 2007 | Delhi, Central India | Hospital based | 5.6:1 | Mean age at injury- 34 years | 48.33% | --- |
| Gupta N et al[11] | 2008 | India | Postal survey involving entire India | 5.4:1 | 18-<25 years and 40-<50 years age group | 25% | 17.4% |
| Manjeet S et al[12] | 2009 | Jammu, North India | Hospital based | 2.9:1 | 2$^{nd}$ -3$^{rd}$ decade of life | 50% | 30.3% |
| ISIC[13] | 2010 | Delhi | Hospital based | 5.6:1 | --- | 38.04% | 43.5% |
| Singh PK et al[14] | 2011 | Maharashtra, India | Hospital based | 4.2:1 | --- | 54.8% | 28.38% |

Road Traffic Accidents (RTA).

This finding reflects the changing social norms in India where females are becoming more active outside the home.[8] There has been little change in age or decade of life at the time of injury between recent studies and those from 20 or 25 years ago; the 2nd-4th decade of life is still the most common age group of injured individuals. Individuals are more active during these decades because of travel related to either their education or occupation; the use of motorcycles is very common among students in this age group and manual laborers at construction sites most commonly belong to this age group. The consistency in the age of students and laborers is likely the reason that the age of injured individuals has not changed.

Fall from a height is the commonest mode of spinal cord injury in most of the studies except in a few studies performed in recent years that showed road traffic accidents to be the major cause of spinal cord injury.

A study performed by the Indian Spinal Injuries Centre, Delhi in 2010 mentioned road traffic accidents as being the major cause of SCI injury, contradicting other studies conducted in India.[13] Gupta N et al found in their study that although fall from a height is the commonest mode of SCI in India, traffic accidents are the major cause of SCI in the 18-25 age group.[11] There is a gradual trend towards an increased incidence of Road Traffic Accidents (RTA) indicating the gradual urbanization of society and an increase in the number of vehicles on the roads in India.

There are epidemiological differences seen in developing countries with respect to developed countries. Fall from a height was found to be the most common mode of injury in most studies in India, Bangladesh, Vietnam, Lao PDR, Cambodia and Nepal. Road traffic accidents are the second most common cause in these countries, including Thailand. Most of the falls from heights take place at home and in a rural/semi-urban setting.[15]

The causes of fall from height are diverse: falls may be from unprotected terraces, trees, electricity poles, overloaded carts, tractors, buses, trucks, trains or other vehicles, falls may be at construction sites, off walls or into an unprotected well. Similarly, factors predisposing to RTA are different - more injuries occur in struck pedestrians or related to the use of two-wheeled vehicles.[15]

*Implications:* An emphasis should be given on preventing the more common modes of injury. Fall from a height, especially in the domestic and rural/semi-urban setting, can be prevented by community awareness and legislation about safety measures related to unprotected terraces, climbing of trees, electricity poles etc. and related to unprotected wells and by improving domestic infrastructure by mandating protected terraces and roofs.[15]

Road traffic accidents can be prevented by optimizing the number of vehicles on the road and by building proper safety infrastructure like roadway lighting, pedestrian pathways and limiting speeds on highways and in all residential areas using camera speed traps. International safety standards must be applied for all vehicles and roads, along with implementation of legislation to enforce safe driving through speed limits, seat belts use, helmets use and by creating community awareness of safe practices.[15]

Trained medical staff at the accident site should practice proper primary care of injured individuals and provide appropriate transportation to dedicated spinal trauma units. Training community volunteers in safe handling techniques and correct transportation methods for patients with SCI15 can be effective at preventing secondary injury which commonly contributes to overall disability.

This could be done through creating trauma care and rehabilitation facilities in cities, towns and in rural areas. Various approaches can be used to raise community awareness programs.

This can be accomplished through group approaches such as lectures, workshops and demonstrations, mass communication methods such as television, radio, newspaper, public posters, public exhibitions, the internet, advertisements in movie halls and concerts or through directed approaches such as safety education provided to children in school.[15]

# MORBIDITY

Morbidity refers to "secondary reasons of ill health not directly due to initial injury." Chacko et al in 1986 found the frequency of decubitus ulceration and urinary tract infections (UTI) unacceptably high and a high percentage of patients with cervical spine injury expired.[5] In a study performed by Shanmugamsundaram, patients admitted within 72 hours and those admitted after that period were called System and Non-System cases, respectively. Nineteen percent of System cases and 45 percent of Non-System cases had pressure sores.[7]

A pattern of emergency urology cases analyzed by Sharma RK et al in 1987 found that 24.2% of patients developed genitourinary dysfunction secondary to spinal cord trauma. They emphasized the necessity of creating a trauma hospital/spinal cord injury centre for the civilian population that could decrease the morbidity and mortality of these patients.[16]

Rath et al in 1993 mentioned in their study that the emotional impact of spinal cord injury could be equated to a "Survivor Syndrome." Psychological consequences and mental morbidity was observed in twenty subjects with spinal cord injury over a period of three months to twelve years. Eight of twenty patients presented with neurotic disorders, five with intense depression, four with depersonalization and four with a paranoid state. Impaired social adjustment was observed in five patients.[17]

A retrospective review of the morbidity associated with 250 consecutive cases of spinal instrumentation was carried out in a neurosurgical spine unit in Indraprastha Apollo Hospital, Delhi in 2005. This study concluded that while, in experienced hands, the neurological complications related to instrumentation was low and infection rate could be kept to a minimum with meticulous sterile technique, the use of instrumentation should be confined to cases where there is a clear indication.[18]

In a study performed by Singh R et al in 2005, key concerns following SCI in women were sexual dysfunction, bladder and bowel dysfunction, bed sores, pain, spasticity, satisfaction of partners and being the subject of cultural taboos.[19]

A cross-sectional survey of caregivers of people with SCI at the Department of Physical Medicine and Rehabilitation was done by Raj JT et al in 2006. This study reported high psychiatric morbidity (53%) with common diagnoses of depression and anxiety. Caregivers who were spouses, women, currently married and had lower educational level had greater psychiatric morbidity and less leisure satisfaction. They did not find any significant association between age, occupation, residence, socioeconomic status, type and duration of SCI with either morbidity or leisure satisfaction.[20] Another study in south India had found significant association between education level and suicidal behavior in people with SCI with psychological distress. [21]

A postal survey performed between August 2004 to May 2006 by Gupta et al revealed a response rate of 46% (n=276). Of all the morbidities related to SCI which were studied, pain was the leading morbidity identified (57.2%) followed by spasticity (39.1%), pressure sores (28.3%), postural hypotension (10.1%), respiratory complications, and fractures (5.8%). There were significant associations between various morbidities and demographics and between the morbidities themselves. Ambulation reduced the incidence of secondary complications.[22] More than half of the subjects complained of pain in the study.[23]

Pain is the leading cause of morbidity irrespective of living environment but the incidence of morbidities overall has been shown to be higher among individuals living in the community.[24] Pain was found to be associated with age, duration of time since injury and ambulation.[23] Pain was most common in the 40-50 year age group followed by the 18-25 year group. This increased rate in older patients could be due to the aging process, greater perception of pain by older individuals, or the decrease in plasticity of the central nervous system with regard to psychological stresses in older patients with SCI. The existing literature supports the hypothesis that there is an association between pain and age as pain often starts within the first six months after injury and continues throughout life. Ambulators experienced less pain, although the frequency of shoulder pain was more among ambulators.[23]

A prospective longitudinal descriptive study was performed by Singh et al in 2008 to evaluate the Quality of Life (QoL) of patients with spinal cord injury in northern India. Fifty persons with SCI were surveyed for medical problems, neurological status and social adjustments. The most common medical problems found in the study were bladder dysfunction (44%), bedsores (36%), gastrointestinal problems (56%), neuropathic pain (42%) and spasticity (60%). The authors did not find any significant association between age, education, marital status and duration of injury and QoL scores. Female sex, employment, mobility, autonomy, cordial partner relations and good social adjustment were associated with higher QoL scores.[25]

Singh et al in 2011 found that among five hundred and forty five patients with SCI, the overall incidence of bacteriuria was 1.70 / hundred person-days and the overall incidence of urinary tract infection was 0.64 / hundred person-days. The incidence of Urinary Tract Infections (UTI) per 100 person-days was 2.68 for indwelling catheterization, 0.34 for Clean Intermittent Catheterization (CIC), 0.34 for condom drainage, 0.56 for suprapubic cystostomy, 0.34 for reflex voiding, and 0.32 for normal voiding. They also reported rates of other urologic complications such as urethritis (14.3%), urethral stricture (12.1%), stress incontinence (11%), periurethral abscess (8.2%), epididymorchitis (8.07%), hematuria (8.07%), lithiasis (4.2%), urethral false passage (4.03%), urethral fistula (2%) and pyelonephritis (1.1%). They concluded in their study that the incidence of UTI and other urological complications was lower in patients performing CIC in comparison to the patients using an indwelling catheter.[26]

In earlier studies, pressure sores and urinary tract infections were the most prevalent morbidities in individuals with SCI while more recently, pain and spasticity were found to be more prevalent (Table 2). The possible reasons for this trend could be inclusion of comprehensive rehabilitation programs, frequent turning of patients, use of clean intermittent catheterization, and improved access to active wheel chair ambulation or orthotics used to assist ambulation.[22]

Rath et al and Raj et al published papers focused on psychological/psychiatric morbidity in patients with SCI. While Rath et al in 1993 described psychological and mental morbidity among individuals with SCI, Raj et al in 2006 studied psychiatric morbidity reported by caregivers of individuals with SCI (Table 2).

Unlike in western countries, mortality and morbidity rates have not come down significantly in India in spite of new technologies and rehabilitation facilities.

Many individuals continue to be re-admitted with preventable complications. The higher incidence of morbidity can be explained by the observation that the majority of persons with SCI live in rural areas, live below the poverty line and are unable to afford the cost of rehabilitation.[22, 23, 24]

**Table 2. Morbidity trend in individuals with spinal cord injury in India**

| Author | Year | Place | Morbidity |
|---|---|---|---|
| Chacko et al [5] | 1986 | Karnataka, South India | Decubitus Ulceration<br>Urinary Tract Infections |
| Shanmuga Sundaram [6,7] | 1987 | Madras, South India | Pressure sores<br>19%-system cases<br>45%-Non system cases |
| Rath et al [17] | 1993 | India | Psychological and Mental Morbidity |
| Singh R et al [19] | 2005 | Haryana, North India | Sexual dysfunction<br>Bladder and Bowel dysfunction<br>Bed sores<br>Pain<br>Spasticity<br>Satisfaction of partner<br>Cultural taboo. |
| Raj JT et al [21] | 2006 | India | Psychiatric Morbidity among informal carers of indidividuals with SCI |
| Gupta N et al [22] | 2007 | India | Pain (57.2%)<br>Spasticity (39.1%)<br>Pressure sore (28.3%)<br>Postural hypotension (10.1%)<br>Respiratory complications (5.8%)<br>Fractures (5.8%) |
| Singh R et al [25] | 2008 | North India | Spasticity (60%)<br>Gastrointestinal problems (56%)<br>Bladder problem (44%)<br>Neuropathic pain (42%)<br>Bed sores (36%) |
| Singh R et al [26] | 2011 | Haryana, North India | Bacteriuria<br>Urinary tract infections |

A survey of 53 centers in India reported that in 37.5% of the institutions, less than 50% of the patients got an adequate rehabilitation during hospitalization whereas 81.82% of the institution had no facilities for a pre-discharge home visit by the staff to suggest home modifications and 73.9% of institutions had no facilities for follow up home care services. [27]

In India, the variation in morbidity among patients with SCI can be attributed to financial resources, health care access (including rehabilitation services, community set ups, follow up home care services) and socio-cultural factors. The support delivery systems vary from centre to centre.[22]

Implications: Emphasis should be given to comprehensive rehabilitation programs. There is a need to have pre-discharge home visits as well as facilities for follow up home care services for the prevention as well as for the timely treatment of such co-morbidities. Educating individuals with SCI and their care takers in India regarding the various causes of morbidities, their prevention and treatment is also necessary.[22]

## COMMUNITY REINTEGRATION/EMPLOYMENT

The term 'employment' by definition, includes any trade, economic activity and profession in the organized and unorganized sector or any trade that may provide monetary remuneration. Employment is one of the most important goals for an individual with SCI, especially in cases in which an individual is the only earning member of the family. Employment not only helps to achieve economic self-sufficiency but is also associated with personal growth, disability adjustment, social integration and life satisfaction.[28]

A study by Sekaran P et al in rural south India showed that there is a decline in community reintegration of SCI patients. Architectural and environmental barriers, poor socio-economic status and co morbidities significantly affected the level of community participation. [29]

Samuelkamaleshkumar S et al found that SCI patients in rural South India who have completed comprehensive, mostly self-financed, rehabilitation with an emphasis on achieving functional ambulation, family support, and self-employment and who attend a regular annual follow-up appointment show a high level of community reintegration, independence, social integration, and cognitive independence. CHART scores in the domains of occupation, mobility, and economic self-sufficiency showed lower levels of community reintegration. [30]

Nalina Gupta et al found that individuals who were employed were living either in centers run by the armed forces or in other specialized centers. None of the individuals living in the community were employed. The centres run by the armed forces provide sheltered workshops for patients with paraplegia to work and give these patietns a monthly salary and a place to live. Specialized centers give vocational training to subjects with SCI and help them with job placement. Community dwelling patients with SCI were not employed in the study, which is probably due to co-morbidities and environmental barriers. [28]

*Implications:* The rehabilitation professional should have a knowledge regarding the various opportunities/policies for people with disability secondary to SCI. There is a need to have a barrier free environment. Emphasis should be given to community reintegration and economic self sufficiency. Government should expand outreach services for poor persons in rural areas. Self-employment through concessional loans by various agencies is required as well as poverty alleviation programs for capacity building. Social security and sustainable livelihood programs need to be applied effectively in an integrated manner to improve the conditions of persons who are poor and disabled. [28]

## SUMMARY

This chapter dealt with the demographics, morbidity and employment of patients with SCI in India. There is a decline in male to female ratio that reflects the changing social norms where females in India are becoming more active and engaged outside the home. There is a gradual trend towards an increased incidence of RTA indicating the gradual urbanization of society and an increase in the number of vehicles on roads in India.

In earlier studies, pressure sores and urinary tract infections used to be the most prevalent morbidities in individuals with SCI while recent studies have demonstrated that pain and spasticity were more prevalent. The possible reasons for this trend could be greater availability of comprehensive rehabilitation programs, frequent turning of patients, use of clean intermittent catheterization, and access to wheel chairs or orthotics to assist ambulation. Psychiatric morbidity reported by caregivers of individuals with SCI is also given greater recognition than in the past. In India, the variation in the rate of morbidities in patients with SCI can be attributed to variation in financial resources, health care access including rehabilitation services, community set ups, types of activities performed in the community, follow up home care services, socio-cultural characteristics and support delivery systems.

There is minimal literature on quality of life, community re-integration and employment of patients with SCI in India. Major barriers for community reintegration are architectural, environmental, socio-economic and related to co-morbidities. The lack of knowledge of medical/paramedical faculty regarding various job opportunities for these individuals is also an important point to consider. Individuals with SCI in centers run by the armed forces or in specialized centers are more likely to be reintegrated than those residing in the community.

## CONCLUSION

This chapter reviewed the demographics, morbidity and employment of patients with SCI in India. Most of the studies are hospital based and there is still no reliable national database existing. Even in India, there are only a few places like in Delhi, Haryana, Jammu, Mumbai and south India where the studies related to epidemiology of SCI are occurring. Thus, there is a need to perform a multi-centric study in India to establish a reliable national database.

## REFERENCES

[1]     Feldman RP, Goodrich JT. 1999. The Edwin Smith Surgical Papyrus. *Child's Nervous System*, 15(6-7):281–284.
[2]     Soubbotina TP. Second edition. Beyond Economic Growth-An Introduction to Sustainable Development: Washington 2000 [cited 2009 Dec 2]. Available from: [http:// www .worldbank .org/depwe /english/ beyond/ global/glossary.html].
[3]     Thanni LO, Kehinde OA. 2006. Trauma at a Nigerian teaching hospital: pattern and docu-mentation of presentation. *African Health Sciences*, 6(2):104-107.
[4]     Awareness and Prevention. Available from: [http:// www. Isiconline .org/aware. htm.].
[5]     Chacko V, Joseph B, Mohanty S.P, Jacob T. Management of spinal cord injury in a general hospital in rural India. *Paraplegia*, 1986; 330-335.
[6]     Rajasekaran S. Prof T K Shanmugasundaram (1929–2008). Indian. J. Orthop., 2,008 Oct–Dec; 42(4): 484–485.
[7]     PL. 480 Paraplegia Project, Madras- IV. Spinal Cord Injury. Rehabilitation Rand D Progress Reports 1985. *Journal of Rehabilitation Research and Development*, 1985:72-73.
[8]     Singh R, Sharma SC, Mittal R, Sharma A. Traumatic Spinal Cord Injuries in Haryana: An Epidemiological Study. *Indian Journal of Community Medicine* 2003; XXVIII (4): 184-186.

[9]     Agrawal P, Upadhaya P, Raja K. A Demographic Profile of Traumatic and Non-Traumatic Spinal Injury Cases: A hospital based study from India. *Spinal cord*, 2007; 597-602.

[10]    Pandey VK, Nigam V, Goyal TD, Chhabra HS. Care of post-traumatic spinal cord injury patients in India: An analysis. *Indian Journal of Orthopaedics*, 2007; 41(4):295-99.

[11]    Gupta N, Solomon J, Raja K. Demographic characteristics of individuals with paraplegia in India: A Survey. *Indian Journal of Physiotherapy and Occupational Therapy*, 2008 July-Sep; 24-27.

[12]    S. Manjeet, S. Siddhartha, W. H. Iftikhar, T. Agnivesh, M. H. Farid, M. Nirdosh and S. Dara. Spine injuries in a tertiary health care hospital in Jammu: A Clinico - Epidemiological Study. *The Internet Journal of Neurosurgery*. 2009; 5(2). Available from: [http://www. ispub.com /journal/the_internet_journal_of_neurosurgery /volume_ 5_number_2_36/article/spine_injuries_in_a_tertiary_health_care_hospital_in_jammu_a _clinico_epidemiological_study.html].

[13]    Road accidents account for the largest number of Injuries including Spinal Cord Injuries in the Country" – Study. Available from: [http:// www. indiaprwire. com/pressrelease/health-care/2010101365098.htm].

[14]    Singh PK, Shrivastva S, Dulani R. Pre-hospital care of spinal cord injury in a rural Indian setting. Rural and Remote Health 2011: 1760. (Online) Available from: [http:/ /www. rrh.org. au/ publishedarticles /article _ print_1760.pdf].

[15]    Guidelines for prevention of spinal cord injuries. Available from: [http://www.ascon. info/100115%20ASCONGuidelines%20on%20prevention.pdf].

[16]    Sharma RK, Sachdeva NK, Vaidyanathan S, Rao MS. Pattern of emergency urology cases in a referral hospital in north-western India (PGIMER, Chandigarh): guidelines for future health care planning. *Indian Journal of Urology*, 1987;4(1):30-33.

[17]    Rath NM, Bag S, Dash PS. A study on emotional aspect of spinal cord injury. *Indian J Psychiat.*, 1993;35(1):51-53.

[18]    Rahmathulla G, Prasad R. Spine Instrumentation: Assessment Of Morbidity Related to 250 Cases. *Apollo Medicine*, 2005;2:37-40.

[19]    Singh R, Sharma SC. Sexuality and Women with spinal cord injury. *Sexuality and Disability*, 2005; 23(1):21.

[20]    Raj JT, Manigandan C and Jacob KS. Leisure satisfaction and psychiatric morbidity among informal carers of people with spinal cord injury. *Spinal Cord*, 2006; 44:676–679.

[21]    Manigandan C, Saravanan B, Macaden A, Gopalan L, Tharion G, Bhattacharji S. Psychological wellbeing among carers of people with spinal cord injury: a preliminary investigation from South India. *Spinal Cord*, 2000;38(9):559-62.

[22]    Gupta N, Solomon J, Raja K. Paraplegia: A postal survey of Morbidity trends in India. *Spinal Cord,* 2007 Oct; 45 (10): 664-70 Epub 2007 Feb.13.

[23]    Gupta N, Solomon J, Raja K. Pain after Paraplegia: a survey in India. *Spinal Cord,* 2010 April; 48(4): 342-346 Epub 2009 Dec. 15.

[24]    Gupta N, Solomon J, Raja K. Characteristics of morbidities in individuals with paraplegia living in various environments in India- a descriptive study. *The Journal Of Indian Association of Physiotherapists*, 2006; 4:28-31.

[25]  Singh R, Dhankar SS, Rohilla R. Quality of life of people with spinal cord injury in
      Northern India. *International Journal of Rehabilitation Research*, 2008; 31(3):247-251.

[26]  Singh R, Rohilla RK, Sangwan K, Siwach R, Magu NK, Sangwan SS. Bladder
      management methods and urological complications in spinal cord injury patients.
      *Indian Journal of Orthopaedics*, 2011;45(2):141-147.

[27]  Chhabra HS. Life after SCI in India- Results of a survey of 53 centers. Available form:
      [http://www.iscos.org.uk/abstract/3.html].

[28]  N Gupta, J Solomon, K raja. Employment after paraplegia in India- a postal survey.
      *Spinal Cord*, Epub 2011 Feb. 22 (in press).

[29]  Sekaran P, Vijayakumari F, Hariharan R, Zachariah K, Joseph SE, Kumar RK.
      Community reintegration of spinal cord-injured patients in rural south India. *Spinal
      Cord*, 2010 Aug; 48(8):628-32. Epub 2010 Feb. 9.

[30]  Samuelkamaleshkumar S, Radhika S, Cherian B, Elango A, Winrose W, Suhany BT,
      Prakash MH. Community reintegration in rehabilitated South Indian persons with spinal
      cord injury. *Arch. Phys. Med. Rehabil.*, 2010 Jul; 91(7):1117-21.

*Chapter 13*

# EPIDEMIOLOGY OF SPINAL CORD INJURIES: INDIAN PERSPECTIVE

## *Roop Singh**

Medical Enclave, PGIMS, Rohtak, Haryana, India

## ABSTRACT

The abrupt onset of spinal cord injury (SCI) is tragic and has a profound impact on the individuals and their families. Knowledge of epidemiology of spinal cord injuries in a given country is important not only for planning of resources, but also for adequate treatment and rehabilitation. In the Indian setup, as in most developing countries, very little is known about the exact incidence of SCI as there is no national database. In India, approximately 1.5 million people live with SCI. Approximate 20,000 new cases of SCI are added every year and 60-70% of them are illiterate, poor villagers. Majority of them are males in the age group of 16-30 years, signifying higher incidence in young, active and productive population of the society. There has been substantial decrease in male female ratio from the past which reflects changing face of social norms where females are becoming more active and outgoing in the modern era. In India fall from height rates highest among the etiological factors. There is a gradual trend towards increasing incidence of road traffic accidents indicating gradual urbanization of society and increase in number of vehicles on roads in India. Seasonal distribution of SCI shows a marked increase during summer, signifying increased movement of people in this season. Head injury is the most common associated trauma. The incidence of secondary medical problems in SCI population is high compared to the western world. There is tremendous lack of basic infrastructure and trained medical personnel, especially in rural areas, involved in initial management of patient. Vast majority of people lack basic knowledge about the initial immobilization and transportation of these patients to higher centers and by the time patient reaches a general or institutional hospital; there may be an extensive damage to neurological status, which could have been prevented.

To conclude, in India, management and rehabilitation of patients with SCI lags far behind. Rescue and retrieval systems for these patients are inadequate. There are few specialized centers for the management of such patents. The frequency of decubitus

---

* Dr. Roop Singh, Professor, 52/ 9-J, Medical Enclave, PGIMS, Rohtak-124001, Haryana, INDIA, E-mail: drroopsingh@rediffmail.com, Ph: +91-1262-213171, Fax: 91-1262-211308.

ulcers and UTI is unacceptably high. There is a strong need to identify the risk factors and to take steps to control them by disseminating information to masses, to train paramedical staff in rural areas about initial handling and transportation of patients having spinal cord injuries. A comprehensive multidisciplinary management and rehabilitation approach is the need of the hour to reintegrate patients with SCI to the community.

# INTRODUCTION

The abrupt onset of spinal cord injury (SCI) is tragic and has a profound impact on the individuals and their families. Knowledge of epidemiology of SCI in a given country is important not only for planning of resources, but also for adequate treatment and rehabilitation. In the Indian set up, as in most developing countries, very little is known about the exact incidence of spinal cord injuries [1]. The incidence as well as the prevalence of SCI has been on the rise with the incidence rate being estimated to be from 15-40 cases per million worlds wide [2]. In India, approximately 1.5 million people live with SCI. Every year, ten thousand new cases add to this group of individuals. Majority of them (82%) are males in age group of 16-30 years. However, this is only an estimate as there is no reliable national database [3]. In our set up, most of these injuries occur due to fall from roofs, fall from hills & trees, or road traffic accidents, which in fact are preventable causes [4,5].

SCI requires specialized surgical intervention initially and a comprehensive rehabilitation afterwards [6]. The developments in the management of SCI have led to decrease in morbidity and mortality rates, thereby increasing the prevalence of patients with varying degree of functional limitation [7]. Most of the SCI patients in west are treated in specialized spinal centers. Unfortunately, in India rescue and retrieved systems for these patients are inadequate [8]. Very few spinal centres have been established in India and hence the acute care of most victims of SCI take place in general hospital instead of specialised spinal centers [8]. There is a lack of team approach to these individuals in various centers all over India. There are some non-government organisations (NGOs) working for these individuals. But there is still lack of team approach to the community from various hospitals to give awareness programme regarding spinal cord injury, its prevention and treatment. There is also lack of regular follow up [9]. All these factors affect prevalence, management and complication in SCI patients.

There is extensive ongoing research on epidemiological aspects of SCI from different parts of the world. There is a dearth of reliable statistics concerning spinal cord injury in India. However, of late there have been individual attempts to collect data on SCI incidence, prevalence and complications. This chapter summarizes the epidemiology of SCI from Indian perspective.

# INCIDENCE OF SCI

In India, approximately 1.5 million people live with SCI. Approximately 20,000 new cases of SCI are added every year [8]. Land transport- related SCI is reported to be much lower than European countries; falls predominate within southern Asia [10]. Highest percentage of falls (58.9%) from India has been reported by Aggarwal et al [7]. Incidence data are inadequate in India as there is no reliable national database.

## PREVALENCE OF SCI

The range of reported global prevalence is between 230 and 1000 per million. Asian countries, particularly China and India are not appropriately represented, with available Asian statistics likely underestimating the overall prevalence with this populous region [10]. Prevalence data only exist for Kashmir region in India with a prevalence rate of 236 per million populations [11]. Among the religions in India more than 70% of people belong to Hinduism. There is no significance regarding the religion vs SCI. More number of patients are from rural areas. Sixty to seventy percent of them are illiterate and poor lacking money to pay for transportation and hospital expenses [8, 12].

## CASE FATALITY OF SCI

Only few of the studies from India have reported mortality rate. Mortality rate has been reported between 1.9 to 20% [4, 7, 12]. It underestimates the true case fatality rate as most of the patients never come for treatment in tertiary care centers and some die at the site of injury due to lack of retrieval and rescue systems.

## CURE RATE AND IMPROVEMENT

Aggarwal et al reported incomplete recovery in 33%, followed by no recovery in 28.8% and complete recovery in 26.3% out of total 207 new cases reporting [7]. Women showed better neurological recovery than men.

## RELATIVE RISK OF SCI

In a study conducted by Jha et al labourer constituted the largest group (29.9%) involved in road traffic accidents (RTA) [13]. The reason may be that the labourers travel in the trucks carrying bricks, stone and other heavy materials and trucks are more commonly involved in accidents [13]. It is important to note that fall from a height posed the greatest risk for SCI, which included falls from trees during manual collection of the produce, fall from buildings during construction as well as workers on electricity posts. Use of safety harness is seldom practiced in these occupations. Although harness has been developed to ensure safety during climbing of trees, they are rarely used by subjects who consider them to be a hindrance to their occupation [7].

Certain preventable risk factors in traumatic SCI (falls, vehicular accidents, improper pre-hospital care and improper transportation) need to be addressed in particular in order to reduce the frequency and morbidity of SCI and the burden on meager financial and health resources in India [14]. There is tremendous lack of basic infrastructure and trained medical personnels, especially in rural areas, involved in initial management of patient [4]. Singh et al observed that 77% patients were transported to their institute by vehicle unsuitable for spinal patients such as car, jeep or maxi cabs which are preventable in our region [4].

# ETIOLOGY OF SCI

Etiology of SCI appears to have a major effect on the level and extent of neurological deficit as well as recovery [2]. Mode of injury in SCI is dependent on local factors. In all Indian series fall from height rates highest among the etiological factors [1, 4, 7, 9, 12, 14, 16]. There is a gradual trend towards increasing incidence of RTA indicating gradual urbanization of society and increase of vehicles on roads in India [4]. Non-traumatic insult to the cord is also one of the etiological factors; but the incidence is less [7].

Table I summarizes the mode of SCI reported in major studies from India. Our socioeconomic, cultural background and occupation are also added factors for the prevalence of SCI [12]. There is remarkable difference in mode of injury among men and women [7]. Various etiological factors are discussed in detail in the following section of the chapter.

**Table 1. Mode of injury reported in different studies from India**

| Series | Falls (%) | RTA (%) | Sports injuries (%) | Burial under mud while digging (%) | Violence (%) | Fall of weight on back (%) | Fall in well (%) | Others (%) | Non-traumatic (%) |
|---|---|---|---|---|---|---|---|---|---|
| Chacko et al (1986) | 55.2 | 12.8 | _ | _ | _ | 18.4 | _ | 13.6 | - |
| Shanmuga Sundram (1987) | 66 | 14 | _ | _ | _ | _ | _ | _ | _ |
| Dave et al (1994) | 49.4 | 36.5 | _ | _ | _ | _ | _ | _ | _ |
| Annamalai and Chinnathambi (Madras Model 1998) | 29.42 | 25.19 | 5.00 | _ | 1.09 | 0.12 | 0.03 | 11.72 | _ |
| Singh et al (2003) | 44.51 | 34.71 | 3.39 | 6.42 | 2.69 | 3.52 | 1.86 | 2.28 | _ |
| Aggarwal et al (2007) | 58.9 | 21.3 | _ | _ | _ | 7.2 | _ | _ | 12.6 |
| Pandey et al (2007) | 48.33 | 43.33 | _ | _ | 1.6 | 6.6 | _ | _ | _ |
| Gupta et al (2008) | 25 | 17.4 | 1 | _ | 4.5 | 6.5 | _ | _ | 8.3 |
| Singh et al (2009) | 50 | 30.3 | 0.7 | 6.9 | 2.7 | 9.2 | 6.2 | _ | _ |

## i.) Traumatic and Non-Traumatic

Most of the series report only traumatic origin of SCI in India and non-traumatic mode of injury is included under heading of others. It makes difficut to estimate true incidence of traumatic vs non-traumatic SCI in India. Aggarwal et al reported an incidence of 12.6% of non-traumatic causes [7] and Gupta et al reported incidence 11.5% of non-traumatic causes [14].

## ii.) Falls

Falls from height rates highest among all the etiological factors in India [4]. Occupational factors lead to spinal injuries from falls. Fall from height include fall from trees, electric poles, buildings and fall into the well [4, 5, 7-9, 12-16]. Literature from developed countries reveals that RTA accounts for the maximum number of spinal injuries [17]. Incidence of falls has been reported between 25-66% [14, 16]. Falls are more common in second and third decades of life [4]. Falls from hill tops and falls into the wells are more common among women [4, 5].

## iii.) Road Traffic Accidents

Road traffic accidents are showing increasing trends compared to three decades back indicating gradual urbanization of society and increase in number of vehicles on roads in India. Chacko et al in 1986 reported RTA incidence of 12.8% and Pandey et al reported the highest rate of 43.33% [8, 18]. Road side accidents are common in third and fourth decade [4, 5]. This shows that the people of most active and productive age groups are involved in RTAs, which add a serious economic loss to community [13]. Lack of strict implementation of traffic rules in various non-metropolitan cities of India along with lack of awareness among general population regarding adherence to traffic rules still prevails as an important cause of RTA and spinal trauma [18].

## iv.) Sports

Incidence of sports related SCI varies between 0.7-5% [4, 5, 14, 15]. Sports related injuries are more common in nothern states of India; in these states maximum number of athletes pursue competitive contact games [4, 15]

## v.) Violence

Violence related data in USA is high in comparison to global data (14% NSCIS) [17]. Incidence of violence related SCI in India varies between 1.09-4.5% [4, 5, 14, 15, 18].

## vi.) Blunt and Penetration Trauma

Gupta et al reported gunshot injuries in 4.5% [14]. We have reported combined rate of 2.69% of blunt and stab injuries from our institute [4]. Annamalai and Chinnalhambi reported 0.2% incidence of gunshot and 0.8% incidence of stab injuries in 1998 [12].

Other few peculiar modes of injuries reported from India include burial under mud while digging (cave-in) (6.4-6.9%) [4,5]; fall of weight on a back (0.12-9.2%) [4, 5, 7, 12, 14, 18]; and fall in wells (0.03-1.86%) [4,5,12]. Fall of object on the head is the common cause in both genders, while fall in well is exclusively seen in females [4]. There is seasonal variation in SCI.

Frequency of SCI shows an increase during summer followed by rainy season [4]. It can be increased on the basis of increased movement of the people in this season; and increase in RTA and roofs collapse during rainy season. In winters people remain confined to their homes [4].

# GENDER

Table 2 shows sex-ratio reported in different series from India. The most common cause for the insult to SCI in males is traumatic and in females, it is non-traumatic [14]. Chacko et al in 1986 reported male: female ratio of 13.5:1 [1] and latest study by Singh et al have shown this ratio decreased to 2.96:1 [4].

Latest data from India are comparable to the western literature [17], it reflect a changing trend when compared to studies conducted 15-20 years back [15, 16]. There has been substantial decrease in male female ratio which reflects changing face of social norms, where females are becoming more active and outgoing. In our region agricuture being the main profession, females are equally participant at work [4]. Etiology in women is same as of men with fall from a height accounting for maximum number of spinal injuries.

This can be due to their participation in high risk jobs like constructions. Biologic factor that is aging with osteoporosis is also found to be a contributing factor for injuries among women [7]. There is still a wide difference in the number of men and women in most series reported from India [4, 5, 8, 14, 15]. Possible explanation for this finding may be most common etiology observed in India.

Women are at risk of fall during construction work. Work involving climbing trees and electric posts are not jobs normally done by women in India [7]. It may also be due to that the move by women into high-risk activities is still too limited to have more than a marginal impact on statistics; aternatively, the women engaged in these activities may perform them more safely than men, thus exposing themselves to lower risk of injury [2]. Conversely women are more likely to carry loads on their head than men [7]. Men being exposed to outdoor risks, poor working conditions, with no regards for worker safety protocols and an increasing number of motor vehicles in India in the last few years are nature's preferred candidates for traumatic SCI. These causes are modifiable with increase in awareness and safety guards [14].

**Table 2. Sex ratio reported in different studies from India**

| Series | Male: Female |
|---|---|
| Chacko et al (1986) | 13.5 : 1 |
| Shanmuga Sundram (1987) | 8.98 : 1 |
| Dave et al (1994) | 3.7 : 1 |
| Annamalai and Chinnathambi (Madras Model 1998) | 7.92 :1 |
| Singh et al (2003) | 2.96 : 1 |
| Aggarwal et al (2007) | 3.6 : 1 |
| Gupta et al (2008) | 5.41 : 1 |
| Singh et al (2009) | 2.98 :1 |

## AGE DISTRIBUTION

As evident from the most series from India majority of victims are in age group of 20-40 years. Incidence of SCI in this age group varies from 37-70.9% [4, 5, 7, 14]. In this age group life is characterized by high risk activities such as rash driving, climbing trees and on moving vehicles resulting in an increased risk for SCI. This age group represents the most productive years of one's life, hence the need for a comprehensive spinal rehabilitation programme to ensure transition back into mainstream society [19]. Fall from a height is the commonest cause for spinal cord insult in all age groups, especially till 40- <50 years. Road traffic accidents are the leading cause in 18- <25 years age group [14]. This is in contradiction to western data where motor vehicle accidents are commonest cause for injury and falls are the leading cause of injury after the age of 45 years [20]. Occupational factors like climbing trees and manual workers are common cause of fall in India. These findings have a notable part to play in increasing awareness. The population most at risk is also that which is contributing the most to the society. Hence, the social impact of these preventable causes of SCI is a cause for concern [14].

## MODE OF TRANSPORTATION

In India there is a poor system of spinal trauma evacuation. Various modes of transportation not suitable for evacuation and transfer of SCI patients are used. In the study by Singh et al in 2003 ambulance was used in transportation only in 23% SCI patients, where as 77% were transported in vehicles unsuitable for SCI patients such as car, jeep or maxi cab [4]. Chacko et al reported that 56% patients were brought recumbent in back seat of a car and 34% recumbent in ambulance. The remainder was brought in smaller vehicles often too small to permit the patient to be recumbent [8]. Improper transportation of a SCI patient can cause secondary trauma and deterioration of neurological status. Annamalai and Chinnathambi reported more than 6 transfers to reach a spinal centre [12]; while Singh et al reported that only 4.7% patients were referred after initial care by qualified doctors [4]. Only 1.86% patients were accompanied by trained personnel during transfer [4]. Pandey et al reported in 81.66% of cases attendants of patients or transporting authorities did not have any knowledge about precautions essential for transportation of SCI patients to prevent neurological deterioration, as evident from the precautions taken during transportation [18].

## TIME LAG BETWEEN INJURY AND ADMISSION

Chacko et al in 1986 reported that 37.6% patients with SCI reported after 48 hours [8]. This scenario is rapidly changing with modern transportation system; in our study in 2003, 76.19% of the patients reported directly to institute and 8.1% reported within 6 hours of injury, 90.3% within 24 hours and only 9.7% reported late [4]. Pandey et al reported a mean 45 days (range 0-188 days) of delay in presentation. A SCI patient was managed at a mean 2.05 hospitals (range 0-6 hospitals) before coming to spinal center [18]. Scivolctto concluded that SCI patients presenting early at spinal unit show better functional outcome after rehabilitation than patient presenting late [6].

## LEVEL OF INJURY

The most common level in individuals with paraplegia is dorsolumbar spine injury with first lumbar being the most common fractured vertebra followed by 12th dorsal vertebra [4, 5, 14]. Next common injury is the cervical spine injury with most common site being 5th and 6th cervical vertebrae [4]. Recently, Aggarwal et al reported cervical spine injury as the most common (36.2%) [7]. The dorsal spine is fixed and less mobile because of rib cage as compared to lumbar spine which is very mobile portion of spine. The sudden transition from fixed to mobile portion makes dorsolumbar area as a precarious site.

## ASSOCIATED INJURIES

Most prevalent associated injuries are head injury (7%), followed by extremities fractures (6.3%), chest injury (3.1%), abdominal injury (0.9%) and pelvic injury (0.7%) [4]. These injuries increase morbidity and mortality of SCI patients.

## HOSPITAL STAY

Singh et al in 2003 reported an average duration of hospital stay of 39.5 days (range 7-93 days) [4]; while Chacko et al in 1986 reported an average stay of 42.3 days [8]. Annamalai and Chinnathambi in 1998 reported that 11.6% of the patients stayed more than 200 days in the hospital. They stated that the stay in the hospital depend upon a number of factors like their socio-economic status, condition of the patient and nature of the treatment [12]. Long hospital stay does reflect the loss of productive hours of the nation, and a financial burden on state as well, which is in fact preventable to certain extent [4].

## EMPLOYMENT

Gupta et al in 2008 reported an employment rate of 41.3% among 276 SCI patients [14]. While a study from our institute in 2008 reported an employment rate of 34% post-SCI [21]. Unemployment in SCI patients can be due to their level of lesion, as individual with lesion at upper thoracic region are more likely to be unemployed. Lack of specialized centers and NGOs in most of the areas, lack of knowledge regarding job opportunities and lack of initiative on the part of medical and paramedical personnels, can be some of the reasons for their unemployment [14]. Employment makes a significant difference in Quality of Life (QoL) of SCI patients. Singh et al reported that patients still employed after SCI had better QoL score (p<0.001) then unemployed patient [21]

## COMPLICATION RATE

**Table 3. Complications reported in SCI persons in different studies from India**

| Series | Singh et al (2003) | Chacko et al (1986) | Annamalai and Chinnathambi (Madras Model 1998) |
|---|---|---|---|
| Pressure ulcers | 36% | 32.4% | 27.8% |
| Urinary tract infections (UTI) | 44% | 64.4% | – |
| Heterotrophic ossification | 20% | – | |
| Orthostatic hypotension) | 68% | – | – |
| Spasticity | 60% | | |
| Muscular atrophy | 42% | | |
| Neuropathic pain | 42% | | |
| Hospital admissions | 48% | – | – |
| Bowel problems | 56% | | |

Spinal cord injury is typically associated with several medical problems that directly result from the loss of sensory, motor and autonomic control [22]. The literature highlights the fact that persons with SCI use medical and/or health- care services at a significant higher rate than the general population and are at increased risk of developing secondary complication and being rehospitalized [23]. Table 3 shows complication rate reported in various studies from India. Singh et al in 2010 reported that at mean 3.7 years post- SCI bladder probems (44%), neuropathic pain (42%), bed sores (36%) and spasticity (60%) were responsible for medical intervention or hospitalization in the participants [24]. They conclude that incidence of secondary medical problems in SCI population is high compared to data collected in western world and this issue needs an urgent attention. They suggested that the persons involved in management and rehabilitation of SCI population can reduce the incidence and intensity of secondary medical problems simply by paying attention to general principles of care for paraplegics and by developing specific strategies targeted to minimize these health-related problems [24]. Singh et al in 2008, reported that bed sores (p<0.001), urinary problems (p<0.01), bowel problems (p<0.01), problematic spasticity (p<0.01) and neuropathic pain (p<0.01) were associated with lower QoL scores [21]. The home visit programme conducted at Ahemdabad by Prabhaka and Thakkar for SCI patients decreased the number of re-admissions by improving the status of rehabilitation, which raises the quality of care for patient with SCI [25].

# CONCLUSION

To conclude, in India, management and rehabilitation of patients with SCI lags far behind. Rescue and retrieval systems for these patients are inadequate. There are few specialized centers for the management of such patents. The frequency of decubitus ulcers and UTI is unacceptably high. There is a strong need to identify the risk factors and to take steps to control them by disseminating information to masses, to train paramedical staff in rural areas about initial handling and transportation of patients having spinal cord injuries. A comprehensive multidisciplinary management and rehabilitation approach is the need of the hour to reintegrate patients with SCI to the community.

# REFERENCES

[1]     Sinha DK. Manual of Patna Model for the care of Spinal cord injury patients. Patna: *SPARSH*. 2000; 9-13.

[2]     Jackson AB. Dijker M. DeVivo M, Poczateek RB. A demographic profile of new traumatic spinal cord injuries: change and stability over 30 years. *Arch Phys Med Rehabil* 2004;85:1740-48.

[3]     Awareness and Prevention. *[http://www.isiconline.org/aware.htm.]*

[4]     Singh R, Sharma SC, Mittal R, Sharma A. Traumatic SCI in Haryana: An epidemiologic study. *Ind J of Community Med* 2005;28 (4): 184-6.

[5]     Manjeet S, Siddhartha S, Iftikhar WH, Agnivesh T, Farid MH, Nirdosh M. Dara S : Spine injuries in a tertiary health care hospital in Jammu: A Clinico - Epidemiological Study . *The Internet J Neurosurg* 2009; 5 (2).

[6]     Scivolctto G, Morganti B, Molinari M. Early versus delayed inpatient spinal cord injury rehabilitation : an Italian study. *Arch Phys Med Rehabil* 2005;86:512-6.

[7]     Agrawal P, Upadhaya P, Raja K. A Demographic Profile of Traumatic and Non-Traumatic Spinal Injury Cases: A hospital based study from India. *Spinal cord* 2007; 597-602.

[8]     Chacko V, Joseph B, Mohanty S.P, Jacob T. Management of spinal cord injury in a general hospital in rural India. *Paraplegia* 1986; 24: 330-5.

[9]     Chhabra HS. Life after SCI in India- Results of a survey of 53 centers. *[http://www.iscos.org.uk/ abstract13.html.]*

[10] Cripps RA, Lee BB, Wing P, Weerts E, Mackay J, Brown D. A global map for traumatic spinal cord injury epidemiology: towards a living data repository for injury prevention. *Spinal Cord* 2011; 49: 493-501.

[11] Razdan S, Kaul RL, Motta A, Kaul S, Bhatt RK. Prevalence and pattern of major neurological disorders in rural Kashmir (India) in 1986. *Neuroepidemiology* 1994; 13:113-9.

[12] Annamalai K, Chinnathambi R. *Spinal cord injuires -The challenges and the achievements.* Chennai: Deptt.of Orthopaedic Surgery, Govt. General Hospital, Chennai 1998; 1-50.

[13] Jha N, Srinivasa DK, Roy G, Jagdish S. Epidemiological study of road traffic accident cases: a study from South India. *Ind J of Community Med* 2004;27 (1): 20-4.

[14] Gupta N, John Solomon M, Raja K. Demographic Characteristics of Individuals with Paraplegia in India- A survey. *Ind J Physio Occup Therapy* 2008-07 - 2008-09; Vol. 2, No. 3.

[15] Dave PK, Jayaswal A, Kotwal PP. Spinal cord injuries –A clinico-epidemiological study. *Ind J Orthop* 1994; 28: 39-45.

[16] Shanmuga Sundram TK. *Final report of Madras Paraplegia Project.* Madras 1987.

[17] National Spinal Cord Injury Statistical Centre Birmingham Alabama. *Spinal Cord Injury facts and figures at a glance.* Alabama, USA, 2008.

[18] Pandey VK, Nigam V, Goyal T, Chabbra HS. Care of post-traumatic spinal cord trauma patients in India: an analysis. *Ind J Orthop* 2007: 41 (4); 295-9.

[19] Rathore MFA, Hanif S, Farooq F, Ahmad N, Mansoor SN. Traumatic spinal cord injuries at a tertiary care institute in Pakistan. *J Pak Med Assoc* 2008; 58: 53-7.

[20] Spinal cord injury information network. *[http://www.spinalcord.org.]*

[21] Singh R, Singh SD, Rohilla R. Quality of life of people with spinal cord injury in Northern India. *Int J Rehab Res* 2008; 31:247-51.

[22] Levi R, Hultling C, Nash MS, Seiger A. The Stockholm spinal cord injury study: 1. medical problems in a regional SCI population. *Paraplegia* 1995; 33: 308-15.

[23] Meyer AR, Branch LG, Cuppler LA, Feltin M, Master RJ. Predictors of medical care utilization by independently living adults with spinal cord injuries. *Arch Phys Med Rehabil* 1989; 471-76

[24] Singh R, Rohilla R, Siwach R, Singh SD, Magu NK, Sangwan SS. Health-related problems and effect of specific interventions in spinal cord injury- an outcome study in Northern India. *Eur J Phys Rehabil Med* 2010; 46: 47-53.

[25] Prabhaka MM, Thakkar TH. A follow-up programme in India for spinal cord injury patients: Paraplegic safari. *J Spinal cord med* 2004; 27: 260-2.

In: Epidemiology of Spinal Cord Injuries
Editors: V. Rahimi-Movaghar, S. B. Jazayeri et al.

ISBN: 978-1-61942-894-2
©2012 Nova Science Publishers, Inc.

*Chapter 14*

# EPIDEMIOLOGY OF SPINAL CORD INJURY IN IRAN

### *Soheil Saadat*

Sina Trauma and Surgery Research Center,
Tehran University of Medical Sciences, Tehran, Iran

Iran is a Middle Eastern country with a surface area of 1,745,150 square kilometers and a population of 74,169,000; 69% living in urban areas (World Bank, 2009). In 2009, the gross national income per capita of Iran was $10,850 USD. Total expenditure on health per capita was $685 USD (Figure 1) and total expenditure on health as percentage of GDP was 5.5%. Life expectancy for male and female was 70 and 75 years.

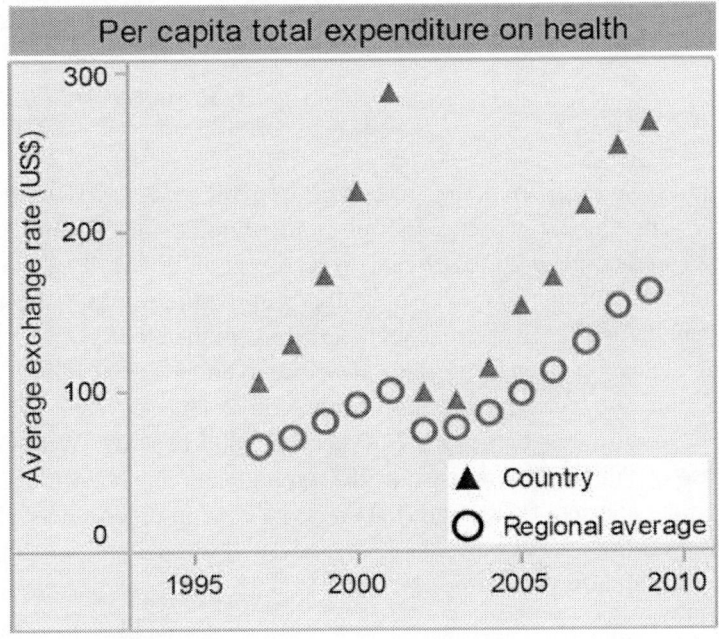

Figure 1. Per capita total expenditure on health, Iran, 2008. WHO.

Trauma is one of the highest burdens of disease in the world and traumatic spinal cord injury (SCI) is a major permanent sequel of trauma (Rahimi-Movaghar et al., 2010). The burden of SCI in Tehran (the capital of Iran) in the year 2008 was 0.7 per 1000 population (Rahimi-Movaghar et al, 2010). By applying this proportion to the country population, the national burden of SCI is estimated as 51,918 DALYs.

# INCIDENCE

The global estimate of SCI incidence from literature lies between 10.4 per million per year and 83 per million per year; the higher rate includes mortalities before hospital admission (Wyndaele et al, 2006). The national rates per annum are quoted as 30–40 per million in America, 40.2 per million in Japan (Burt, 2004), 14.5 per million in Australia (O'Connor, 2002) and 57.8 per million in Portugal (pre-hospital mortalities included)(Martins, 1998).

There are few studies reporting incidence of SCI in Iran. The estimates tend to be hospital based and therefore underestimate the true incidence. Based on a population-based study, the annual incidence of traumatic SCI in Tehran was 44 (12–114) per million population (Rahimi-movaghar et al 2009). This estimate was based on a household survey and was not able to capture severe cases that had to live in nursing facilities. Also, the pre-hospital mortality rate of SCI in different countries is estimated as 15 to 56% (Wyndaele et al, 2006). By applying this estimate of pre-hospital mortality to the above-mentioned estimation of incidence (44 per million) the incidence of all SCI cases including pre-hospital mortality, is estimated as 52-100 per million in Tehran.

A hospital-based study estimated the incidence of spine fracture as 160 per million and the incidence of SCI as 30 per million in Kashan, a town with a population of 350,000 (Fakharian et al, 1383).

# AGE

Different studies have reported the mean age of patients referred to Iranian hospitals because of spine fracture as 27-39 years. In reports involving countries with a high incidence of SCI, the average age range is 20 to 40 years (Ackery et al, 2004). It seems that developed communities report an older age range for individuals at the time of SCI, possibly because of longer life expectancies and the greater frequency of falls in the elderly.

In the United States, between 1973 and 1979, the average age at injury was 28.7 years, with most of the injuries occurring between the ages of 16 and 30 years. The average age is steadily increasing to an average age of 37.6 years in 2000 to 2003. With the exception of violence as a cause of injury, this increase in the average age has been found in all etiology groups (motor vehicle crashes, falls, sports). The prevalence in older adults above the age of 65 years has increased from 4.7% between 1973 and 1979 to 10.9% since 2000, whereas the prevalence among children between the ages of 0 and 15 years has decreased from 6.4% to 2.0% (ho et al, 2007).

There are no published studies to assess the age trend in SCI occurrence in Iran.

# ETIOLOGY

Among all etiologies of SCI, motor vehicle crashes is the leading cause, accounting for 38.5% to 59.4% of all traumatic SCIs worldwide (Rasouli et al., 2011). Tator et al reported a change in the trend of SCI injuries from 1947 to 1981 in Toronto, Canada. More motor vehicle and sport-recreational accidents and fewer, less severe work-related accidents were reported.

In the United States, the most common cause of SCI between 2000 and 2003 continued to be motor vehicle crashes. They account for 50.4% of all cases, with a similar rate of 48.7% between 1973 and 1979. However, the rates for falls have progressively increased over the last 3 decades, from 16.5% in the 1970s to 23.8% between 2000 and 2003. Even though falls were still the second most common cause of SCI across all age groups, it has been the only cause with a rate that has steadily increased over the last 3 decades. When stratified by age group, it was apparent that falls were the most common cause of SCI in people over age 60. The SCI rates associated with sports have decreased over the decades, from 14.4% between 1973 and 1979 to 9% between 2000 and 2003 (ho et al, 2007).

According to McKinley et al, 39% of adult SCI admissions in a level I rehabilitation center were non-traumatic in etiology (spinal stenosis: 54%; tumor: 26%). Compared to subjects with traumatic SCI, those individuals with non-traumatic SCI were older and more likely married, female, and retired. Injury characteristics revealed significantly more paraplegia and incomplete SCI within the non-traumatic SCI group. Both non-traumatic and traumatic SCI individuals had significant Functional Independent Measure changes from rehabilitation admission to discharge. They suggest that non-traumatic SCI patients can achieve rehabilitation outcomes similar to patients with traumatic SCI.

In a retrospective, cross-sectional study evaluating patients with complete and incomplete SCIs (American Spinal Injury Association Grades A and B) under the coverage of the financial, medico-social, and rehabilitative support provided by the State Welfare Organization of Iran (SWOI), there were 3791 cases of traumatic SCI (63.2%) and 2110 cases of non-traumatic SCI (35.2%) (Taghipoor et al., 2009).

Road Traffic Collision, RTC, is the leading cause of traumatic SCI in Iran (Moini et al) and Australia (O' Connor) and the USA (ho et al, 2007). Rasouli et al reported that 59.4% of blunt trauma SCI patients who were transferred to a trauma center in the south of Iran have been injured due to RTC (Rasouli et al, 2007).

Fall has been reported as the second cause of SCI in Iran. However, there is not enough data to study the causes of SCI.

# ANATOMICAL DISTRIBUTION OF SCI

Throughout all the time periods observed, cervical injuries occurred more often than thoracic and lumbar injuries, in the United States (ho et al, 2007).

In Iran, thoracolumbar (Taghippor et al, 1384) and cervical spine (Yousefzadeh et al, 2010) have been reported as the most common anatomical regions of trauma among SCI patients.

The most frequent region of injury among SCI patients injured due to RTC was the thoracolumbar junction (Rasouli et al, 2007).

There is not enough data to assess a trend in the anatomical distribution of injury among SCI patients in Iran.

# SPINE FRACTURE ASSOCIATED WITH SPINAL CORD INJURY

Spine fractures are frequently seen in association with trauma, particularly among younger individuals. These injuries, which exist on a spectrum from minor avulsion fractures to significant fractures in association with spinal instability and spinal cord injury (SCI), can exert an enormous direct financial toll on the health care system. The even greater significance of these injuries is because of the indirect losses from lost productivity, especially in young patients who sustain complete SCIs. The overall incidence of cervical spine fractures among US military has been reported as 290 per million person-years. The incidence of fracture-associated SCI has been reported as 70 per million (Schoenfeld et al, 2011).

In Iran, SCI was reported as 5.6% to 60% in all patients with spine fractures. The lowest percentage is based on the Iranian national trauma registry database from 1999 to 2004 (Heidari et al., 2010). The highest percentage was reported from a referral neurosurgical center in Shiraz (Taghippor et al, 2005).

# MORTALITY

The in-hospital mortality of SCI was reported as 8% in Canada. Older age is a risk factor of death; mortality was 18% in patients 60 years and older, compared with 5% for patients younger than 60 years (Picket et al, 2006). Pre-hospital mortality of SCI is reported as ~16% (Dryden et al, 2003, Martins et al, 1998). The survival rate for SCI patients discharged from a hospital, is reported as 81% after 10 years, 75% after 20 years and 62% after 30 years. It was inversely associated with age and high level of injury (Catz et al, 2002). Neither pre-hospital nor in-hospital mortality of SCI are studied in Iran.

# A REVIEW OF LOCAL STUDIES IN IRAN

No published nationwide study was found about the epidemiology of SCI in Iran. Instead, there are local studies that reflect the epidemiology of SCI and/or spinal fracture in single cities in Iran. A brief review of some of them are presented as follows:

## Tehran (Rahimi-Movaghar et al, 2009)

In a population-based study that took place in 2007-8, the incidence of SCI was estimated as 44 per million. The mean age of the patients was $31 \pm 7$ years.

The National Welfare Organization had provided financial support to 25% of the cases.

As in other studies on the incidence of SCI in Iran (Rasouli et al, 2007), this study demonstrated that road traffic collisions are the leading cause of SCI and falls were the second major cause.

Regarding the level of SCI, 50% of cases had a SCI involving the upper lumbar region. This is in agreement with a report from southeastern Iran (Rasouli et al, 2007).

This study is the only population-based survey aimed to describe the epidemiology of SCI in Iran in the literature.

## Zahedan

In another study of 64 cases of SCI involving the poorest socioeconomic state of Iran in the southeast of the country, 95% were male and the mean age was 27 ± 9 years. Motor vehicle crashes (68%) and fall (32%) were the most common etiology of SCI. Of all SCI cases, 84% presented as ASIA-A, 3% as ASIA-B, and 13% as ASIA-C, with no ASIA-D. Thoracolumbar junction was the most common level of injury at 45% (Rasouli et al., 2007). This was similar to a report from Germany that estimated the incidence of complete motor and sensory deficit in spine fracture as 11% and that of incomplete deficit as 13.5% (Leucht et al, 2009).

Some degree of motor score improvement occurs following SCI with or without operative surgery in the follow-up period (Rahimi-Movaghar et al., 2005; 2006; 2009).

## Kashan (Fakharian et al, 2004)

In a survey in Kashan, patients admitted to the neurosurgery ward of a university hospital with a history of spine trauma, from 1995 to 1999, were included. The mean age of patients was 39±18 years and the male to female ratio was 3.7.

SCI was reported in 17% of all patients with a spine fracture and 40% of patients who had a cervical spine fracture. The most common mechanism of trauma in this survey was falls followed by RTC that was different from other studies from Shiraz and Tehran. However, there are reports from India and Bangladesh that indicate falls as the most common cause of SCI (Burt, 2004).

Only patients who survived long enough to be admitted to the neurosurgery ward were studied. Therefore, this study neither reflects the true incidence of SCI nor the incidence of SCI among spine fracture cases.

## Shiraz (Taghippor et al, 2005)

All patients referred to a hospital in Shiraz with a history of spine fracture were included. Sixty percent of these patients had experienced spinal cord injury.

The mean age of patients was 35±12 years with 80% male. The male to female ratio was 10:1 in 50-59 years age group and 1:1 in 0-9 years age group. The most frequent age group was 20-29 (36%) followed by 30-39 (21%).

RTC was the leading cause of injury (54%) followed by falls (42%).

The anatomical regions of spinal fracture were cervical followed by lumbar, thoracolumbar and thoracic region. Interestingly, the distribution of anatomical region of spinal cord injury was: thoracolumbar followed by cervical, thoracic and lumbar spine.

Again, the severe SCI patients with pre-hospital mortality were not included. Therefore, this study neither reflects the true incidence of SCI nor the incidence of SCI among spine fractures.

## Guilan (Yousefzadeh et al, 2010)

In a descriptive study of all traumatic spine injury cases admitted to Poursina Hospital, located in the north of Iran, 17% of patients had abnormal neurological findings. The mean age of patients was 38.2 years; the most common age group at which spinal injury occurred in males was 25-44 years and in females was 45-64 years. The male to female ratio was 2.6.

The most common mechanism of injury was RTC (52%) followed by falls (43%); however, fall was the most common cause in the ≥45 age group.

The most common site of injury among spine fracture patients was thoracolumbar region (47%); nevertheless, cervical spine was the most affected region in SCI patients (39%).

Again, the severe SCI patients who had not survived to hospital had not been included. Therefore, this study neither reflects the true incidence of SCI nor the incidence of SCI among spine fractures.

## EARTHQUAKE

Disasters including earthquakes are one of the mechanisms that cause SCI. Patients who develop SCI during a disaster have particular needs that are hardly provided. This may increase the mortality and morbidity of SCI. To worsen the situation, patients who suffer from SCI during a disaster are less likely to receive family support, as the family is affected by the disaster too.

On December 26, 2003, a 12-second earthquake in Bam resulted in 36,000 dead and 23,000 injured among a population of about 100,000. After a few months, approximately 100 individuals with SCI due to earthquake were identified in Bam and the surrounding area. However, the exact incidence of SCI due to the earthquake was not completely clear.

The demographic characteristics of these patients were different from other studies. In contrast to a mainly male predominance, half of SCI patients detected after the earthquake were female with some pregnant. The male to female ratio in Portugal is reported as 3.4:1 and in Japan as 4:1, when earthquake has not been the cause of injury (Burt, 2004).

There were a few children as young as 1.5 years old (Raissi, 2007). Normally, SCIs in children are uncommon, particularly before the age of 12 (Burt, 2004).

The SCI patients suffered from unexpectedly low standards of care. For example, although there were some facilities for physical therapy, of the 34 patients visited during the first months after the disaster, only 3 had received education regarding bladder care and only 1 had received education regarding bowel care. Many patients had pain syndromes, but there was little attention to pain management. Transportation was another major problem, particularly for individuals with SCI needing access to rehabilitation services. Although a few mobile teams consisting of a physiotherapist and sometimes an occupational therapist were partly effective, the medical and nursing problems of these patients remained largely untreated (Raissi, 2007).

Ninety percent of patients sustained injury at the thoracolumbar level, 8% at thoracic level and 2% in cervical spine (Karamouzian et al, 2010). The frequency of burst fractures, fracture-dislocations and wedge fractures, were 49%, 30% and 13% respectively. Patients sustaining fracture dislocations had worse neurological conditions. One-fourth of patients who had ASIA-A impairments at the time of the earthquake recovered sufficient hip and knee strength to ambulate with the use of conventional orthoses after 18 months (Karamouzian et al, 2010). The authors concluded that the neurological outcome of patients with SCI due to earthquakes is better than other etiologies of SCI (Karamouzian et al, 2010).

# REFERENCES

Ackery A, Tator C, Krassioukov A. A global perspective on spinal cord injury epidemiology. *J Neurotrauma*.2004;21(10):1355–1370.

Burt AA. (iii) The epidemiology, natural history and prognosis of spinal cord injury. *Current Orthopaedics* (2004) 18, 26–32

Catz A, Thaleisnik M, Fishel B, Ronen J, Spasser R, Fredman Bet al. Survival after spinal cord injury in Israel. *Spinal cord* 2002;40: 595–598.

Dryden DM, Saunders LD, Rowe BH, et al. The epidemiologyof traumatic spinal cord injury in Alberta, Canada. *Can J Neurol Sci*. 2003;30(2):113–121.

Fakharian E, Tabesh H, Masoud SA. (An epidemiologic study on spinal injuries in kashan). *Guylan medical university journal*.1383;49:79-85.

Heidari P, Zarei MR, Rasouli MR, Vaccaro AR, Rahimi-Movaghar V. Spinal fractures resulting from traumatic injuries. *Chinese Journal of Traumatology* 2010; 13(1):3-9.

Ho CH, Wuermser LA, Priebe MM, Chiodo AE, Scelza WM, Kirshblum SC. Spinal Cord Injury Medicine. 1. Epidemiology and Classification. *Arch Phys Med Rehabil* 2007;88(3 Suppl 1):S49-54.

Karamouzian S, Saeed A, Ashraf-Ganjouei K, Ebrahiminejad A, Dehghani MR,Asadi AR. The Neurological Outcome of Spinal Cord InjuredVictims of the Bam Earthquake, Kerman, Iran. *Archives of Iranian Medicine*, Volume 13, Number 4, July 2010

Leucht P, Fischer K, Muhr G, Mueller EJ. Epidemiology of traumatic spine fractures. Injury, *Int. J. Care Injured* 40 (2009) 166–172

Martins F, Freitas F, Martins L, Dartigues JF, Barat M. Spinal cord injuries: epidemiology in Portugal's central region. *Spinal Cord*. 1998;36(8):574–578.

McKinley WO, Seel RT, Hardman JT. *Nontraumatic Spinal Cord Injury: Incidence, Epidemiology, and Functional Outcome Arch Phys Med Rehabil* Vol 80, June 1999

Moini M, Rezaishiraz H, zafarghandi MR. Characteristics and outcome of injured patients treated in urban trauma centers in Iran. *J Trauma* 2000; 48:503-507.

O'Connor P. Incidence and patterns of spinal cord injury in Australia. *Accid Anal Prev*. 2002;34(4):405–415.

Pickett GE, Benitez MC, Keller JL, Duggal N. Epidemiology of Traumatic Spinal Cord Injuryin Canada. *SPINE Volume 31*, Number 7, pp 799–805

Rahimi-Movaghar V, Moradi-Lakeh M, Rasouli MR, Vaccaro AR. Burden of spinal cord injury in Tehran, Iran. *Spinal Cord.* 2010; 48, 492–497

Rahimi-Movaghar V, Rasouli MR, Smith H, Vaccaro AR. Chapter 24: An evidence-based review of spinal cord injury decompression in experimental animals and human studies. In: Berkovsky TC. *Handbook of spimnal cord injuries: Types, treatments and prognosis.* Nova Science Publishers, Inc. New York; 2010, pp. 635-663.

Rahimi-Movaghar V, Vaccaro AR, Mohammadi M. Efficacy of surgical decompression in regards to motor recovery in the setting of conus medullaris injury. *J Spinal Cord Med.* 2006; 29: 32-38.

Rahimi-Movaghar V. Efficacy of surgical decompression in the setting of complete thoracic spinal cord injury. *J Spinal Cord Med.* 2005; 28: 415-420.

Rahimi-Movaghar[a] V, Saadat S, Rasouli MR, Ganji S, Ghahramani M, Zarei MR, Vaccaro AR. Prevalence of Spinal Cord Injury in Tehran, Iran. *J Spinal Cord Med.* August 2009;32(4):428–431

Rahimi-Movaghar[b] V, Vaccaro AR, Mohammadi M. The efficacy of non-operative and operative Intervention in regards to motor recovery in the setting of cervical spinal cord injury. *Iran J Psychiatry* 2009; 4: 131-136.

Raissi GR. Earthquakes and Rehabilitation Needs: Experiences From Bam, Iran. *J Spinal Cord Med.* 2007;30:369–372

Rasouli MR, Nouri M, Rahimi-movaghar R. Spinal cord injuries from road traffic crashes in southeastern Iran. *Chinese journal of traumatology* 2007; 10(6):323-326

Rasouli MR, Rahimi-Movaghar V, Vaccaro AR. Chapter 5: Safety promotions for motor vehicle crashes-related spinal column and cord injuries. In: Ferraro CN. *Traffic safety.* Nova Science Publishers, Inc. New York; 2011, pp. 161-180.

Schoenfeld AJ, Sielski B, Rivera KP, Bader JO, Harris MB. Epidemiology of cervical spine fractures in the US military. *The Spine Journal 2011*; (Article in press)

Taghipoor KD, Arejan RH, Rasouli MR, Saadat S, Moghadam M, Vaccaro AR, Rahimi-Movaghar V. Factors associated with pressure ulcers in patients with complete or sensory-only preserved spinal cord injury: is there any difference between traumatic and nontraumatic causes? *J Neurosurg Spine.* 2009 Oct;11(4):438-44.

Taghippor M, Sherafatkazemzadeh E. [Traumatic vertebral column and spinal cord injuries in shiraz nemazi hospital, an epidemiological study]. *Armaghan e danesh.* 2005; 4: 55-62 [Persian]

Tator CH, Duncan EG, Edmonds VE, Lapczak LI, Andrews DF.Changes in Epidemiology of Acute Spinal Cord Injury from 1947 to 1981.*Surg Neurol.* 1993;40:207-15

World Health Organization.*http://www.who.int/countries/irn/en/*

Wyndaele Mand Wyndaele JJ.Incidence, prevalence and epidemiology of spinal cord injury:what learns a worldwide literature survey?*Spinal Cord* 2006 44, 523–529

Yousefzadeh Chabok S, Safaee M, Alizadeh A, Ahmadi Dafchahi M, Taghinnejadi O, Koochakinejad L. Epidemiology of Traumatic Spinal Injury: A Descriptive Study. *Acta Medica Iranica* 2010; 48(5): 308-311.

In: Epidemiology of Spinal Cord Injuries
Editors: V. Rahimi-Movaghar, S. B. Jazayeri et al.

ISBN: 978-1-61942-894-2
©2012 Nova Science Publishers, Inc.

*Chapter 15*

# DEMOGRAPHICS OF SPINAL CORD INJURIES IN PAKISTAN

## *Farooq A. Rathore*[*,1] *and Sahibzada Nasir Mansoor*[2]

[1] Department of Rehabilitation Medicine,
Combined Military Hospital, Panoaqil Cantt, Sindh, Pakistan
[2] Department of Rehabilitation Medicine,
Combined Military Hospital, Kohat Cantt, Pakistan

## ABSTRACT

Epidemiological research on Spinal Cord Injuries (SCI) in Pakistan is limited to hospital based surveys. Further limitations are the absence of a national trauma registry, a small sample size in reported studies, under-representation of certain regions and a lack of focus on non-traumatic spinal cord injuries (NTSCI). The demographics of SCI in Pakistan described in this chapter are based on a diverse research methodology. It comprises of a electronic and manual literature search, interviews with professional colleagues throughout the country who manage SCI patients and the personal experience of the authors working at the largest spinal rehabilitation unit in Pakistan.

Fall from height is the most common etiology for Traumatic SCI (TSCI) followed by road traffic accidents (RTA) and acts of violence. The majority of the patients are young males in their second and third decade. Pre-hospital care and evacuation from the site of trauma is inadequate most of the time due to the lack of widespread implementation of cervical spine precautions following injury. This is likely because of a deficiency of trained emergency personnel throughout the region. Paraplegia is the most frequent presentation and most of the patients have a complete neurological injury at admission. Surgical interventions are carried out in most of the cases of TSCI but rehabilitation referrals are often delayed and multidisciplinary SCI rehabilitation is not widely available. Spinal Tuberculosis is the most common cause of NTSCI followed by transverse myelitis and degenerative spinal disorders. NTSCI is more common in males in their fifth and sixth decades. The complication profile of SCI patients in Pakistan is similar to the reported complications in developed countries with a notably increased

---

[*] Corresponding Author: Dr Farooq Azam Rathore, Department of Rehabilitation Medicine, Combined Military Hospital, Panoaqil Cantt, 65130 Sindh, Pakistan farooqrathore@gmail.com.

incidence. Social support systems and community re-integration programs for SCI patients are not well established and patients face social, financial and mobility barriers while attempting community re-integration.

There is a need to establish a national trauma registry, improve pre-hospital care for SCI, improve the existing neurosurgical services, and develop multidisciplinary SCI rehabilitation and social services for SCI patients in Pakistan.

**Keywords:** Spinal Cord injury, Pakistan, Paraplegia, epidemiology, demographics

# INTRODUCTION

Spinal Cord injury (SCI) is a devastating neurological trauma that most commonly affects the young, active male population throughout the world. It leads to life long disability in most cases, reduces life expectancy [1] and quality of life (QOL) [2, 3], predisposes the individual to late complications and is a major economic burden to the society. [4, 5] A better understanding of the epidemiological and demographics of SCI leads to better prevention and management strategies. There is no comprehensive comparative data on SCI in Pakistan available in the literature and this chapter aims to address this issue.

# HEALTH CARE SYSTEM IN PAKISTAN

Pakistan is located in South Asia and is the sixth largest country in the world with a population of over 170 million. [6, 7] The majority of the population is between 15 to 64 years old and lives in rural areas [2] with inadequate access to health care facilities. While there has been noticeable improvement in health care over recent years, in general, Pakistan ranks poorly with regard to health care access. Overall, life expectancy in Pakistan remains lower than many south Asian countries, while infant as well as maternal mortality rates are amongst the highest. [8].

In Pakistan, health care is being provided to the public through a vast infrastructure of health facilities consisting of hospitals, dispensaries, basic health units and maternity child health centers. In addition there are private hospitals, clinics and philanthropic institutes providing health care services. The number of health care providers is inadequate, with 139,555 registered doctors, 9,822 registered dentists and 69,313 nurses. [8] There are 916 hospitals [9] and the number of patients per bed is 1592. [8] Access to health care varies among different regions with urban population having better access to quality health care facilities. There are dozens of medical colleges all around the country with affiliated teaching hospitals and accredited universities. [10]

# DATA COLLECTION

The data for this chapter was collected from different sources. An electronic and manual literature search was performed with the parameters and key words specified in Table 1. Because the purpose of this work was essentially descriptive, no attempt was made to weigh the quality of the articles that were identified. The results from the electronic literature search have been summarized in Table 2. Colleagues and experts working with SCI in the fields of neurology, neurosurgery, spinal orthopedic surgery and rehabilitation medicine were interviewed. They were asked about their experiences and opinions about the current situation of SCI in Pakistan. These semi-structured interviews were analyzed for extraction of useful information for this chapter. In addition, authors had more than five years' experience of working at the largest rehabilitation institute in the country (Armed Forces Institute of Rehabilitation Medicine) with the only dedicated SCI Rehabilitation unit in Pakistan. AFIRM admits around one hundred patients of traumatic and non-traumatic SCI annually and patients are admitted for follow up of complications.

**Table 1. Literature search methodology**

| Electronic literature search | Medline, Google scholar, Science Direct, OVID, CINAHL, Springer link, Informaworld and Pakmedinet (Pakistani biomedical journals database). |
|---|---|
| Limitations | English language and human studies only with data bases searched from earliest possible date to June 2011. |
| Gray Literature search | Online and manual search for thesis and dissertations of CPSP Websites of Govt. of Pakistan for statistics related to health care Newspapers and relevant articles on SCI online |
| Key Words | Spinal cord injury, spinal injuries, spinal trauma, paraplegia and quadriplegia combined with following in different combinations Pakistan, epidemiology, demographics, ASIA score, assessment, pre-hospital management, developing countries, complications, pressure ulcers, urinary tract infections, neurogenic bladder, neurogenic bowel, deep vein thrombosis, spasticity, depression, follow up, aging , mortality, pediatrics, child hood SCI, community reintegration, support groups etc. |

# LIMITATIONS OF SPINAL CORD INJURY RELATED RESEARCH IN PAKISTAN

SCI is an important cause of long term disability in young adults in Pakistan. Multiple manuscripts have been published in the past two decades in the national and international biomedical literature. [11- 21]

These manuscripts primarily address the epidemiological pattern and demographics of SCI in particular settings. Some address complications like deep vein thrombosis (DVT)[22, 23], pressure ulcers [24] and bowel care management. [25]

A review of these studies reveals a few limitations in the SCI related research of Pakistan.

- First is the lack of a national trauma or SCI registry in Pakistan. This makes the exact estimates of the epidemiology and demographics difficult to collect and analyze.
- All available studies on SCI in Pakistan are hospital based surveys mostly covering only one unit or hospital with the exception of the study by Raja et al [11], which was a nationwide survey of different neurosurgical departments and units. There is no information available about demographics of SCI patients living in the community.

# Table 1. Demographics of SCI in Pakistan: Results of electronic literature search

| S/No | Authors | Year of Publication | Study Design | Duration of Study | Type of SCI | Sample size | M:F ratio | Average age or range (years)$^\mu$ | Neurological Level (%) Paraplegia(P) Quadriplegia(Q) | Management Surgical(S) Non-Surgical(NS) | Avg LOS | Mortality |
|---|---|---|---|---|---|---|---|---|---|---|---|---|
| | Butt RM et al | 1997 | Prospective, Single center | 1 year | TSCI | 173 | 7:3 | 41%(21-40) | P: 41.1% Q: 58.9% | NR | NR | 12.5% |
| | Qureshi AA et al | 2001 | Prospective, Single center | 3 years | TSCI | 156 | 2.6:1 | 79% (20-30) | P: 100% | S: 77.82% NS: 22.18% | 2-4 wks | 12% |
| | Raja IA et al | 2001 | Retrospective, Multi center | 4 years | TSCI | 2654 | 2.5:1 | NR | P: 32% Q: 68% | S: 68% NS: 32% | NR | NR |
| | Malik F | 2005 | Retrospective, Multi center | NS | Non Traumatic | 150 | 7:3 | 28.8 | P: 2.7% Q: nil | NR | NR | NR |
| | Brohi SR et al | 2006 | Prospective, single centre | 5 years | Non Traumatic | 248 | 1: 1.91 | <40 years (66.9%) | P:88.29% Q:11.69% | S: 100% | NR | NR |
| | Butt RM et al | 2006 | Retrospective, Single center | 1 year | TSCI | 37 | 3.6:1 | 15-70 | P:100% | S:100% | NR | NR |
| | Devrajani et al | 2006 | Prospective, Single center | 1 year | Non Traumatic | 44 | 1.5:1 | 18-62 | P:95.5% Q:4.54% | S: 11(25%) NS: 29(75%) | NR | NR |
| | Siddique ZR et al | 2007 | Prospective, single centre | 3 months | TSCI | 32 | 3:1 | 20-50 (72%) | P:75% Q:25% | S:18.8% NS:81.2% | 6% | NR |
| | Rathore MFA et al | 2007 | Prospective, Single center | 3 months | TSCI | 187 | 8.0:10.7 | 28.3 | P: 89.3% Q: 4.8% | S: 75.4% NS: 24.6% | NR | NR |
| | Ali MN et al | 2007 | Prospective, single centre | 2.5 years | TSCI | 32 | 2.6:1 | 23 | P: 100% | S: 100% | NR | NR |
| | Rathore et al | 2008 | Prospective, Single center | 1 year | TSCI | 83 | 4.5:1 | 29.3 | P: 71.1% Q: 29.9% | S: 51.8% NS: 48.2% | NR | NR |
| | Rehman et al | 2008 | Prospective, single centre | 10 months | TSCI | 106 | 3:1 | 20-30 (41%) <20 (21%) | P:81.2% Q:18.8% | S: 100% | NR | NR |
| | Masood et al | 2008 | Retrospective, Single center | 4 years | TSCI | 214 | 7.5:1 | 32.7 | P: 57.5% Q: 47.2% | S: 23.4% NS: 76.6% | 8.4 ± 7.6 days | NR |
| | Arif et al | 2009 | Retrospective, Single center | 4 years | TSCI | 76 | 4.9:2.7 | 32 | P:100% | S: 100% | NR | NR |

| S/No | Authors | Year of Publication | Study Design | Duration of Study | Type of SCI | Sample size | M:F ratio | Average age or range (years)μ | Neurological Level (%) Paraplegia(P) Quadriplegia(Q) | Management Surgical(S) Non-Surgical(NS) | Avg LOS | Mortality |
|---|---|---|---|---|---|---|---|---|---|---|---|---|
| | Qureshi et al | 2010 | Retrospective, (Case series) Single center | 7 years and 8 months | TSCI | 521 | 3.3:1 | 39.1 | P: 70.9% Q: 27.5% | S: 70% NS:30% | NR | 4 |
| | Raja RA et al | 2010 | Prospective, Single center | 1 year | TSCI | 50 | 4.3:0.7 | 30.7 | P:80% Q:NR | S: 57.4% NS: 42.6% | NR | NR |
| | Bukhari MA et al | 2010 | Prospective, Single center | 3 years | TSCI | 37 | 4.2:1 | | P: 78% Q: 22% | S: 100% | NR | NR |

NA; Not applicable, NR; Not reported, LOS; Length of stay, TSCI; Traumatic Spinal cord injury, NTSCI; Non traumatic SCI, P;paraplegia, Q; Quadriplegia.

μ Range has been mentioned where average age was not calculated by the authors.

- Many of these studies were based on retrospective, chart based data collection. Accurate record keeping is a problem in many of the hospitals around the country, especially in the public sector.[26, 27]. SCI mostly presents in the emergency department and the data collection and documentation is sometimes deficient and inaccurate. [28]Many hospitals have implemented improved record keeping systems including electronic health management system in the last few years but gray areas still exist. This can be a possible source of bias when describing the demographics of SCI in Pakistan.
- Most of these studies use different assessment tools (Frankel's and American Spinal Injury Association (ASIA) impairment scales) while describing the patients with SCI. This makes comparison between studies difficult.
- The data collection techniques, study periods (more than 3 years [11,16,20] to less than three months[29]) and the sample population among studies vary widely. (2654 to 32)
- Pakistan has four provinces. All of these studies were conducted in three provinces of Pakistan; namely Punjab, Khyber Pakhtunkwa and Sindh. The study population in Oct 2005 related SCI was primarily from Kashmir [14,22], but there is no information about SCI in one of the largest provinces in Pakistan by area; Baluchistan.

It is important to note that many of these limitations are also encountered while studying the demographics of SCI in other countries throughout the world. [30].

# ETIOLOGY

Motor vehicles accidents are the leading cause of traumatic SCI (TSCI) in developed countries, while falls and acts of violence are more frequent in the developing countries and low socioeconomic groups in the developed countries. [30,31] Falls are the most frequent cause of TSCI reported in most of the studies from Pakistan. [15,16,20, 29,32, 33, 34]] These falls are mostly from trees, roof tops and the work place (electricity poles, construction workers etc). These highlight the general lack of awareness in the public about the hazards of unsafe climbing and the lack of work laws and prevention strategies to reduce the incidence of work related falls.

There has been an exponential increase in the number of motorized vehicles (passenger cars, commercial vehicles and motorcycles) in the last decade in Pakistan. [35] Motor vehicle accidents (MVA) are the second commonest cause of TSCI in Pakistan. We have observed that in contrast to falls, a person sustaining a MVA is more liable to get a high and neurologically worse SCI with more complex associated injuries and a lesser chances of recovery.

Another important cause of SCI in Pakistan is related to the use of fire arms and terrorist bombing attacks. A recent report described the pattern of SCI related to terrorist suicide bombings which was different from the pattern reported from non–terrorism related SCI. [36]

The October 2005 earthquake was the worst natural disaster in Pakistan's history. It resulted in hundreds of SCI patients which added to the pre-existing burden of SCI in

Pakistan. The demographic pattern of this particular subset was different from the pattern observed before and will be discussed at the end of this chapter.

Non traumatic SCI is also an important contributor to the overall burden of SCI patients in Pakistan. The three most frequent causes of NTSCI in Pakistan in order of decreasing frequencies are Spinal Tuberculosis (TB), [37, 38, 39] Transverse Myelitis [40] and metastatic cord compression. Many times there is a delay in the diagnosis especially with spinal TB when the patient presents with a major neurological deficit and abscess formation along with gibbous deformity. Spinal TB more commonly involves the thoracic spine.

Sporting events have been documented in the developed countries as an important etiological factor of TSCI. [41, 42, 43] Sports related SCI is rarely seen in Pakistan and mostly occurs in the context of a young male diving in a shallow village pond or swimming pool and sustaining a cervical spinal injury.

## GENDER DISTRIBUTION

The general trend of gender distribution of SCI in Pakistan follows the global trend of male preponderance. All studies show an increased incidence of SCI in males in Pakistan (See Table 1). Males in Pakistan usually are the source of primary income for their families, and are therefor engaged in occupations and outdoor activities that expose them to falls and other occupational hazards. In addition, all commercial and heavy vehicles in Pakistan are operated primarily by male drivers. Moreover, males are more likely to be involved in acts of violence and firearm use. All of these factors increase the risk among males of sustaining SCI. The only notable exception to this trend was during Oct 2005 earthquake, when more females were injured in the disaster. [14] A possible explanation is that during the time of the disaster, females were at home doing their household chores and the earthquake resulted in collapse of buildings and homes leading to SCI in a large number of females.

## AGE DISTRIBUTION

SCI in Pakistan, like all other countries mainly occur in young males between 20 to 40 years of age. In any society, this age group makes up the majority of the work force. These are the most productive years of one's life. This highlights the importance of an effective SCI rehabilitation program that would give these young individuals the potential to reintegrate into society. [15]

Spinal TB and metastatic spinal cord compression tends to occur more in patients in their fifth and sixth decades of life.

Pediatric SCI has been reported in developed countries. [44, 45] It is rarely seen in Pakistan, except during the Oct 2005 earthquake which resulted in a relatively large number of children with SCI[14]. The reason for this large number is likely because most children were in schools when the earthquake struck at 08:52 AM resulting in widespread collapse of school buildings and serious injuries. [14]

There was an interesting trend observed at AFIRM in the last five years regarding traumatic cervical spine injury in the elderly. Many of these patients came from mountainous and rural areas where they regularly climbed trees to cut branches for fuel or collect fruit. Most of them presented with incomplete cervical spine injury (Central cord syndrome variant), were managed conservatively and improved neurologically within 2 to 4 months.

## MARITAL AND EDUCATIONAL STATUS

SCI not only affects the patient but also the entire family. Marital status after SCI correlates with life satisfaction [46], pain [47] and employment status [48] Many times, the involved male is the only family member earning an income and is the head of the household. After the injury he finds himself in a position where he cannot contribute financially and is dependent upon others for his needs. There is a general trend of getting married in the second and third decades in Pakistan. Moreover, family centered values and a sense of responsibility towards serving the disabled husband is well entrenched in Pakistani females. Therefore, even after the injury the wives usually stay with their husbands and act as a long-term care giver, [15] despite the fact that this is a lifelong physical and psychological burden. [49] The divorce rates after SCI in the West are higher than the normal population [50, 51] in the developed countries. This is in contrast to the general trend seen in Pakistan where the husband and wife stay together and carry on with their lives. The possible factors for this positive trend could be the strong religious influences in Pakistani culture which promote valuing family/ community need over personal needs, presence of strong family networks which share the burden of care (at least in the initial phase of the injury and rehabilitation) and a cultural stigmatization associated with divorcing a partner when he/ she was in need of support.

The education level of the SCI patient correlates positively with a better marital status [52] , satisfaction with life [46] and early return to work. [53, 54] The literacy level (defined as individuals age 15 and over who can read and write) in Pakistan is around 50 % [7]. Most people sustaining SCI are from the low socioeconomic strata of society and have issues with reading and understanding the grave nature of SCI. [15, 55]. It is very difficult to counsel these patients and administer different SCI assessment tools to monitor progress and predict outcomes. The majority of these patients are only interested in knowing when they might be able to walk again [15].

## TYPES OF INJURIES

There is a wide variation among the descriptions used in studies to describe the level and completeness of SCI. Most of the studies show that the thoracic and thoracolumbar level injuries are more common than cervical spinal injuries.[12,14,15,19,20,36,38,39,16] This could be explained on the basis of a relatively inadequate pre-hospital and trauma care system in Pakistan and falls being the leading etiology of SCI. As in many other developing countries, emergency medical services, especially pre-hospital emergency care, has long been neglected in Pakistan. [56] Consequently, patients are brought to the emergency departments by relatives or bystanders in private cars, taxis or any other readily available mode of transportation. Ambulances, where they exist, lack spinal boards and staff are not familiar with log roll transfer and immobilization precautions in suspected cases of SCI. [15] It is very unlikely that a patient with a cervical spine injury would survive the delayed and often improper handling at the trauma site, thus leading to an increase in number of paraplegics presenting at the emergency department. The pre-hospital trauma care has improved in Pakistan in the last decade with the establishment of Rescue 1122 and Rescue 15 services in certain parts of the country [56, 57] but there is still room for improvement and expansion of these services.

The other possible factor for an increased number of paraplegics relates to the mechanism of falls. Most of the documented falls are from a height of less than 30 feet and patients usually land on their backs rather than heads, resulting in more thoracic traumas.

All types of vertebral injuries are encountered, with fracture dislocations being more common in MVA and burst fractures in falls.

## MANAGEMENT PROTOCOLS

All patients sustaining an acute SCI in Pakistan are initially admitted to the neurosurgical or orthopedic spinal wards. There is currently only one dedicated SCI Rehabilitation unit in the country at the AFIRM, Rawalpindi. Therefore, most of the patients under the initial neurosurgical or orthopedic care undergo surgical interventions (Table 1). All types of surgical decompression and stabilization procedures are performed in Pakistan.

Conservative management of neurologically intact thoracolumbar burst and compression fractures is an effective means of management [58, 59] but requires expertise that is available in only a few locations in Pakistan. Hence there is a trend towards surgical intervention even if the patient presents after weeks or months [16]. In addition, many of cases of Spinal TB present at a stage when there is already an abscess with vertebral body erosion and resulting instability. These cases require surgical debridement and stabilization to optimize patient care.

## COMPLICATIONS PROFILE

There are no studies that specifically address the secondary complications in SCI. The complication profile reported in the SCI population from Pakistan [13,14,15,17,20,22,24,21] is similar to reports from different developing nations of the world [60, 61, 62] The only exception to this trend is the low rate of DVT in a cohort of Pakistani population [22] as compared to the data reported from developed countries [63, 64, 65]. The possible factors for this low incidence could include activated protein C resistance, an increase in the inhibitor of plasminogen activator-1, hyper-homocysteinemia or a lower prevalence of factor V leiden mutation, which is more common in the western population. [66, 67, 68] Another possible explanation proposed was the high rate of passive range of motion exercises three times per day and frequent massage of lower limbs due to the availability of large number of care givers and attendants.[22]

The other documented complications include a larger number of pressure ulcers (Fig 1 and 2), contractures (Fig 3), muscle wasting, heterotrophic ossification (Fig 4), Urinary tract infections, depression and pulmonary infections. An important observation is the significantly reduced incidence of complications in patients who are under the care of a physiatrist. [14,15]

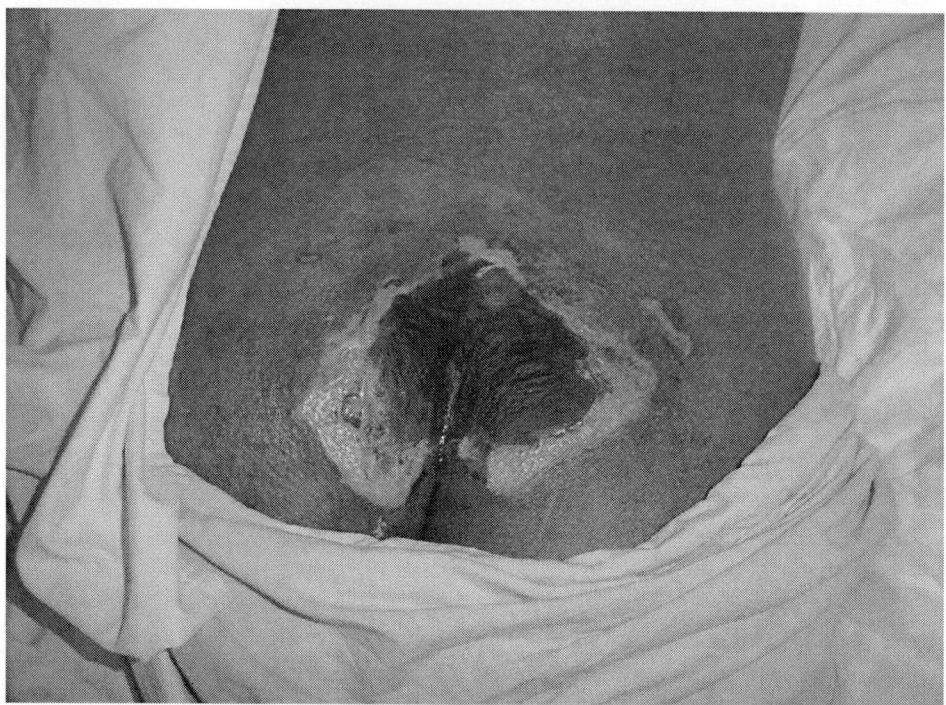

Figure 1.

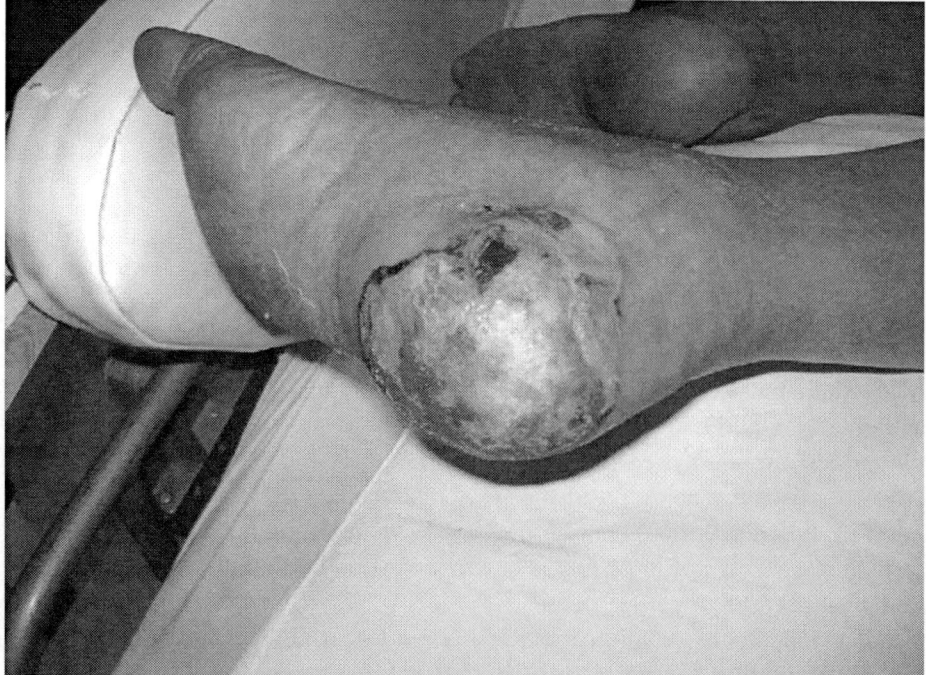

Figure 2.

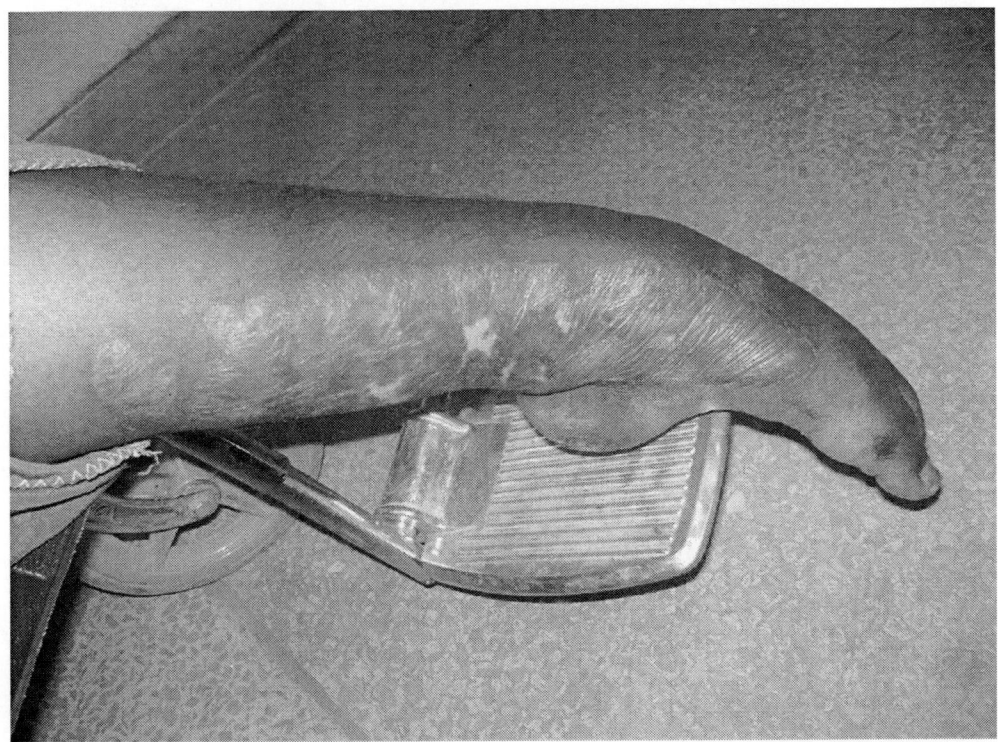

Figure 3.

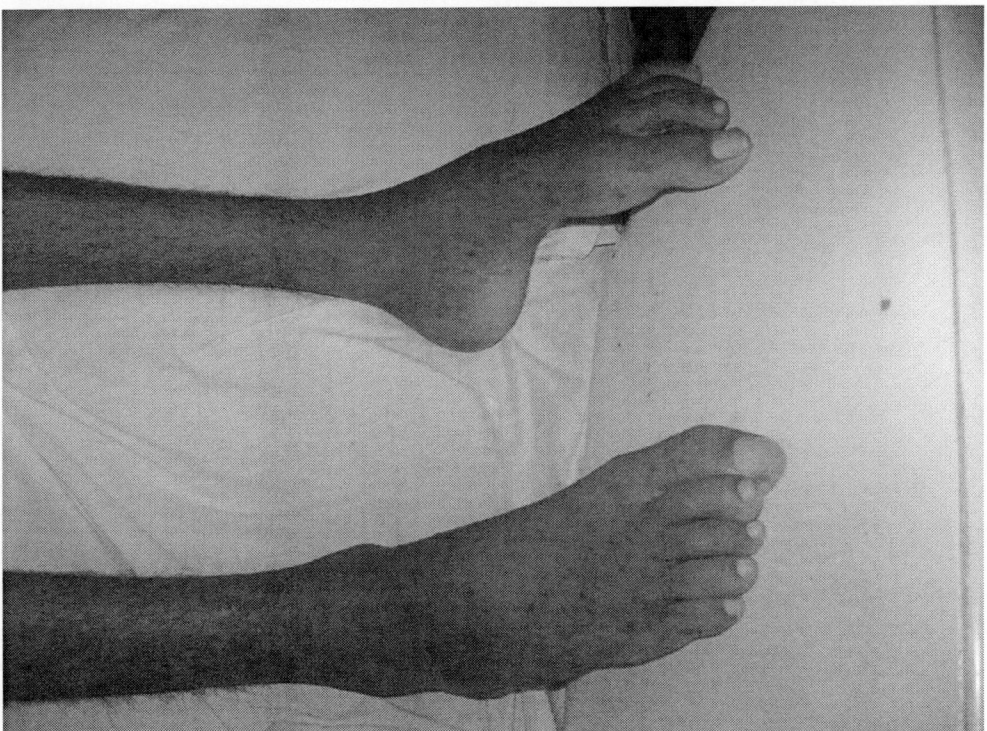

Figure 4.

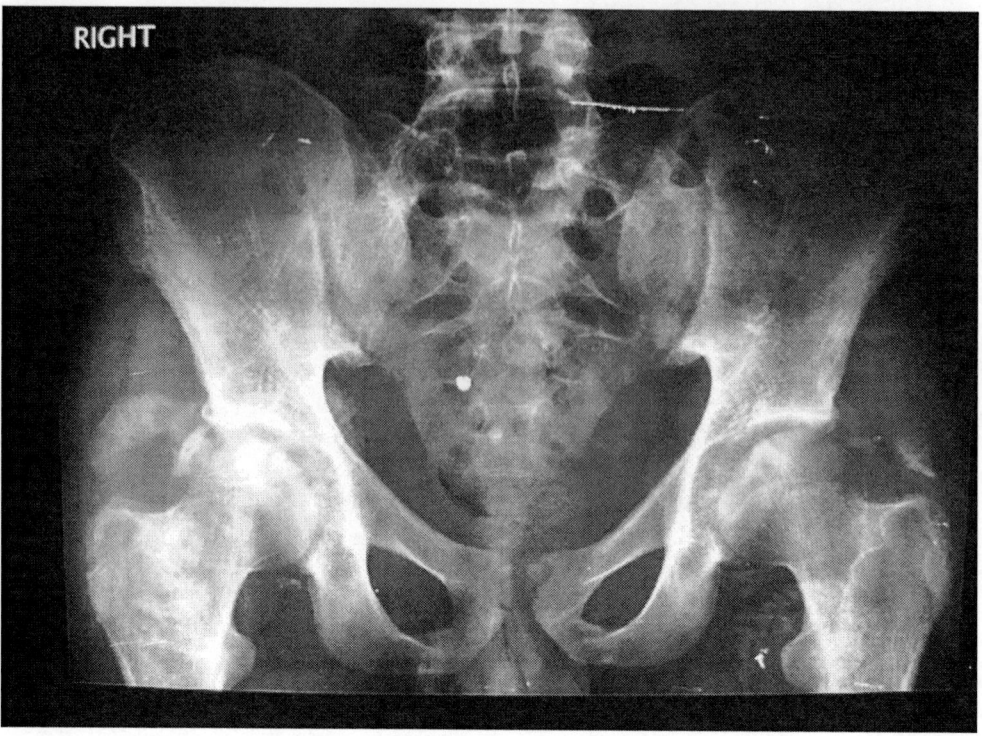

Figure 5.

# CONCLUSION

SCI is an important cause of neurological disability in young Pakistani males and adversely affects the individual, family and the society as a whole. The lack of a national trauma registry and accurate record keeping makes it difficult to make precise estimates of the current burden of SCI in the country. There is a need for an awareness campaign targeting safer working conditions and better road safety protocols. Government also has a role by enforcing legislation aimed at reducing the incidence of MVA and trauma in the country.

There is a need to develop SCI rehabilitation services so that patients can be reintegrated into society, rather than being confined to their homes for the rest of their lives. Different aspects of SCI care such as complication profile, functional outcomes, post injury employment and barriers to community reintegration should be studied to formulate better policies for the future. The health care professionals involved in the SCI care in Pakistan (Physiatrists, Orthopedic surgeons, Neurosurgeons and Spinal surgeons) should take a leading role in promoting awareness about this disability and conduct large scale nationwide epidemiological surveys to assess the true burden of the disease.

It is also imperative that the SCI patient communities in Pakistan rally together for their rights to fight against discrimination and address social barriers and ways to optimize community re-integration.

# REFERENCES

[1] Ahoniemi E, Pohjolainen T, Kautiainen H. Survival after spinal cord injury in Finland *J Rehabil Med.* 2011 ;43:481-5.

[2] Migliorini CE, New PW, Tonge BJ. Quality of life in adults with spinal cord injury living in the community. *Spinal Cord.* 2011 ;49:365-70.

[3] Hu Y, Mak JN, Wong YW, Leong JC, Luk KD. Quality of life of traumatic spinal cord injured patients in Hong Kong. *J Rehabil Med.* 2008 ;40:126-31.

[4] Kawu AA, Olawepo A, Salami AO, Kuranga SA, Abdulhameed S, Esenwah VC. *A cost analysis of conservative management of spinal cord-injured patients in Nigeria. Spinal Cord.* 2011 Jun 21. doi: 10.1038/sc.2011.69. [Epub ahead of print]

[5] Tator CH, Duncan EG, Edmonds VE, Lapczak LI, Andrews DF. Complications and costs of management of acute spinal cord injury. *Paraplegia.* 1993 ;31:700-14.

[6] Population census Organization. Government of Pakistan. Available from *http://www.census.gov.pk/* ( Accessed 15th July 2011)

[7] The Central Intelligence Agency: The World Fact book online. Pakistan. Available from *https://www.cia.gov/library/publications/the-world-factbook/geos/pk.html* (Accessed 15th July 2011)

[8] Khan A. Health and Nutrition in Pakistan Economic Survey 2009-10. Government of Pakistan. Available from *http://www.finance.gov.pk/survey/chapter_10/11_Health.pdf* (Accessed 15th July 2011)

[9] Basic Facts. Ministry of Information and Broadcasting. Government of Pakistan. Available from *http://www.infopak.gov.pk/BasicFacts.aspx* ( Accessed 15th July 2011)

[10] Recongnized Medical Colleges in Pakistan. Pakistan Medical and Dental Council. Available from *http://www.pmdc.org.pk/AboutUs/RecognizedMedicalDentalColleges /tabid /109/Default.aspx* ( Accessed 15th July 2011)

[11] Raja IA, Vohra AH, Ahmed. M. *Neurotrauma in Pakistan World J. Surg* 2001 ;25: 1230–1237.

[12] Qureshi AA, Irfan A, Memon MA. *Spinal Injuries: A Prospective Study. Biomedica* 2001;17:27-29.

[13] Butt RM, Shams S, Habib A, Raja IA, Sarwar A, AhmedA. Epidemiology of Spinal Injuries. *Pak J Neurol* 1997; 3:20-25.

[14] Rathore MFA, Rashid P, Butt AW, Malik AA, Gill ZA, Haig AJ. Epidemiology of spinal cord injuries in the 2005 Pakistan earthquake. *Spinal Cord* 2007; 45: 658–663

[15] Rathore FA, Hanif S, Farooq F, Butt AW, Ahmed N. Traumatic Spinal Cord Injuries At A Tertiary Care Rehabilitation Institute In Pakistan. *J Pak Med Assoc* 2008;58:53-57

[16] Qureshi MA, Khalique AB, Pasha IF, Asad A, Malik AS, Shah MQ, Ahmed A. Epidemiology of non-disaster spinal injuries at a spine unit. *J Coll Physicians Surg Pak.* 2010;20:667-70.

[17] Rathore FA , Muzammil S.( letter to Editor) Epidemiology of Non-Disaster Spinal Injuries at a Spine Unit. *J Coll Physicians Surg Pak.* 2011 ;21:384.

[18] Khattak MJ, Syed S, Lakdawala RH. Operative management of unstable thoracolumbar burst fractures. *J Coll Physicians Surg Pak.* 2010 ;20:347-9.

[19] Riaz AR. Management of thoracolumbar spine injuries at a tertiary care hospital. *J Ayub Med Coll.* 2010; 22(1): 171-75.

[20] Masood Z, Wardug GM, J A. Spinal Injuries: Experience of a local neurosurgical centre. *Pak J Med Sci* 2008;24:368-71

[21] Bashir F, Malik A, Abaidullah S. Complications Developed in Spinal Cord Injured and Physiotherapy. *Ann King Edward Med Uni.* 2001; 7:61-3.

[22] Rathore MF,, Hanif S, Rashid P, Butt AW, New P, S-U Khan. The incidence of Deep Vein Thrombosis in a cohort of patients with Spinal Cord Injury following the Pakistan earthquake of October 2005. *Spinal Cord.* 2008; 46:523–526

[23] Rathore FA, Farooq F. (Letter to editor) Physical therapy versus heparin for prevention of deep venous thrombosis. *Spinal Cord* 2010 :765.

[24] Rathore FA, New PW, Waheed A. Pressure ulcers in spinal cord injury: at an unusual site with an unusual etiology. *Am J Phys Med Rehabil.* 2009;88:587–590

[25] Yasmeen R, Rathore FA, Butt AW, Ashraf K. How do chronic spinal injury patients in Pakistan manage their bowels? A cross sectional survey of 50 patients. *Spinal Cord* 2010; 48:872-5.

[26] Ali M, Kuroiwa C. Accurate record keeping in referral hospitals in Pakistan's North West frontier province and Punjab: a crucial step needed to improve maternal health. *J Pak Med Assoc.* 2007; 57:443-6.

[27] Aziz S, Rao MH.Existing record keeping system in government teaching hospitals of Karachi. *J Pak Med Assoc.* 2002 ;52:163-74.

[28] Bhatti MA, Ajaib MK, Masud TI, Ali M. Road traffic injuries in Pakistan: challenges in estimation through routine hospital data. *J Ayub Med Coll Abbottabad.* 2008 ;20:108-11.

[29] Siddiqui ZR, Ahmed E, Ud din N, Zaman KU. Preventing Spinal cord Injuries: Is this the best we can do? *Ann Pak Inst Med Sci* 2007;3:148-151

[30] Ackery A, Tator C, Krassioukov A. A global perspective on spinal cord injury epidemiology *J Neurotrauma.* 2004 ;21:1355-70.

[31] Chiu WT, Lin HC, Lam C, Chu SF, Chiang YH, Tsai SH.Review paper: epidemiology of traumatic spinal cord injury: comparisons between developed and developing countries. *Asia Pac J Public Health.* 2010 ;22:9-18

[32] Rehman L, Nasir A, Illias M, Khattak A, Siddique M, Mushtaq. Pattern of Traumatic Spinal Injury: Expereince at Hayatabad Medical Complex (HMC), Peshawer . *Ann Pak Inst Med Sci* 2008; 4:85-87.

[33] Raja RA. Management of Thoracolumbar spine Injuries at a tertiary care hospital. *J Ayub Med Coll Abbottabad* 2010;22:171-175

[34] Mohammed All Bukhari, Waqar Aziz Rahman, Ahmed Nadeem Tahir, Ali Manzoor, Hussain Abid. A three years prospective study of spinal injuries treated by internal fixation with adjustable titanium cage *J Sheikh Zayed Med Coll* 2010;1:21-7.

[35] Ahmad A. Road Safety in Pakistan.2007 Available from *http://www.unescap.org/ttdw /common/Meetings/TIS/EGM%20Roadsafety%20Country%20Papers/Pakistan_Roadsa fety.pdf* ( Accessed on 18th July, 2011)

[36] Rathore FA, Ayub A, Farooq S, New PW. Suicide bombing as an unusual cause of spinal cord injury: a case series from Pakistan. *Spinal Cord.* 2011; 49:851-4.

[37] Devrajani BR, Ghori RA, Memon N, Memon MA. Pattern of spinal Tuberculosis at Liaquat University Hospital, Hyderabad / *Jamshoro J Liaquat Uni Med Health Sci* 2006;5:33-9.

[38]  Naveed M. *Tuberculosis of spine; Pattern of the disease in PaksitanProfessional Med J* 2001;8:221-5.

[39]  Brohi SR, Memon GN, Brohi AR, Lakhair M, Memon RA. Experience with spinal instrumentation for Tuberculosis spine at PMCH Nawabshah *Med Channel* 2006;12(1):71-4.

[40]  Kahloon AA, Arif H, Baig SM, Khawaja MR.Characteristics of acute transverse myelitis at Aga Khan University Hospital, Karachi. *J Pak Med Assoc.* 2007 Apr;57(4):215-8.

[41]  Hermanus FJ, Draper CE, Noakes TD. Spinal cord injuries in South African Rugby Union (1980 - 2007). *S Afr Med J.* 2010 30;100:230-4.

[42]  Tator CH, Provvidenza C, Cassidy JD. Spinal injuries in Canadian ice hockey: an update to 2005. *Clin J Sport Med.* 2009 ;19:451-6.

[43]  Spinecare Foundation; Australian Spinal Cord Injury Units .Spinal cord injuries in Australian footballers. *ANZ J Surg.* 2003 ;73:493-9.

[44]  Parent S, Dimar J, Dekutoski M, Roy-Beaudry M. Unique features of pediatric spinal cord injury. *Spine* (Phila Pa 1976). 2010 Oct 1;35(21 Suppl):S202-8.

[45]  Parent S, Mac-Thiong JM, Roy-Beaudry M, Sosa JF, Labelle H. Spinal Cord Injury in the Pediatric Population: A Systematic Review of the Literature. *J Neurotrauma.* 2011 Jun 9. [Epub ahead of print]

[46]  Dowler R, Richards JS, Putzke JD, Gordon W, Tate D.Impact of demographic and medical factors on satisfaction with life after spinal cord injury: a normative study. *J Spinal Cord Med.* 2001 ;24:87-91.

[47]  Putzke JD, Richards JS, DeVivo MJ.Predictors of pain 1 year post-spinal cord injury. *J Spinal Cord Med.* 2001 ;24(:47-53.

[48]  Jang Y, Wang YH, Wang JD.Return to work after spinal cord injury in Taiwan: the contribution of functional independence. *Arch Phys Med Rehabil.* 2005;86:681-6.

[49]  Dickson A, O'Brien G, Ward R, Allan D, O'Carroll R.The impact of assuming the primary caregiver role following traumatic spinal cord injury: An interpretative phenomenological analysis of the spouse's experience. *Psychol Health.* 2010 ;25:1101-20.

[50]  Arango-Lasprilla JC, Ketchum JM, Francis K, Premuda P, Stejskal T, Kreutzer J.Influence of race/ethnicity on divorce/separation 1, 2, and 5 years post spinal cord injury. *Arch Phys Med Rehabil.* 2009 ;90:1371-8.

[51]  DeVivo MJ, Hawkins LN, Richards JS, Go BK.Outcomes of post-spinal cord injury marriages. *Arch Phys Med Rehabil.* 1995 ;76:130-8.

[52]  Karana-Zebari D, de Leon MB, Kalpakjian CZ.Predictors of marital longevity after new spinal cord injury. *Spinal Cord.* 2011 ;49:120-4.

[53]  Ramakrishnan K, Mazlan M, Julia PE, Abdul Latif L.Return to work after spinal cord injury: factors related to time to first job. *Spinal Cord.* 2011 Mar 8. [Epub ahead of print]

[54]  Ramakrishnan K, Loh SY, Omar Z.Earnings among people with spinal cord injury. *Spinal Cord.* 2011 May 10. [Epub ahead of print]

[55]  Kazi ZK, Qureshi A.Psychological and social problems of paraplegics in Pakistan. *Paraplegia.* 1972 ;10:107-10.

[56] Waseem H, Naseer R, Razzak JA.Establishing a successful pre-hospital emergency service in a developing country: experience from Rescue 1122 service in Pakistan. *Emerg Med J.* 2011; 28:513-5.

[57] Ali M, Miyoshi C, Ushijima H.Emergency medical services in Islamabad, Pakistan: a public-private partnership. *Public Health.* 2006 ;120:50-7

[58] Dai LY, Jiang LS, Jiang SD.Conservative treatment of thoracolumbar burst fractures: a long-term follow-up results with special reference to the load sharing classification. *Spine* (Phila Pa 1976). 2008 1;33:2536-44.

[59] Weninger P, Schultz A, Hertz H.Conservative management of thoracolumbar and lumbar spine compression and burst fractures: functional and radiographic outcomes in 136 cases treated by closed reduction and casting. *Arch Orthop Trauma Surg.* 2009 Feb;129(2):207-19.

[60] Hoque MF, Grangeon C, Reed K Spinal cord lesions in Bangladesh: an epidemiological study 1994 - 1995. *Spinal Cord.* 1999 ;37:858-61

[61] Iwegbu CG.Traumatic paraplegia in Zaria, Nigeria: the case for a centre for injuries of the spine. *Paraplegia.* 1983 ;21:81-5.

[62] Idowu OK, Yinusa W, Gbadegesin SA, Adebule GT.Risk factors for pressure ulceration in a resource constrained spinal injury service. *Spinal Cord.* 2011 May;49(5):643-7.

[63] Germing A, Schakrouf M, Lindstaedt M, Grewe P, Meindl R, Mügge A.Do not forget the distal lower limb veins in screening patients with spinal cord injuries for deep venous thromboses. *Angiology.* 2010 ;61:78-81.

[64] [1] Sugimoto Y, Ito Y, Tomioka M, Tanaka M, Hasegawa Y, Nakago K, Yagata Y.Deep venous thrombosis in patients with acute cervical spinal cord injury in a Japanese population: assessment with Doppler ultrasonography. *J Orthop Sci.* 2009 ;14:374-6.

[65] Furlan JC, Fehlings MG.Cardiovascular complications after acute spinal cord injury: pathophysiology, diagnosis, and management. *Neurosurg Focus.* 2008;25(5):E13.

[66] Bagaria V, Modi N, Panghate A, Vaidya S. Incidence and risk factors for development of venous thromboembolism in Indian patients undergoing major orthopedic surgery: results of a prospective study. *Postgrad Med J* 2006; 82: 136–139

[67] Kalstky AL, Armstrong MA, Poggi J. Risk of pulmonary embolism and/or deep vein thrombosis in Asian Americans. *Am J Cardiol* 2000; 85: 1334–1337.

[68] Aito S, Abbate R, Marcucci R, Cominelli E. Endogenous risk factors for deep-vein thrombosis in patients with acute spinal cord injuries. *Spinal Cord* 2007; 40: 627–631.

In: Epidemiology of Spinal Cord Injuries
Editors: V. Rahimi-Movaghar, S. B. Jazayeri et al.

ISBN: 978-1-61942-894-2
©2012 Nova Science Publishers, Inc.

*Chapter 16*

# PATTERN OF SPINAL CORD INJURY IN FIJI ISLANDS IN OCEANIA

## *Jagdish C. Maharaj*

Lourdes Hospital & Community Health Service, Dubbo NSW, Australia

## ABSTRACT

Spinal cord injuries also afflict inhabitants of Oceania islands countries and territories. Selected data from the region is presented. Fiji has a well developed healthcare sector with post-acute rehabilitation of all spinal cord injury (SCI) being provided at the rehabilitation hospital.

The incidence of new SCI admitted to the rehabilitation hospital was 18.7 per million population per year comprising 53.6% traumatic and 46.4% non-traumatic causes. The incidence varied according to gender and ethnicity with Fijian males being at the highest (41.85) risk. Among traumatic SCI, 38.7% were due to falls, 25.3% motor vehicle accidents, 20% sports, 8% shallow water dive and 4% each deep sea diving and others, whereas among non-traumatic SCI, 52.3% were due to unknown causes, 32.3% infections, 9.2% neoplasms and 6.2% others. The male/female ratio was 4:1. The 16-30 year age group accounted for 35% of SCI. 31% had tetraplegia and 52.1% had complete lesions.

The subset of the sample that experienced traumatic SCI were more likely to be employed, aged between 16-30 years at the time of injury and to sustain complete tetraplegia. Those who experienced incomplete paraplegia were more likely to be unemployed, aged 46-60 years and educated to primary level at the time of injury. There was a high proportion of complete spinal lesion when compared with other studies. The incidence of secondary complications such as pressure sores and UTI were also found to be high when compared with other studies.

The data support the view that young Fijian males are most prone to sustaining traumatic spinal cord injury, and that there is a high incidence of secondary preventable complications.

**Keywords:** Spinal cord injury, Fiji Islands, Oceania, epidemiology, aetiology, incidence

# INTRODUCTION

Spinal cord injury results in profound and long-term disability or death. It is one of the most catastrophic lesions suffered by modern man, often leading to permanent paralysis. Spinal cord injury is defined here as traumatic or non-traumatic lesion of the spinal cord resulting in any degree of sensory or motor loss or bowel or bladder dysfunction. Multiple medical, social and vocational complications affect the victims who usually are young and in their most productive stages of life. This causes burden and suffering not only to the victim but to their families, to the healthcare system and to the community as a whole. The humanitarian and financial cost and implications of spinal cord injury are enormous. Sir George Bedbrook reiterated that "although spinal medicine has made much advances persons afflicted with injury (traumatic or non-traumatic) of the spinal cord origin constitute a major area of disability in every country and were neglected by most communities until the mid forties (and later) of last century, and this disability is today still the greatest handicap man can sustain" [1]. Some low income countries and regions within countries are still not able to sufficiently care for persons with spinal cord injury.

During years of experience in the Oceania region, the author observed a high incidence of spinal cord injuries of both traumatic and non-traumatic aetiologies, causing many young person's to suffer extensive disabilities and sometimes death. Often limited personal as well as community resources results in further activity limitations and participation restrictions. Although the aetiology of spinal cord injuries varies from population to population within countries and between countries, it is observed that trauma probably accounts for most of the spinal cord injury. It is important to have detailed knowledge of the pattern of spinal cord injury and its sequelae to be able to best prevent such conditions. This chapter discusses available spinal cord injury data from the Oceania island countries and territories.

# OCEANIA REGION

The Oceania region in the western Pacific is one of the largest and most diverse regions in the world. The 36 million people of the Oceania region are scattered across one-third of the earth's surface with 96% of the area being sea in the form of the Pacific Ocean. Although there are some similarities, the cultural and economic variation across the Oceania region is as diverse as the nations are dispersed. Some of the country specific socio-demographic characteristics are provided below. Oceania encompasses Australasia (Australia and New Zealand) and the Pacific Islands (Melanesia, Micronesia and Polynesia). The boundaries of Oceania are essentially political. In the Pacific Ocean it excludes Taiwan, Japan, the Philippines, islands associated with the mainland countries of Asia and the Americas, the western half of the island of New Guinea (claimed successively by Portugal, the Netherlands and Indonesia) and the whole of Indonesia; but does include the French possessions, New Caledonia, French Polynesia (aka Tahiti), Wallis and Futuna Islands. There is a very wide variation in Gross Domestic Product (GDP) per capita ranging from only US$600 for Solomon Islands to US$37,500 for that of Australia. Similarly, the sizes of their national dry landmasses in square kilometres, populations and densities all vary greatly. The continent of Australia alone constitutes nine-tenth of the Oceania's landmass and has the largest population size, but the lowest population density, while Nauru with the smallest landmass has the highest population density. Healthcare delivery services are varied across the Oceania countries and territories.

# FIJI ISLANDS

Fiji is an archipelago of 330 islands of different sizes, some of which are only islets and reefs, scattered in the south western Pacific. Only about 100 of these islands are permanently inhabited while many more are used for planting food crops or as temporary residence. The two principal islands are Viti Levu (covering 10,400 sq km) and Vanua Levu (which is 5,630 sq km). Altogether the archipelago covers an area of about 650,000 sq km, with only 18,272 sq km made up of dry land. Straddling the international dateline and lying between 15 degrees and 22 degrees south of the equator, Fiji lies 3,100 km north east of Sydney, Australia and 2,100 km north of Auckland, New Zealand.

Fiji has a multi-ethnic population. The first inhabitants were Melanesians who are thought to have reached the Pacific by way of New Guinea. It is believed that the Spaniards may have visited it, but the first record of a European sighting of Fiji was that by Abel Tasman in 1643. The first recorded visit to the archipelago was not until 1774 when Captain James Cook anchored off Vatoa Island in southern Lau. Captain William Bligh of HMS *Bounty* made rough charts of most of the islands in 1789, during his epic voyage in a small boat after being cast adrift following mutiny. On 10th October 1874, Fiji became a British colony when it was formally ceded to Britain. The economic development of the island for the next hundred years under British colonization resulted in a multi-ethnic society. In 1879 the first indentured labourers were brought from India to work on the sugar cane plantations. When the indenture system ended in 1916 some 64,000 Indians were brought of which 40,000 chose to stay on after their 5-year work agreements expired. Subsequently Fiji gained independence in 1970. The two main ethnic groups being Fijians and Fiji-Indians, and other ethnic groups include Rotumans, Pacific Islanders, Europeans, part-Europeans, and Chinese. The total population of Fiji at the last census conducted in 2007 was 837,271 [2].

The socio-economic developments have resulted in a rapid increase in the size of urban communities and nuclear families. The shift from an agricultural-based subsistence economy to a cash economy has influenced the lifestyles of many. Accompanied with the economic changes has been the breakdown of the extended family system which was taken for granted in such a culture. Several factors contribute to this vigorous economic climate, not the least of which is the Government's commitment to create and support an export-based economy. Over the years, as a developing country, Fiji has managed to contain most of the infectious diseases through its very successful immunization program, improved hygiene and living conditions, sanitation and water supply. The non-communicable diseases have emerged with their resultant chronic and disabling effects. The gradual ageing of the population also contributes to the emergence of chronic and disabling conditions, changing the disease pattern albeit at a younger age compared to the developed countries. Although Fiji is regarded as a developing nation the disease pattern resembles that of developed nations. Persons who sustain spinal cord injury are usually first admitted to one of the three base hospitals before being transferred to the rehabilitation hospital. The Fiji data presented in the following sections is extracted from previous research [3-4] and updated with local and regional available data from literature excluding Australasia.

## INCIDENCE OF SPINAL CORD INJURY

The incidence of new spinal cord injury admitted to the rehabilitation hospital in Fiji was 18.7 per million population per year. The incidence due to traumatic causes was 10.0 and non-traumatic causes 8.7 per million population per year. Wyndaele and Wyndaele reported the incidence of spinal cord injury between 10.4 and 83 per million inhabitants per year from worldwide literature review [5]. Reviewing publications from 1975 to 1990 Shingu et al reported the incidence of the newly hospitalised patients with traumatic spinal cord injury to range from 9.2 to 53.4 per million population per year [6]. In a study by Lan et al in Hualien county Taiwan, which excluded the patients who died before hospitalisation, the incidence was still very high as 56.1 per million population per year [7]. The incidence of 10.0 for traumatic cases for Fiji lies at the lower end of the 9.2 to 53.4 range with only the incidence of Denmark being less than that of Fiji. The incidence of traumatic spinal cord injury varies from 24 to 50 per million population per year for hospital data to 28 to 54.8 per million population per year when pre-hospital facility figures are included for United States of America (USA) [8]. The incidence in Japan was similar to that of studies from Australia, the Federal Republic of Germany and the USA, which were reported to range from 27.6 to 36.0. The incidence of 8.7 for non-traumatic spinal cord injury is also low compared to that found by Murray and Kusior in a three year retrospective review of 150 cases of new spinal cord injury admitted to hospitals in Monroe county in New York of 23.8 per million population per year due to cancer, 15.2 due to spondylotic myelopathy, 12.9 due to benign tumour, intraspinal abscess, vascular injury, transverse myelitis and epidural haematoma [9]. The authors suggest the differences in the incidence rates to be due to the socio-economic situations in each region as the leading probable cause, with the definition of spinal cord injury and the epidemiological methods used, to at least contribute in part to the differences [9]. The Fiji figures are rehabilitation facility rates which is expected to yield a low incidence as people with spinal cord injury who were referred and admitted to the facility only are taken into account. Those who died pre-hospital reported to be approximately 20% [10] or at the other hospitals before being admitted for rehabilitation are not included. Price et al estimated that the reporting sensitivity of spinal cord injury at hospital level was only 77% in the United States [8]. There is no study from the region to estimate the reporting sensitivity of spinal cord injury at acute hospitals. Thus the true incidence of spinal cord injury could be higher than estimated from this sample.

## CAUSES OF SPINAL CORD INJURY

In Fiji, the traumatic causes accounted for 53.6% and non-traumatic for 46.4% of spinal cord injuries. The combined traumatic and non-traumatic data shows that the most frequent cause of spinal cord injury was from 'unknown causes' 24.3%; followed by falls 20.7%; infectious causes 15.0%; motor vehicle accidents 13.6%; sports injuries 10.7%; shallow water dive and tumours 4.3% each; others (non-traumatic) 2.9% and deep sea diving and others (traumatic) 2.1% each. A different research showed 27.3% traumatic and 72.7% non-traumatic causes of spinal cord injury [9]. This could be explained by the higher mean age of 54.4 ± 21.6 years for their sample. On the other hand, a study of 616 cases with majority in the age group 20-29 years in South Africa showed that 89% were due to traumatic and only 11% non-traumatic causes [11]. In this series, acts of violence had accounted for 55% of the cases. In Denmark, research estimated the incidence of traumatic spinal cord injury of 9.2 per million population per year over a 10 year period from 1975-1984 from rehabilitation hospital data [12]. Among all the spinal cord injuries admitted for rehabilitation 74.4% were newly sustained traumatic and 25.6% were non-traumatic in nature. It is observed that, in Fiji although non-traumatic 'unknown cause' accounted for the highest proportion (24.3%) as a single category, overall, there are more cases of spinal cord injury due to trauma. Falls are the leading cause of traumatic spinal cord injury followed by motor vehicle accidents and sports, whereas infections are second only to 'unknown cause' of non-traumatic spinal cord injury. The following sections provide further analysis of traumatic and non-traumatic causes.

## TRAUMATIC CAUSES

Amongst the traumatic causes the figures show that falls (38.7%) accounted for the highest proportion of traumatic spinal cord injury followed by motor vehicle accidents (25.3%), sports injuries (20%), shallow water dive (8%), deep sea diving (4%) and (4%) other causes. Falls from a height and falls at ground level were not distinguished. Majority of the falls were from breadfruit, mango and coconut trees, and buildings and houses. The status of victims being passenger, driver or pedestrian in motor vehicle accidents was also not distinguished. All the cases resulting from sports were males due to rugby except one that was due to soccer. The shallow water dives were from rivers, sea and swimming pools. All the injury due to deep sea diving comprised of spinal Decompression Sickness from diving for *beche-der-mer* in deep waters with the "Hookah" or scuba diving apparatus. Shingu et al also compared the causes of spinal cord injuries as reported in the literature for the 1975-1990 period for Australia, Florida, and Taipei with that of Japan [6]. They showed that road traffic accident consistently comprised the main cause of spinal cord injury with falls as the next highest cause. Research by Campo da Paz et al [13] in Brazil (traffic accident 41.7%, falls 14.8%), Lan et al [7] in Taiwan (traffic accident 61.6%, falls 23.3%), and Thurman et al [14] in Utah, USA (motor vehicle crashes 49.3%, falls 21.1%) show motor vehicle accidents as the leading cause of traumatic spinal cord injury followed by falls. Other research in India (falls 55.2%, road traffic accidents 12.8%) [15], Nigeria (falls 48%, road traffic accidents 36%) [16] and Romania (falls 59%, road traffic accidents 13%) [17] show falls as the leading cause of spinal cord injury. Okonkwo has suggested that falls from trees in Nigeria may be related to seasonal weakening of the tensile strength of jigs woven from palm fronds and used for climbing palm trees [16]. Fiji has largely an agricultural based economy and an abundance of seasonal fruiting which probably explains the high incidence of spinal cord injury due to falls (38.7%) from trees; and a well developing road network which contributes to motor vehicle accidents (25.3%) as another cause. Other authors have similarly reported spinal cord injury resulting from falls from tress in the Oceania countries including in Fiji [18], Solomon Islands

[19] and other serious injuries in Papua New Guinea [20]. In India falls from a height is reported as the commonest cause of spinal cord injury accounting for 54.8%, followed by road traffic accidents and then farm-related injuries [21]. In general, causes of spinal cord injury probably reflect the state of industrialisation and economic development of a nation.

## SPORTS-RELATED SPINAL CORD INJURIES

Large numbers of the catastrophic cervical spinal cord injuries resulting in tetraplegia or death seemed to be from rugby injuries in Fiji. Rugby is almost exclusively played by native Fijians. An increasing trend of spinal cord injury from rugby union was reported in Fiji [22]. When all the people with spinal cord injury due to rugby, who were admitted to the rehabilitation hospital, are excluded from the calculation, the overall incidence rate for Fijians decreases from 41.85 to 33.48 per million population per year which is less than the rate of 35.93 for all the other ethnic groups combined. Thus just one sport contributed significantly to the incidence of spinal cord injury among Fijians as compared to the other ethnic groups in Fiji. This sample does not include the fatal cases who were not admitted to the rehabilitation hospital, so the actual incidence will be higher. Spinal cord injuries in rugby union has been reported to range from as low as 0.8/100,000 per year for England to a high of 13/100,000 per year for Fiji with other countries falling in between [23]. The author of these figures Fuller, argues that a rate of 0.1-2/100,000 per year is 'acceptable' and 2-100/100,000 per year 'tolerable' for rugby union and suggests that "although catastrophic injuries in rugby union cause public concern and generate strong emotive reactions, the magnitude of society's concern about this type of injury is often dominated by people's perceptions rather than by actual levels of risk" [23].

Cantu and Mueller reported that a total of 128 players incurred permanent cervical cord injuries playing rugby from 1977 through to 1989 with the defensive players being greater at risk for tetraplegia than the offensive players and most injuries happening during tackling [24]. It had been reported that while the incidence of rugby injuries to the cervical spinal cord had dropped in certain countries like the United Kingdom and New Zealand this did not appear to be the pattern in South Africa [25]. Further analysis of 40 rugby players sustaining injuries to the spinal cord during the period 1985 to 1989 the authors found that high tackles and dive tackles were responsible for more cases of complete permanent tetraplegia than the scrum [25]. In a survey of 35 traumatic spinal cord injury patients resulting from sports accidents from 1975 to 1991 and admitted to the Hakone National Hospital in Japan, Noguchi showed that 88.6% were under the age of 30 years, the most common sports was swimming (51.4%) followed by gymnastics (22.8%) and that the injuries were predominantly at the C4-5-6 level [26]. He concluded that the most common factor leading to spinal cord injuries in sports was lack of skill. The increased awareness and rigorous implementations of preventative rules seems to have reduced the incidence of spinal cord injuries happening in sports, including that in Fiji.

## NON-TRAUMATIC CAUSES

Amongst non-traumatic causes of spinal cord injury in Fiji the 'unknown cause' category accounted for the highest proportion of 52.3%. This was followed by infectious causes (32.3%), tumours (9.2%) and (6.2%) for all other non-traumatic causes. Most of the spinal cord injuries from the 'unknown causes' were investigated at the acute hospitals but no aetiology was established. Some of these could have constituted cases of Transverse Myelitis. However, all the infectious cases were established as such. Most of these were epidural abscesses surgically decompressed and confirmed with microbiology. Cases of spinal epidural abscess resulting in spinal cord paralysis are admitted to rehabilitation facility annually. There was an increasing trend over the years of the numbers of spinal cord injury from epidural abscess presenting for rehabilitation reported in Fiji [27]. An increase in epidural abscesses with residual neurological deficits is possibly secondary to increasing intravenous drug abuse and cases of metastatic paraspinal abscess causing paraplegia following simple dental extraction and subsequent bacteraemia from neglected mouth hygiene have been reported in literature [28-29]. Cases of spinal cord injury with paraspinal tuberculosis (Potts Disease) are not an uncommon feature in Fiji. Some were diagnosed as Mycobacterium infection through radiological evidence and concomitant pulmonary disease. If recognised and treated early the prognosis is good. Cases of intramedullary tuberculomas causing spinal cord compression have been reported in young patients of 28.6 years average age and 69% of them having pulmonary tuberculosis [30].

There were other non-traumatic causes of spinal injury that were evident in Fiji. Kippax and Maharaj reported a series of four patients with conversion disorder presenting as spinal cord injury that met the diagnostic criteria of the *Diagnostic and Statistical Manual III* and came from a single hospital (Colonial War Memorial Hospital, Suva, Fiji) within the same year [31]. A twelve month prospective study at the Prince Henry Hospital in Sydney, Australia found a high proportion of 9.8% of acute spinal cord injuries diagnosed as conversion disorder [32]. In this series the mean age was 23 ± 8 years, the male/female ratio 8:1 and more than 50% had a previous history of conversion disorder.

The cases due to tumour included both primary as well as secondary metastatic tumours. Primary intraspinal neoplasm (meningioma being the most common followed by ependymoma and neurilemoma) as well as metastatic diseases results in spinal injury [33-34]. Choucair argued that with advances in cancer therapy and consequent extension of survival, the overall incidence of neurological complications of cancer is on the rise, and that, second to brain metastases, metastasis to the spinal cord and its roots constitute the most common neurological complication of cancer with an estimated 5-10% of patients developing spinal cord involvement that leads to serious impairment of function [35]. The spinal cord dysfunction, while usually nonfatal, leaves the patient with a major neurological disability. In a study of patients with prostate carcinoma and suspected spinal cord compression, 74% were confirmed as having epidural spinal cord compression [36]. All patients were initially treated with radiation, steroids and androgen deprivation therapy. Overall, 27% had recurrent compression and the average survival of patients who either presented with paraplegia or in whom paraplegia developed secondary to recurrent spinal compression was 3.9 months versus 18 months for the group as a whole. A retrospective research of 253 cases in Senegal over 16 years (January 1972 to December 1987) revealed extradural compression in 65% with secondary cancer of the spine and epiduritis followed by extramedullary intradural cause (70 cases) [37]. This was predominantly in men aged between 40 and 50 years.

Howlett et al studied an epidemic of spastic paraparesis, similar to that caused by Human T-cell lymphotropic virus type I (HTLV-1), affecting 39 cases aged 4 to 46 years with uniform clinical findings of abrupt and permanent but not progressive damage to the upper motor neurons in a drought-affected rural area of Tarine district in northern Tanzania [38]. The authors report that due to the failure of other crops, the diet at the onset of paraparesis consisted almost exclusively of bitter cassava roots, a drought-tolerant starchy root crop widely cultivated in Africa. It is believed that high levels of dietary cyanide exposure which, was confirmed by very high serum levels of thiocyanide was the causative agent. Tests for HTLV-1 antibodies were negative. Cassava root is a common food crop utilised in Fiji and the Pacific Islands.

## AGE-RELATED DIFFERENCE

The age at the onset of spinal cord injury in Fiji ranged from 6 to 76 years with a mean of $38.3 \pm 17.3$ years. The mean age for males was 38.7 and that of females was 37.0 years. Other studies reported age range from 6 to 56 years with a mean of $30.3 \pm 1.1$ years and 75.9% cases were in the 11 to 40 year age group in Brazil [13], whereas in Japan the age ranged 6 to 96 years with a mean of $48.3 \pm 19.5$ years with males $48.3 \pm 19.6$ and females $49.2 \pm 19.3$ years [6]. The rate of spinal cord injury in different age groups in Fiji was as follows: 0-15 years: 5.7%; 16-30 years: 35%; 31-45 years: 24.3%; 46-60 years: 22.1% and 61+ years: 12.9% . The age group 16-30 years accounted for highest proportion of people with spinal cord injury for both genders. The age group 16-45 years accounted for 59.3% of all people with spinal cord injury. There was a significant association ($p<0.001$) between age and causes of spinal cord injury with the younger age group more likely to sustain traumatic and the older age group non-traumatic spinal cord injury.

Haffner et al in a review of 277 patients under the age of 16 years admitted to the Pediatric spinal injury unit at Rancho Los Amigos Medical Center, USA from 1960 to 1989 found that complete and incomplete injuries were about equal and that the aetiology of the most recent 5 year period had changed to a more violent nature like gunshot wound [39]. On the other hand, research of 62 consecutive acute spinal cord injury patients who were aged 55 years and older compared to 296 spinal cord patients of age less than 55 years found that there were more incomplete tetraplegic patients (63%), significantly more females (29%) and with pre-existing medical conditions (87%) and associated injuries (55%) [40].

In Fiji the 0-15 year age group had 62.5% affected by infectious causes. The 16-30 year age group has a bi-modal pattern with sports and falls accounting for 24.5% of people with spinal cord injury each. In the age group 31-45 years 23.5% were due to motor vehicle accidents, 17.6% from falls followed closely at 14.3% each for infection and 'unknown causes'. The 'unknown causes' accounted for the highest proportion of 38.7% and 35.5% in the 46-60 and 61+ year age groups respectively. The 16-30 year age group accounted for 50.7% of traumatic causes and 46-60 year age group for 35.4% of non-traumatic causes of spinal cord injury. There is a definite pattern to aetiology and incidence associated with age.

# GENDER AND ETHNICITY

The rate of spinal cord injury varies according to gender and ethnicity. With Fiji being a multi-ethnic nation, an ethnic breakdown of people with spinal cord injury is presented. There were 80% male and 20% female with spinal cord injury, the male/female ratio being 4:1 in Fiji. This ratio is similar to that reported in the literature from Taiwan and South Africa (4:1), Brazil (3.9:1) and Turkey (11:3) [7,11,13,41]. Eighty seven percent male and 13% female had traumatic while 72% male and 28% female non-traumatic spinal cord injury. Fijian males had the highest rate of 41.85 per million population per year followed by 35.93 for males of other races, 19.91 for Fiji-Indian males, 12.34 for Fijian females, 11.18 for other females and 3.47 for Fiji-Indian females. There were twice as many Fijian males and more than three times Fijian females compared to that of Fiji-Indians.

The unadjusted available data shows that there were 64.3% Fijians, 29.3% Fiji-Indians, and 6.4 % others who sustained spinal cord injury. There were equal numbers of Fijians with spinal cord injury due to traumatic and non-traumatic causes each. There were almost twice the number of Fiji-Indians with spinal cord injury due to traumatic compared with non-traumatic causes. Fijians had the highest incidence followed by other ethnic groups and Fiji-Indians. Fiji has a unique ethnic mix and only a couple of studies found in the literature reported the ethnic difference in the incidence. Dixon et al from New Zealand reported that although spinal cord injury occurs most often in young Caucasian as a result of motor vehicle accidents, ethnicity adjusted rates showed high rates for Maori males [42] and in Oklahoma, USA report stated that spinal cord injury among blacks (as compared to the whites) as a result of violence, was "remarkable" [8]. The authors suggest that more complete reporting of spinal cord injury among blacks than among whites could account for some discrepancy as violence related spinal cord injury is more completely reported and that socio-economic status may have a role. There is no study from a similar ethnic mix to Fiji to compare with. Nonetheless, in Fiji, the nature of activities of different ethnic groups could possibly explain the differences in incidence rates.

# EDUCATIONAL, OCCUPATIONAL AND MARITAL STATUS

The majority of the people with spinal cord injury (61.4%) had primary school level education, 28.6% secondary and only 10.0% had tertiary level of education at the time of injury in Fiji. There was a significant association between level of education and whether the spinal cord injury was due to traumatic or non-traumatic cause. Campo da Paz et al found that in Brazil majority of spinal cord injury in their sample had "lower education level", whereas DeVivo et al studying the trend in USA from 1973 to 1986 showed that the incidence of spinal cord injury had increased significantly amongst high school graduates [13,43]. They suggested that this trend could be due to increase in average age at injury.

The occupational status of persons sustaining spinal cord injury in Fiji at onset showed that 17.1% were students, 30.0% were employed, 42.1% were unemployed and 10.7% had retired. The significant association (p<0.001) of occupational status and whether the spinal cord injury was due to traumatic or non-traumatic cause could be a reflection of age distribution related to occupation. A research from Romania reported that 40% of the patients were manual workers, 12% intellectuals and 18% retired [17]; and from Turkey report stated that the highest incidence was amongst housewives, followed by agricultural workers and private industry workers with the agricultural workers' wives group most at risk [41]. Again these proportions may be explained by national proportions of the variable.

At the time of spinal cord injury in Fiji 59.3% were married, 37.1% (including children and adolescents) were never married and 3.6% were widowed at the time of injury. A follow up study of spinal cord injuries in Iceland found that 35.6% were married before injury [44] and in a large USA research for trend between 1973 and 1986 found that an average of 54.3% were single at the time of the injury [43]. The USA sample had a lower mean age of 29.5 years compared to that of Fiji sample of 38.3 years.

## NEUROLOGICAL LEVEL OF LESION

There were 30.7% spinal cord injury above the first thoracic nerve (T1) resulting in tetraplegia/paresis and 69.3% below T1 resulting in paraplegia/paresis. The figures show that there was only 0.7% with high (C1-4) level tetraplegia, 30.0% with low level (C5-T1) tetraplegia/paresis and amongst the paraplegic/paretic 10.0% were with high thoracic (T2-6) level, 37.9% lower thoracic (T7-12) level and 21.4% lumbosacral (L-S) level spinal cord injury admitted for medical rehabilitation in Fiji. The percentages of tetraplegics and paraplegics vary in different reports from only 8.1% tetraplegics and 91.9% paraplegics in Turkey [41], 28% and 72% in Nigeria [16], 38% and 62% in Spain [45], 51% and 49% in Denmark [12] to 71.7% and 28.3% in Naples, France [46]. DeVivo et al reported a slightly increasing percentage of tetraplegics in a multi-centre study in the USA [43]. There was a significant association (p<0.001) between the level of the lesion and whether the lesion was due to traumatic or non-traumatic cause. Tetraplegia is more likely to result from trauma. The ratio of tetraplegia to paraplegia seems to be related to the cause of injury and will be affected by the survival rate of high tetraplegics in different healthcare settings.

## COMPLETENESS OF LESION

In Fiji, 52.1% sustained complete and 47.9% incomplete spinal cord injury. There was a 2.23 times higher risk of having a complete lesion due to traumatic causes. There was no significant association between the completeness and level of the lesion, however was significantly associated (p<0.01) with whether the lesion was caused by trauma or non-trauma. Again the ratio of complete to incomplete lesions, vary in the literature. Different reports in literature indicate 50% each; 72.8% and 27.2%; 48% and 52%; 43.4% and 56.6%; and 8% and 92% complete and incomplete spinal cord lesions respectively [12,15,39,42,47]. Completeness of the lesion seems to be related to the cause of injury with complete lesions more likely to result from trauma. Immediate first aid and pre-hospital care as well as the acute management must play a role in preserving or sparing of neurological function. This could be an area for further investigation and intervention as an incomplete lesion indicated a better survival rate and higher rehabilitation potential.

# MEDICAL COMPLICATIONS

Medical complications related to spinal cord injury are not uncommon. The secondary medical complications can consume extensive resources, delay rehabilitation and cause further impairments and activity limitations. Maynard reported 67% of traumatic spinal cord injured developed spasticity with 37% needing antispasticity medication [48]. There can be increased participation restrictions due to depression and psychological distress in the spinal cord injured 2 to 7 years since injury [49]. Heterotopic ossification is shown to occur in the more severely neurological injured and young at the rate of up to 20% [50]. In a follow up self-reported study (1973-1989) in Iceland of 59 spinal cord injury patients comprising 55.6% tetraplegic and 44.4% paraplegic, the most common complications were pain (64.4%), urinary tract infection (UTI) (62.2%), spasticity (60%) and pressure sores (58%) [44]. The incidence of non-traumatic shoulder pain and associated disability during the first 18 months after spinal cord injury was found to be 78% in tetraplegics and 35% in paraplegics in the first six months [51]. When re-examined 6 to 18 months later 33% of the tetraplegics and 35% of the paraplegics continued to have pain. The functional limitations resulting from the shoulder pain was not a significant problem for the paraplegics; however, 84% of the tetraplegics having pain had either moderate or severe functional disability during the first six months after spinal cord injury, and this impairment persisted in patients with shoulder spasticity at follow-up evaluation between six and 18 months post injury.

In Fiji 29.3% of people with spinal cord injuries were free from any complications and the rest of the 70.7% were admitted to rehabilitation with various complications. These included 15% pressure sores alone, 5.7% urinary tract infection (UTI) alone, 2.9% spasticity alone and total of 47.1% had combinations of multiple medical complications. Several authors report varying incidences of these complications [11,13,15,17,44,45]. The most consistent of these seem to be pressure sores and urinary tract infection followed by respiratory infection, spasticity, pain and others. Jackson et al in a study of 261 patients from 1985 to 1990 from five Model Regional Spinal Cord Injury Care Systems in the USA showed that 67% experienced respiratory complications. Of these 36.4% had atelectasis, 31.4% pneumonia and 22.6% ventilatory failure within an average of 15.6 days post injury [52]. In the Fiji research there was a highly significant association (p<0.001) between completeness of the lesion and the presence of complications. The most commonly reported complications of pressure sore and urinary tract infection are largely preventable and every effort should be made to prevent these from developing in acute, rehabilitative as well as after care phases.

# NEUROLOGICAL/FUNCTIONAL IMPROVEMENT

On discharge from rehabilitation 31.4% of people with spinal cord injury were found to have had neurological/functional improvement compared with their admission status and the rest of 68.6% remained the same. Biering-Sorenson et al reported that 41% of traumatic spinal cord injury patients had an improvement in their neurological status after their admission to rehabilitation hospital [12]. Fiji data demonstrated a significant association (p<0.001) between improvement and completeness of the lesion with incomplete lesions 19 times more likely to show improvement. There was no significant association between neurological/functional improvement and whether the spinal cord injury was due to traumatic or non-traumatic cause. Ditunno et al in a study of 150 motor complete tetraplegic subjects recruited within one week of their injuries showed that the pattern of recovery in the key muscles of the 67 subjects with some motor power in the zone of partial preservation (incomplete lesion) was significantly (p<0.001) greater than the 83 subjects with no motor power (complete lesion) at three to six months post injury [53]. It has been demonstrated that although the motor recovery rapidly declined in the first 6 months and then subsequently plateaued, 4% showed "late conversion" (more than 4 months after injury) from complete to incomplete spinal cord injury status [54-55]. Hart and Williams reported recovery in 42% of their sample with stab wounds and non-traumatic lesions showing better rates of recovery than motor vehicle accidents and gunshot wounds [11]. This is probably related to the extent of tissue damage caused by different aetiological agents. Although prevention is better than cure, when spinal cord injury does occur it is most important to have first aid, pre-hospital and acute care facilities geared towards preserving whatever neurological sparing that may be present as an incomplete lesion has a much greater chance of neurological/functional recovery than a complete lesion.

# MORTALITY

The mortality rate of spinal cord injured persons admitted to the rehabilitation hospital in Fiji was 10.7% which is similar to that reported in literature [7] and compared to an 8% mortality rate in Oklahoma, USA [8]. The mortality subgroup comprised of 93% complete lesion, 60% paraplegics, equal proportions of traumatic and non-traumatic spinal cord injuries, majority male and Fijians in the older age group. Soopramanien noted a mortality rate of 22% in 1985-1991 period decrease to 10.1% in 1992 in Romania [17]. In Fiji and as reported in the literature majority of the deaths were due to renal, pulmonary and pressure sore complications. Elderly (61+ years) Fijians with complete injury were at the highest risk of mortality from spinal cord injury.

# CONCLUSION

The overall incidence of spinal cord injury in Fiji is 18.7 per million population per year with Fijian males (41.85) being at the highest risk. Spinal cord injury due to rugby football injuries accounted for this high rate among young Fijian males. The highest proportion of injury is among the 16 to 30 year age group for both gender and persons with only primary level education, married and unemployed at the time of injury. Age (p<0.001), gender (p<0.03), level of education at the time of injury (p<0.001), occupational status at the time of injury (p<0.001), level of spinal lesion (p<0.001), completeness of lesion (p<0.01) and complications (p<0.06) were significantly associated with whether the cause of injury was traumatic or non-traumatic, whereas ethnicity (p<0.30), marital status (p<0.37) and neurological/functional improvement (p<0.87) were not. Improvement in neurological /functional state (p<0.001) and the incidence of complications (p<0.001) were both significantly associated with completeness of the lesion.

There was a higher incidence of complete spinal cord lesions as compared to some other reports in the literature. The true incidence of complete lesions could be even higher when the samples for pre-hospital and acute hospitals are taken into account. Methods aimed at reducing complete lesions by improving immediate first-aid, pre-hospital and acute medical care are important as incomplete spinal cord lesions have a much better survival and rehabilitation potential.

The incidence of some preventable secondary complications such as pressure sores and urinary tract infection are also high, further increasing impairments, activity limitations and mortality. These and other complications of spinal cord injury must be prevented to reduce impairments and activity limitations and improve survival.

Most of the data discussed is from a medical rehabilitation facility sample thus reflecting the characteristics of only the people with spinal cord injury who are admitted for rehabilitation. It is likely that the picture would be different when pre-hospital and acute hospital data were taken into account. Nonetheless, this accurately reflects the population of people with spinal cord injury in Fiji who survive and utilise medical rehabilitation health services and are re-integrated back into the community.

In this region, apart from the Australasian countries, there seems to be scarcity of spinal cord injury research data from the smaller Oceania countries.

# REFERENCES

[1]     Bedbrook, G. M. (1987). Keynote Address. In W. Refshauge (Ed.), Towards Prevention of Spinal Cord Injury - *The Menzies Foundation Technical Report (No. 1, 9-12). Melbourne.* The Menzies Foundation.

[2]     Fiji Islands Bureau of Statistics. (2008). 2007 Census of Population and Housing. Fiji Islands Bureau of Statistics, *Statistical News* No 45.

[3]     Maharaj, J. C. *Pattern of Spinal Cord Paralysis in Fiji: A descriptive analytical ten year (1985-1994) retrospective study. Masters (MPH) thesis 1995.* University of New South Wales, Sydney.

[4]     Maharaj, J. C. (1996). Epidemiology of spinal cord paralysis in Fiji: 1985-1994. *Spinal Cord*, 34, 549-559.

[5]     Wyndaele, M. & Wyndaele, J. J. (2006). Incidence, prevalence and epidemiology of spinal cord injury: what learns a worldwide literature survey? *Spinal Cord*, 44, 523–529.

[6]     Shingu, H., Ikata, T., Katoh, S. & Akatsu, T. (1994). Spinal cord injuries in Japan: a nationwide epidemiological survey in 1990. *Paraplegia*, 32, 308.

[7]     Lan, C., Lai, J. S., Chang, K. H., Jean, Y. C. & Lien, I. N. (1993). Traumatic spinal cord injury in rural region of Taiwan: an epidemiological study in Hualian County, 1986-1990. *Paraplegia*, 31, 398-403.

[8]     Price, C., et al. (1994). Epidemiology of Traumatic Spinal Cord Injury and Acute Hospitalisation and Rehabilitation Charges for Spinal Cord Injuries in Oklahoma, 1988-1990. *American Journal of Epidemiology*, 139(1), 37-47.

[9]     Murray, P. K. & Kusior, M. F. (1984). Epidemiology of nontraumatic and traumatic spinal cord injury, *Arch Phys Med Rehabil*, 65, 634.

[10]  Sekhon, L. H. S. & Fehlings, M. G. (2001). Epidemiology, demographics, and pathophysiology of acute spinal cord injury. *Spine*, 26(24S), S2-S12.

[11]  Hart, C. & Williams, E. (1994). Epidemiology of spinal cord injuries: a reflection of changes in South African society. *Paraplegia*, 32, 709-714.

[12]  Biering-Sorensen, E., Pedersen, V. & Clausen, S. (1990). Epidemiology of spinal cord lesion in Denmark. *Paraplegia*, 28(2), 105-18.

[13]  Campos da Paz, A., Beraldo, P. S. S., Almeida, M. C. R. R., Neves, E. G. C., Alves, F. & Khan, P. (1992). Traumatic injury of the spinal cord. Prevalence in Brazilian hospitals. *Paraplegia*, 30, 636-640.

[14]  Thurman, D. J., Burnett, C. L., Jeppson, L., Beaudoin, D. E. & Sniezek, J. E. (1994). Surveillance of spinal cord injuries in Utah, USA. *Paraplegia*, 32, 665-669.

[15]  Chacko, V., Joseph, B., Mohanty, S. P. & Jacob, T. (1986). Management of spinal cord injury in a general hospital in rural India. *Paraplegia*, 24, 330-335.

[16]  Okonkwo, C. A. (1988). Spinal cord injuries in Enugu, Nigeria - preventable accidents. *Paraplegia*, 21, 12-18.

[17]  Soopramanien, A. (1994). Epidemiology of spinal injuries in Romania. *Paraplegia*, 32, 715-722.

[18]  Gupta, A. & Reeves, B. (2009). Fijian seasonal scourge of mango tree falls. *ANZ Journal of Surgery*, 79, 898–900. doi: 10.1111/j.1445-2197.2009.05141.x

[19]  Mulford, J. S., Oberli, H. & Tovosia, S. (2001). Coconut palm-related injuries in the pacific islands. *ANZ Journal of Surgery*, 71, 32–34. doi: 10.1046/j.1440-1622.2001.02021.x

[20]  Barss, P., Dakulala, P. & Doolan, M. (1984). Falls from trees and tree associated injuries in rural Melanesians. *Br Med J (Clin Res Ed)*, 289, 1717. doi: 10.1136/bmj.289.6460.1717.

[21]  Singh, P. K., Shrivastva, S. & Dulani, R. (2011). Pre-hospital care of spinal cord injury in a rural Indian setting. Rural and Remote Health [Online serial], 11(1760). (Accessed 20 June, 2011). Available from: *http://www.rrh.org.au*

[22]  Maharaj, J. C. & Cameron, I. D. (1998). Increase in spinal injury among rugby union players in Fiji [letter]. *Med J Aust.*, 168, 418.

[23]  Fuller, C. W. (2008). Catastrophic Injury in Rugby Union: Is the Level of Risk Acceptable? *Sports Medicine*, 38(12), 975-986.

[24]  Cantu, R. C. & Mueller, F.O. (1990). Catastrophic spine injuries in football (1977-1989). *Journal of Spinal Disorders*, 3(3), 227-31.

[25]  Scher, A. T. (1991). Catastrophic rugby injuries of the spinal cord: changing patterns of injury. *British Journal of Sports Medicine*, 25(1), 57-60.

[26]  Noguchi, T. (1994). A survey of spinal cord injuries resulting from sports. *Paraplegia*, 32, 170-173.

[27]  Maharaj, J. C. (2002). "Dramatic increase in incidence of Spinal Epidural Abscess in Fiji: a 10 year survey". International Spinal Cord Society Australasian Branch Conference 2002 - "Total Care" *An Interdisciplinary Approach Proceedings*, Auckland, New Zealand.

[28]  Weingarden, S. I. & Swarczinski, C. (1991). Non-granulomatous spinal epidural abscess : a rehabilitation perspective. *Paraplegia*, 29(9), 628-31.

[29]  Larkin, E. B. & Scott, S. D. (1994). Metastatic paraspinal abscess and paraplegia secondary to dental extraction. *British Dental Journal*, 177(9), 340-2.

[30] MacDonnell, A. H., Baird, R. W. & Bronze, M. S. (1990). Intramedullary tuberculomas of the spinal cord: case report and reviews. *Reviews of Infectious Diseases, 12*(3), 432-9.

[31] Kippax, D. & Maharaj, J. C. (1986). Conversion disorder presenting as spinal cord injury or disease. *Fiji Medical Journal, 14*(1&2), 13-16.

[32] Dickson, H., Cole. A., Engel, S. & Jones, R.F. (1984). Conversion reaction presenting as acute spinal cord injury. *Medical J. of Aust., 141*, 427-429.

[33] Helseth, A. & Mork, S. J. (1989). Primary intraspinal neoplasms in Norway, 1955 to 1986. A population-based survey of 467 patients. *Journal of Neurosurgery, 71*(6), 842-845.

[34] Stanley, P. & Suminski, N. (1988). The incidence and distribution of spinal metastases in children with posterior fossa medulloblastoma, *American Journal of Pediatric Hematology-Oncology, 10*(4), 283-7.

[35] Choucair, A. K. (19991). Myelopaties in the caner patient: incidence, presentation, diagnosis and management. Part 1 (Review). *Oncology, 5*(6), 71-80.

[36] Smith, E. M., Hampel, N., Ruff, R. L., Bodner, D. R. & Resnick, M. I. (1993). Spinal Cord Compression Secondary to Prostate Carcinoma: Treatment and Prognosis. *The Journal of Urology, 149*, 330-333.

[37] Ndiaye, I. P., Ndiaye, M. M., Gueye, M., Mauferon, J. B., Kone, S. & Gueye, L. (1989) Etiological spects of non-tubercular spinal cord compression in Senegal (report of 253 cases). *Dakar Medical, 34*(1-4), 64-7.

[38] Howlett, W. P., Brubaker, G. R., Mlingi, N. & Rosling, H. (1990). Konzo, an epidemic upper motor neuron disease studied in Tanzania. *Brain, 113*(Pt 1), 223-35.

[39] Haffner, D. L., Hoffer, M. M. & Wiedbusch, R. (1993). Etiology of children's spinal injuries at Rancho Los Amigos. *Spine, 18*(6), 679-84.

[40] Roth, E. J., Lovell, L., Heinemann, A. W., Lee, M. Y. & Yarkony, G.M. (1992). The older adult with spinal cord injury. *Paraplegia, 30*(7), 520-6.

[41] Dincer, F., Oflazer, A., Beyazova, M., Celiker, R., Basgoze, O. & Altioklar, K. (1992). Traumatic spinal cord injury in Turkey. *Paraplegia, 30*, 641-646.

[42] Dixon, G. S., Danesh, J. N. & Caradoc-Davies, T. H. (1993). Epidemiology of spinal cord injury in New Zealand. *Neuroepidemiology, 12*(2), 88-95.

[43] DeVivo, M. J., Rutt, R. D., Black, K. J., Go, B. K. & Stover, S. L. (1992). Trends in Spinal Cord Injury Demographics and Treatment Outcomes Between 1973 and 1986. *Arch Phys Med Rehabil, 73*, 424-30.

[44] Knutsdottir, S. (1993). Spinal cord injury in Iceland 1973-1989. A follow up study. *Paraplegia, 31*, 68-72.

[45] Garcia-Reneses, J., Herruzo-Cabrera, R. & Martinez-Moreno, M. (1991). Epidemiological Study of Spinal Cord Injury in Spain 1984-1985. *Paraplegia, 28*, 180-190.

[46] Palma, V., et al. (1992). Spinal cord injury: some epidemiological data. A review of 233 cases. *Acta Neurologica, 14*(1), 29-38.

[47] Kiwerski, J. E. (1993). The causes, sequelae and attempts at prevention of cervical spine injuries in Poland. *Paraplegia, 31*, 527-533.

[48] Maynard, F. M., Karunas, R. S. & Waring, W. P. (1990). Epidemiology of spasticity following traumatic spinal cord injury. *Arch Phys Med Rehabil, 71*(8), 566-9.

[49] Tate, D., Forchheimer, M., Maynard, F. & Dijkres, M. (1994). Predicting Depression and Psychological Distress in Persons with Spinal Cord Injury based on indicators of Handicap. *Am J Phys Med Rehabil*, 73, 175-183.

[50] Wittenberg, R. H., Peschke, U. & Botel, U. (1992). Heterotopic ossification after spinal cord injury. Epidemiology and risk factors. *Journal of Bone & joint Surgery - British Volume*, 74(2), 215-8.

[51] Silfverskiold, J. & Waters, R. L. (1991). Shoulder Pain and Functional Disability in Spinal Cord Patients. *Clinical Orthopaedics and Related Research*, 272, 142-5.

[52] Jackson, A. B. & Groomes T. E. (1994). Incidence of Respiratory Complications Following Spinal Cord Injury. *Arch Phys Med Rehabil*, 75, 270-5.

[53] Ditunno, J.F., Stover, S.L., Freed, M.M. & Ahn, J.H., Motor Recovery of the Upper Extremities in Traumatic Quadriplegia: A Multicenter Study, *Arch Phys Med Rehabil* 73:413-6 (1992).

[54] Waters, R. L., Yakura, J. S., Adkins, R. H. & Sie, I. (1992). Recovery Following Complete Paraplegia. *Arch Phys Med Rehabil*, 73, 784-9.

[55] Waters, R. L., Adkins, R. H., Yakura, J. S. & Sie, I. (1994). Motor and Sensory Recovery Following Incomplete Tetraplegia. *Arch Phys Med Rehabil*, 75, 306-11.

In: Epidemiology of Spinal Cord Injuries
Editors: V. Rahimi-Movaghar, S. B. Jazayeri et al.

ISBN: 978-1-61942-894-2
©2012 Nova Science Publishers, Inc.

*Chapter 17*

# REVIEW OF EPIDEMIOLOGY OF ADULT AND PEDIATRIC SPINAL CORD INJURY IN SOME SELECTED COUNTRIES FROM ALL OVER THE WORLD

*Mohammad R. Rasouli[1], Seyed Behzad Jazayeri[2], Amirali Sayadipour[1] and Alexander R. Vaccaro[1]*

[1] Department of orthopedic surgery, Rothman Institute of orthopedics,
Thomas Jefferson University, Philadelphia, PA, US
[2] Sina Trauma and Surgery Research Center,
Tehran University of Medical Sciences, Tehran, Iran

## INTRODUCTION

In this chapter, the available literature is reviewed on epidemiology of spinal cord injuries (SCI) from countries that have not been covered in other chapters. The epidemiology of SCI in pediatrics based on available evidence is also appraised.

## EUROPE

The incidence of SCI in Western Europe is 16 per million; which is slightly higher than Australia (15 per million) and much lower than North America (39 per million). Motor vehicle accidents (MVA), mainly four-wheeled, are the major cause of SCI in these regions. However, other etiologies of SCI vary between these areas. The highest rate of fall etiology is seen in the Western Europe (37%); probably resulting from older population of Western Europe. Australia (20%) and North America (20%) follow with respect to incidence of fall-related SCI. Incidence of SCI resulting from violence/ self-harm is estimated to be 6% in Western Europe and 2% in Australia versus 15% in North America. [1] Figure 1 displays incidence of SCI in some European countries. The epidemiology of SCI in selected European countries is further delineated.

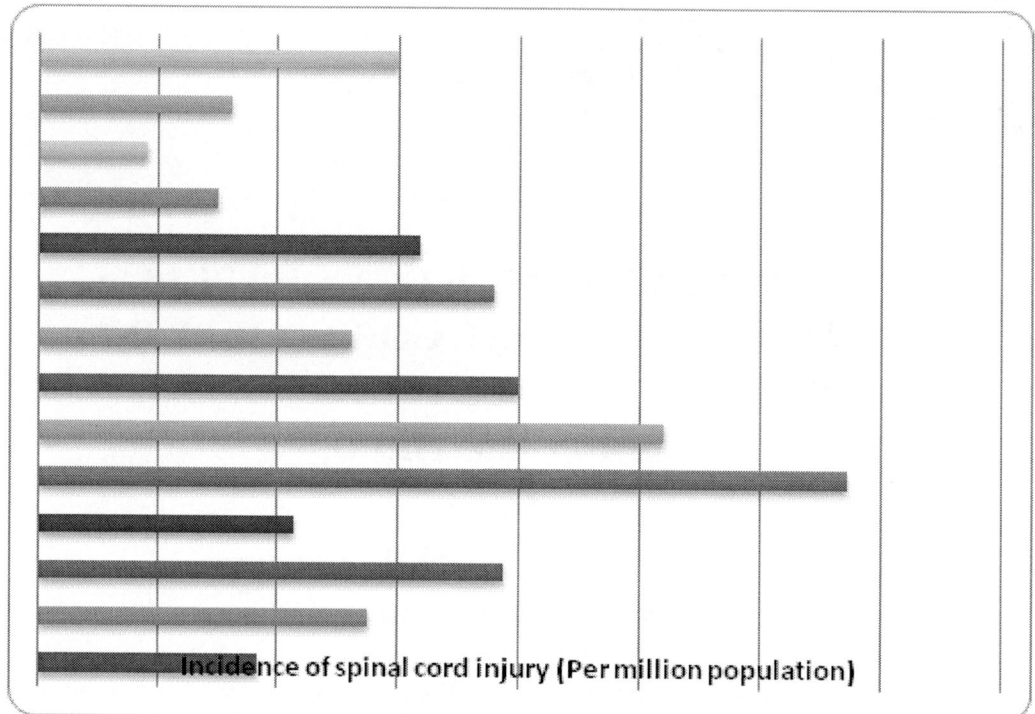

* Incidences varies in different reports. The numbers in the figure are based on the paper by Cripps et al.

Figure 1. Incidences of spinal cord injury in selected European countries. [1]

## Denmark

The annual incidence of SCI was estimated to be 9.2 cases per million during 1975-1984. [2] The etiological range was MVA (47%), falls (23%), attempted suicides (8%), shallow water diving (6%) and sporting accidents (6%). Among cases with traumatic SCI, 40% were sustained at 15-24 years of age. Incomplete tetraplegia was the most common form of SCI at 29% followed by 26% motor complete paraplegia, 23 % incomplete paraplegia, and 22% motor complete tetraplegia. There was a decreasing trend in number of MVA-related SCI with the introduction of general speed limits and seat belt regulations.

## Estonia

During 2003 to 2007, the annual incidence of SCI in Estonia was estimated at 27.9 cases per million population; 83.2% of cases were male. [1] Falls (42%), MVA (27%), sports/recreation (15%), violence (4%) and self harm (1%) were known causes of SCI. SCI resulted in 50.2% tetraplegic and 49.8% paraplegic.

## Greece

In a study conducted by Divanoglou and Levi in Thessalonik, the annual incidence of SCI was estimated at 33.6 per million during 2006 to 2007. [3] This study only included cases older than 15 years who survived 7 days after the initial injury. Annual age-adjusted and gender-adjusted incidences were calculated as 33.6 and 33.2 per million. Among the 81 enrolled cases, 71 subjects (88%) were male. The mean age was 43 years with standard deviation of 19. The age distribution was >40% ages 16–30, 11% ages 31–45, 27% ages 46–60, 16% ages 61–75 and 5% in the > 75 year age group. MVA was the most common cause of SCI and was responsible for 51% of injuries. Fall (37%), sports/ recreation (4%) and violence (2%) followed. SCI resulted in 48% tetraplegic and 52% paraplegic.

In another study carried out at Chios island of Greece, SCI cases were included from the capital and 52 villages. [4] The study included both traumatic and non-traumatic cases with 67.6% male and a mean age of 43 years. MVA was the most common cause of SCI (44.8%) followed by work-related accidents. The level of SCI was also classified, with thoracic-lumbar injuries as the most frequent at 23.5% of cases, followed by thoracic (20.6%), lumbar (14.7%) and lumbar-sacral (14.7%).

## Greenland

Greenland is the world's largest island and is an autonomous country within the Kingdom of Denmark. In the study performed by Pedersen et al. during the 22-year period from 1965 to 1986, 27 patients (20 males) with SCI from Greenland were admitted to the department of neurosurgery at a hospital in Copenhagen, Denmark. [5] Fall and attempted suicide were major causes of SCI and were observed in 9 and 7 cases; accidental gunshot trailed. Two thirds of the patients were paraplegic and one third were tetraplegic; 13 cases were complete SCI. The authors concluded that it is difficult to precisely estimate incidence of SCI in Greenland. However, by considering the 27 SCI admissions during 22 years and population of about 50,000, they estimated an annual incidence of 26 per million for Greenland, which was relatively high compared to other reports.

## Iceland

In a study during the time period from 1973 to 1989, a questionnaire was sent to 59 out of 79 patients with SCI in Iceland. [6] Of these 59 cases, 55 (76.3%) including 29 males answered the questionnaire. Among these subjects, 55.6% and 44.4% were quadriplegic and paraplegic and 29% had a complete SCI. The most frequent age group was 21-30 followed by ages 10-20. Pain 64.4%,, urinary tract infection (UTI) 62.2% and spasticity 60% were the most common complications. Twenty-four cases were wheelchair-bound, and 50% cases developed pressure ulcers. According to this study, the annual incidence of SCI in Iceland was estimated to be 316 per million. [1]

## Ireland

During 2000, a study was performed at Ireland's National Spinal Cord Injury Centre to examine the epidemiology of SCI. [7] Forty-six patients (40 males) with SCI were admitted with a median age of 37 years, range 6 to 82 years. MVA was the most frequent cause of SCI at 50%, followed by falls and sport injuries which were observed in 37% and 9% of cases. There were no injuries caused by assaults or gunshot wounds. Cervical and thoracic SCI were found in 23 and 19 cases. The American Spinal Injury Association (ASIA) class breakdown was 18 A, 8 B, 5 C, and 15 D. According to this study, the annual incidence of SCI in Ireland estimated to 13.1 per million.

## Poland

In a study conducted by Jankowski et al. from 1979 to 1992, 511 cases of spinal injury including 449 males were evaluated.[8] MVA (41%), sports/recreation (19%) and work-related injuries (15%) were common causes of injuries. SCI resulted in 50.3% tetraplegic and 49.7% paraplegic. According to other reports, it appears that falls from a horse cart and diving were frequent causes of SCI; particularly injuries of cervical spine. [9, 10] Kiwerski reported that predictors of mortality in patients with SCI in Poland were: the level and degree of the spinal cord lesion, etiology, advanced age, associated injuries and type of treatment. [9]

## Portugal

Martins et al. assessed the epidemiologic pattern of SCI in the central region of Portugal between 1989 and 1992.[11] During the study period, 398 new cases of SCI were identified which provided an annual incidence rate of 57.8 per million; this study included pre-hospital fatalities. The mean age of cases was 50 (range 1 to 92 years) and 77% were male. MVA and fall were responsible for 57.3% and 37.4% of SCI. Neurological lesion was complete in 220 cases (55.6%) and incomplete in 176 cases (44.4%). The annual rate was 25.4 new cases per million.

## Romania

In retrospective (1975-1991) and prospective (1992-1993) studies conducted at Bucharest, 262 patients with SCI were evaluated with a male-to-female ratio 3.3. [12] The annual incidence of SCI was 17.3 per million. Falls were the most common etiology at 59% followed by MVA (13%) and diving accidents (7%). Frankel classification was used to assess the severity and neurological level of the injury: 33% grade A, 6% grade B, 6% grade C, 18% grade D and 37% grade E. SCI resulted in 53% complete and 47% incomplete injuries. The level of injury distribution was 40% thoracolumbar and 60% cervical.

## Russia

Unfortunately there are few articles on the epidemiologic properties of spinal cord injuries (SCI) in Russia. The majority of the papers are in Russian, and only one detailed article of SCI epidemiology is available in English. Below is the summary of two full texts and one abstract. Although this chapter is based on limited data, it can represent enough demographic properties of three largest cities of Russia: Moscow, Saint Petersburg and Novosibirsk (table 1).

**Table 1. Epidemiologic data of Moscow, Saint Petersburg and Novosibirsk**

|  | Novosibirsk [14] | Saint Petersburg [15] | Moscow [13] |
|---|---|---|---|
| Incidence (per million) | 29.7 | 44 | - |
| Male | 21.8 | 30.5 | - |
| Female | 7.9 | 13.5 | - |
| Male/Female | 78.1%/21.9% | 69.4%/30.6% | 84%/16% |
| Mean age (years) |  | - | 30.8±11.5 |
| Male | 34.7 |  | ? |
| Female | 32.3 |  | ? |
| Etiology |  | - |  |
| Traumatic | 26.7% |  | 100% |
| Non-traumatic | 73.3% |  | - |
| Site of injury |  | - |  |
| Cervical | 49% |  | 48% |
| Thoracic | 27.5% |  | ? |
| Lumbar | 23.5% |  | ? |

### 1. Moscow

In Moscow, the largest city of Russia, the epidemiologic data of 50 SCI patients referred to a rehabilitation center after 12.36±15.45 months following SCI is documented. However, it is not mentioned whether this is the first course of rehabilitation or if there had been an earlier rehabilitation program as well. Data representing the number of staff providing care for the patients is shown in table 2. There were no social workers or psychologists in the treatment team.

**Table 2. Staff data of Moscow rehabilitation center**

| Staff | Positions | Positions per bed |
|---|---|---|
| Physicians | 6 | 0.13 |
| Nurses | 20 | 0.44 |
| Nurses' aids | 6 | 0.13 |
| Physiotherapists | 2 | 0.04 |
| Occupational therapists | 5 | 0.11 |

The Hospital in Moscow, compared to the hospitals in Lithuania, Denmark and Israel, was been more crowded and staffed with fewer providers with less training and less rehabilitation equipment. However, the hospital was equipped with a unique neurostimulator and special equipment for prevention of bedsores.

The patients were referred to the rehabilitation center with the following goals:

1. Restoration of impaired function that can be achieved during a predetermined limited rehabilitation period.
2. Voiding by trigger or Crede maneuver or by contracting abdominal muscles.
3. Maximal mobility that can be achieved during a predetermined limited rehabilitation period.

As shown in table 1, the mean age of the patients was 30.8±11.5 years, including 42 males and 8 females. All patients had history of traumatic SCI. Of the patients, 76% had grade A, 4% grade B, 2% grade C and 18% grade D on the American Spinal Injury Association impairment scale (AIS).

The average length of stay was 46.92±20.50 days. After the hospital stay, 56% of patients were discharged home, 26% to nursing home, and the others (18%) were discharged to another hospital or institution. Neurological improvement of at least one AIS grade was observed in 16%, and useful recovery, upgrading from AIS grade A, B or C at admission to D or E at discharge, was detected in 5%. In addition to less staff and equipment, injuries were more severe in Moscow compared to Lithuania, Denmark, and Israel, with 76% of patients grade A at admission. As such, the useful recovery rate of only 5% could be expected in advance. [13]

## 2. Novosibirsk

Novosibirsk, with population of around 1.5 million, is the third largest city in Russia after Moscow and Saint Petersburg. The department of Spine and Spinal Cord Injuries (SCI) of Novosibirsk was founded in 1989.

In a study during the first five years after creating the SCI center, data were collected and reported by Silberstein. [14] Two hundred and eight cases of SCI were recorded in their database between 1989 and 1993. Based on the population of Novosibirsk at that time (1.4 million), the incidence of SCI was about 29.7 per million. The injuries were frequently seen in males with a male to female ratio of 3.5 to 1. The mean age of injured males was 34.7 and 32.3 in females. Fall from a height (40.4%) and traffic injuries (25.1%) were the most common causes of injury. Diving was also a common cause in young patients, accounting for 23.2% of cases. The other etiologies included sports injuries (gymnastic and wrestling), stab wounds, and shotgun injuries. Alcohol abuse was detected in 20.3% of males and 9.3% of females at the time of injury. The most common types of lesions were wedge-shaped fractures and fracture-dislocations, and the most common site of injury was the cervical spine (49%). Injuries to C3-7 were 5.4 times more frequent than C1-2 injuries. Thoracic injuries had occurred in 27.5% and lumbar injuries in 23.5% of cases. Of the patients who died, 84% had cervical injuries at the C4 or above, and there was a 16.8% mortality rate associated with SCI. In a comparison to other countries at the time of study, patients of Novosibirsk were much younger. This may have been due to the low number of recorded cases or because of different SCI etiologies in Novosibirsk: about half of the cases were due to sports injury and diving, activities in which a younger population tends to participate. On the other hand, traffic injuries, a main cause of SCI in other countries, were less common in Novosibirsk. This may be explained by the low per capita number of cars in Russia at that time. Additionally, Russia had a speed limit 60 KmH$^{-1}$ and no high speed motorways. Generally, older people are more likely to be injured in traffic accidents, and Russian life expectancy is lower than other countries such as Japan. Both of these factors may have contributed to the lower average age of SCI patients in Russia. [14]

### 3. Saint Petersburg

There is a short report of SCI incidence in Saint Petersburg from 1994 to 1996 which reported an SCI incidence of 44 cases per million. [15]

In conclusion:

- Russian SCI patients are young.
- Traffic accidents, although a major cause of SCI, are not as common of an etiology as in other countries.
- Most Russian SCI etiologies are traumatic.
- Russian patients suffer from more severe SCI.
- Although about half of the patients returned to home after rehabilitation, the other half still needed to be discharged to a nursing home or other hospital.

## Spain

An epidemiologic study was performed in Spanish hospitals during 1984 to 1985; 1100 SCI cases (both traumatic 61% and non-traumatic) were evaluated. [16] Based on this study, the annual incidence for traumatic SCI is 0.8 per 100,000. The average age of individuals was 41 years and the highest incidence of SCI was between 20 and 30 years. Males comprised 72% of cases. MVA was the most frequent cause of SCI followed by falls.

Van Den Berg reported the epidemiologic pattern of SCI in Arago´n, Spain during 1972 to 2008. [17] A total of 540 SCI cases were identified over the 36-year study. Crude annual incidence rates of SCI per million were calculated as 8.2 during 1972–1980, 13.8 during 1981–1990, 12.9 during 1991–2000, and 13.4 during 2001–2008. Mean age of cases was 39.6 years with standard deviation of 17.7 and males comprising 79% of cases. The two peak age ranges were 20 to 29 years and 60 to 69 years. MVA was the most common cause of SCI and was responsible for 57% of lesions however, in cases older than 60 years, fall was the most common etiology of SCI. Thoracic (37.4%) and cervical (36.9%) lesions were the most prevalent levels of injury. ASIA grade A was most commonly observed.

## Switzerland

In a study conducted by Gehrig and Michaelis in Switzerland which covered the time period from 1960 to 1967, 584 cases (461 males) with SCI were evaluated. [18] An annual SCI incidence of 15 per million was estimated in Switzerland based on this study. MVA (36%), work-related injuries (35%) and sports/recreation (19%) were common causes of injuries. SCI resulted in 33% tetraplegic and 66% paraplegic.

## PEDIATRIC SCI IN EUROPE

Results of a survey performed in 19 European countries, showed that pediatric SCI is rare in Europe. [19] The study demonstrated the incidence of pediatric SCI in Portugal (27/million children/year) and Sweden (4.6/million children/year). Fatal injuries were included in the calculation of these incidences. The estimated incidence of pediatric SCI in other countries without considering fatal injuries varied from 0.9 to 21.2/million children/year in the age group of 0–14 years.

In a study conducted by Martin et al., the UK Trauma Audit and Research Network Database was utilized to identify children with spine injury during 1989 to 2000. [20] Within the trauma registry there were 527 cases of spine fracture/ dislocation (2.7%) and 109 cases (0.56%) of SCI; 16.5% of spine fractures had SCI. Spinal cord injury without radiological abnormality (SCIWORA) was found in 30 children, constituting 0.15% of all trauma cases and 4.5% of spine injuries.

## ASIA

### Afghanistan

A study conducted in two towns of Afghanistan (Kabul and Herat), estimated the incidence of SCI as 128.5/million and 108.7/million[21]. Incidence rates of SCI were 59/million for Enjeel and 100/million for Gozara, two rural regions of Herat. Males comprised 90% and 94% of cases in Kabul and Herat with a mean age of 25 ±11.5 and 28 ±12.4 years. In Kabul, 7% of lesions were cervical while the corresponding percent in Herat was 6%. In each town, 80% of lesions were complete.

Pressure ulcers (30% in Kabul and 43% in Herat), contractures (41% in Kabul and 54% in Herat), spasticity (58% in Kabul and 41% in Herat), pain (77% in Kabul and 56% in Heart), spine deformity (35% in Kabul and 32% in Herat), recurrent UTI (49% in Kabul and 76% in Herat), constipation (70% in Kabul and 80% in Herat), negative feelings (61% in Kabul and 51% in Herat) and dissatisfaction with sex (71% in Kabul and 74% in Herat) were reported as secondary complications.

### Bangladesh

In a prospective study conducted at a rehabilitation center from January 1994 to June 1995, 179 patients with traumatic SCI were included with a male-to-female ratio of 7.5. Fall from height was the most common cause of SCI (43%) followed by fall while carrying heavy load (20%) and MVA (18%). SCI resulted in 40% tetraplegic and 60% paraplegic. In traumatic cases, the most common injury levels were C5 and T12/L1. Development of pressure ulcers was the major cause of delay in discharging from the center.

## China

In a retrospective study carried out from 1982 to 2002 in Beijing, 1079 were estimated to have a SCI which provided an incidence of 60.6 per million. [22] The previous reported incidence, between 1982 and 1986, was 6.7 per million. The mean age of patients was 41 years with a male to female ratio of 3.1. Fall from height (37.5%), MVA (26.9%), struck by object (16.3%) and fall on ground (8.3%) were common causes. The proportion of cervical, thoracic and lumbar injuries was 4.9%, 28.0% and 65.9%.

According to another study which was performed in Tianjin from 2004 to 2008, the incidence of SCI was estimated as 23.7 per million. [23] The male to female ratio was 5.6:1 and the mean age was 46± 14.2 years. Falls were the leading cause of SCI and MVA was next. The lesion level was cervical in 71.5%, thoracic in 13.3% and lumbosacral in 15.1%. The frequency of tetraplegia (71.5%) was higher than paraplegia (28.5%).

## Japan

In the study conducted by Ide and colleagues during 1988 to 1989 in Okayama prefecture, the annual incidence of SCI was estimated at 28.6 per million.[24] The majority of cases (45 out of 55) were male. In this small study, work-related injuries were the leading cause of SCI(38%), followed by MVA (33%) and fall (16%). SCI resulted in 69% tetraplegia and 31% paraplegia.

Based on a survey performed on traumatic SCI in all 47 prefectures of Japan from January 1990 to December 1992, 7471 cases with neurologic deficits (Frankel A-D) were identified that provided an incidence of 40.2 per million.[25] The incidences of SCI were estimated to be 39.4/million during 1990, 40.1/million during 1991 and 40.2/million during 1992. The mean age was 48.6 years and ranged from 11 months to 96 years. Two peaks in age distribution were found; 59 (main peek) and 20 year. The male to female ratio was 4.1. A cervical lesion was found in 75% of cases. MVA was the leading cause of SCI and was observed in 43.7% of cases followed by falls from height, which occurred in 28.9%. Frankel grade A was the most frequent observed grade of injury at 25.8%, followed by E (23.8%) and C (20.3%).

In another study, which was carried out at the National Rehabilitation Center for the Disabled, 1047 patients with SCI (both traumatic and non-traumatic) who were treated during a 15-year period from 1980 - 1994 were evaluated. [26] The % of male patients was 88.3%. Mean age was 33 years with standard deviation of 13.3. MVA including motorbike accidents (28%) and car accidents (16.9%) was the most common etiology followed by falls and sports injuries. The level of injury was: cervical (35.5%), thoracic (52.2%) and lumbar (12.3%). Complete cervical SCI was seen in 68.8% of cervical cases.

## Jordan

In a study performed at Amman, capital of Jordan, and covered the time period from 1988 to 1993, 151 SCI cases admitted to a hospital were reviewed. [27] Mean age was 33 and 85.4% were male. MVA was the leading cause of SCI (44.4%) followed by ballistic injuries

(25.8%) and falls (21.2%). There were 31.8% cervical SCI's, and 68.2% thoraco-lumbar injuries. These injuries resulted in 68% paraplegic and 32% tetraplegic (n=103). The annual incidence of SCI was estimated to be 18 per million.

## Kuwait

In a retrospective study conducted at Physical Medicine and Rehabilitation Hospital from1991 to 1999, 90 patients were included with male-to-female ratio 7.1. [28] The incidence of SCI was 7.8 per million. MVA was the most common etiology accounting for 63.3% followed by fall from height (24.7%), hit by falling object (6.7%), diving (2.2%), and stabbing (2.2%). The severity of the injury was determined as: 29% grade A, 22.7% grade B, 38.3% grade C, and 9.9% grade D. There were 56.02% paraplegic and 43.98% tetraplegic. UTI was the most common complication (60%) followed by digestive complications (18%), pressure ulcer (16%), autonomic dysreflexia (4%), deep vein thrombosis (4%), ectopic ossification (4%) and respiratory complications (3%).

## Qatar

In a retrospective study conducted at a hospital from 1987 to 1996, 75 patients were included with male-to-female ratio 8.3. [29] Annual incidence of SCI was 12.5 per million. MVA was the leading cause of SCI accounting for 72% of injuries, followed by fall (13.3%), falling heavy object (9.3%) and penetrating wounds (2.7%). The severity of SCI was 58.7% complete injury and 41.3% incomplete injury. Thoracolumbar and cervical SCI were found in 42.7% and 57.3%.

## Nepal

In a study by Mukhida and colleagues, pediatric cases with acute neurological trauma admitted to a teaching hospital in Katmandu between 2001 and 2004 were reviewed. [30] Among 416 children with neurotrauma, only 4% had spinal injuries. Lumbar fractures were observed in 47% of spinal injuries while cervical trauma was responsible for 35% of spinal injuries. ASIA grade of A, B, C, D, and E were observed in 24, 6, 12, 29, and 24% of cases. Vertebral fracture and subluxation were detected in 59% and 6% of cases; the cause of injury was not specified in the remaining cases. The leading etiology for neurological injuries was falls at 61%. MVA's were responsible for increasing the proportion of injuries in school-aged children; the majority of these cases were pedestrians.

## Saudi Arabia

In two separate reports, Al-Jadid et al. evaluate quality of life in males and females with SCI in Saudi Arabia [.31, 32] In the first study that covered a 20-year time period, 57 males with SCI were evaluated. The most frequent age groups were 21-30 years and 31-40 years. [31] The lesion was cervical in 43.9%, thoracic in 40.35% and lumbar in 23.5% of cases. The most common lifetime complication was UTI (80.7%) and followed by pressure ulcers (50.9%). In the second study that covered the same period of time, 50 females with SCI were evaluated. [32] The most frequent age groups were the same as the preceding study. The majority of injuries were at the thoracic level (82%). Lifetime complications of recurrent UTI (80%) and pressure ulcer (76%) were also seen.

## Singapore

In a prospective study carried out at four main hospitals during a 2-year period, 70 patients were enrolled. [33] More than 50% of cases were in the age group of 15 to 35 year. Male to female ratio was 9. The incidence of SCI was 13.7%. The two most common causes of SCI were MVA (34.3%) and industrial accident (34.3%) followed by domestic accident (18.6%), crime (7.1%) and sports injuries (5.7%). In elderly patients, cervical spine injuries were more common while younger patients had more frequent thoracolumbar injuries.

## South Korea

In a study conducted at a rehabilitation hospital in South Korea, 590 patients with traumatic and non-traumatic SCI's were admitted during the time period from 1987 to 1996. [34] There was a male predominance of 79.6% with the most common age group of 20 to 29 years. The majority of cases were traumatic SCI (91.2%) and among all etiologies, MVA and fall accounted for 57.6% and 26.4% of cases. With regard to the type of SCI, 20.5% had complete tetraplegia, 23.9% had incomplete tetraplegia, 38.8% had complete paraplegia and 16.5% had incomplete paraplegia. In tetraplegics, incomplete injuries increased from 40% during 1987-1991 to 56.7% during 1992-1996. The authors concluded that the incidence of SCI resulting from MVA and sports, as well as the incidence of female incomplete injuries were increasing.

## Thailand

A retrospective study was carried out at Siriraj Hospital in Bangkok from 1989 to 1994. [35] Records on 219 SCI patients were reviewed. Male to female ratio was 5.6. The annual incidence of SCI was reported as 5.8 per million, however, another study from Thailand that covered the time period from 1985 to 1991 in Chiang Mai, estimated the annual incidence of SCI as high as 23 cases per million. [36] MVA was the leading cause of SCI and was responsible for 51% of injuries followed by fall (30.6%), assault (8.2%) and hit by moving objects (7.8%). Another study conducted later from 1997 to 2000, showed that MVA related SCI increased and was responsible for 74.7% of injuries followed by falls accounting for 16.9% SCI. [37] There were 49.8% thoracolumbar injuries while 50.2% were cervical injuries. The leading cause of death was respiratory complications in 89% of cases. [35]

## Taiwan

Multiple studies have been carried out to determine the epidemiologic pattern of SCI in Taiwan. [38-40] A retrospective study was performed during the time period from 1986 to 1990 in four local general hospitals in Hualien county, Taiwan. During the study period, 135 traumatic SCI patients were identified which provided an estimated annual incidence of 56.1 per million. The male to female ratio was 4:1 and mean age of male patients was lower than female patients (44 vs. 46 years). There were 36 tetraparetic, 33 tetraplegic, 12 paraparetic and 18 paraplegic patients. MVA was the major cause of injury in 61.6% of SCI's while accidental falls were responsible for 23.3% of SCI. [39]

Based on another study conducted by Chen et al., the annual incidence of SCI in Taiwan was estimated to be 18.8 per million population. In the geriatric population, the estimated incidence was much higher at 47.7 cases per million.[38] Tetraplegia was more common in geriatrics (54.1% versus 42.8%) while paraplegia was more prevalent in young cases (57.2% versus 45.3%). MVA etiology was more frequent in young individuals compared to geriatrics (49% versus 33%) whereas fall related SCI was more common in geriatrics than younger subjects (62% versus 41%).

More recently, Yang et al. used the National Health Insurance database to calculate annual incidence of hospitalized acute spinal trauma during 2000 to 2003 in Taiwan. [40] The study calculated average incidence of hospitalized acute spinal trauma including both injuries with or without neurologic deficits as 61.61 per 100,000 population. Figure 2 demonstrates percent of SCI cases in various groups of spine fractures based on the study by Yang and colleagues. [40] In that study, there was a decreasing incidence of spine fractures with neurological deficit compared to spine fractures without neurological deficit.

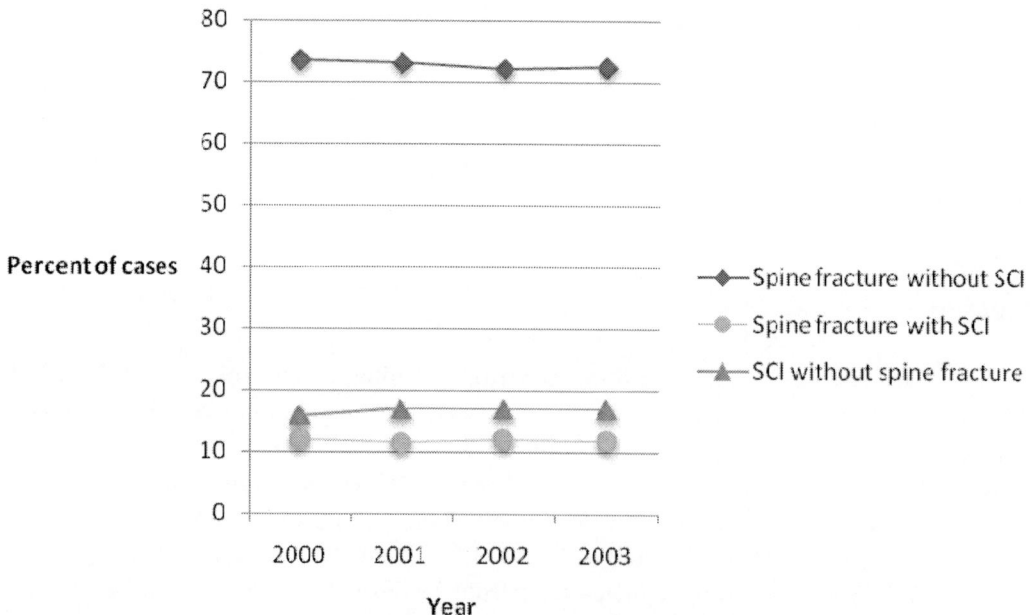

Figure 2. Percent of cases in various groups of spine fracture and spinal cord injury (SCI) [37].

## Vietnam

Prevalence of SCI in Vietnam was estimated to be 464 per million during 2006-2007. [1]

# AFRICA

## Nigeria

In a retrospective study conducted at a teaching hospital from 2004 to 2006, 71 patients were included with a male to female ratio of 2:1.[41] The most common cause was MVA accounting for 51% of patients followed by fall (30.6%), violence (8.2%), hit by moving objects (7.8%) and other (1.4%). Within these cases, 23.7% were tetraplegic, 28.8% were paraplegic, 21% were paraparetic and 26.5% were tetraparetic. In another prospective study conducted at Calabar University between 2005 to 2006 the male to female ratio was 4:1 and the number of MVA related SCI was significantly higher (85.7%).[42] The most frequent site of injury was lumbar (43%). Associated injuries were limb, head and rib fracture, splenic rupture, bowel injury and soft tissue laceration. The most common complication was pressure ulcer (29%) followed by paralytic ileus (14.3%), hyperpyrexia (7%), UTI (21.4%), respiratory difficulty (7%) and loss of sexual function (male impotence) (7%).

## South Africa

In a retrospective study from 1988 to 1992, 551 patients were included with a male to female ratio of 3.4:1. [43] The estimated annual incidence of SCI in South Africa was 48.5 per million. Gunshot injuries were the leading cause of SCI (35%) followed by MVA (30%) and stab wounds (26%). The study showed a shift from stab wounds to gunshot injuries during these years. The level of injury was cervical in 26%, thoracic in 59% and lumbar in 15% of cases. Of these SCI's 9.7% and 90.3% were tetraplegic and paraplegic.

In another study that covered the time period of 1988 to 1993, 492 males and 124 females were evaluated. [44] The most frequent age group was 20-29 years. Gunshot injuries were the most cause of SCI (36%), followed by MVA (25%), stab wounds (20%) and falls from heights (2.4%). There were 25% and 75% tetraplegic and paraplegic cases. In South Africa, there is a disproportionately high incidence of violent injuries as the cause of SCI, particularly in terms of gunshot wounds, compared to other countries.

## Sierra Leone

A SCI epidemiology study was conducted in Sierra Leone, one of the poorest countries in the world. [45] During an 18-month period, 24 patients (22 males and 2 females) were evaluated. Average age of the patients was 30 years (range 4 to 55 year). Complete and partial SCI were found in 21 and 3 cases. MVA was the most frequent cause of SCI (12 cases) followed by fall from tree (10 cases) and crush by collapsed wall (2 cases). Seven patients died during hospitalization. Of 17 cases discharged from the hospital, 12 had thoracolumbar injury and 5 had cervical injuries. Of the survivors, 13 out of 17, were followed for an average of 17.4 (range 10 to 28) months after discharge. During the follow up period, only 5 cases were still alive.

## Zimbabwe

In a prospective study conducted at a National Rehabilitation Center from 1988 to 1994, 136 patients were included with a male to female ratio 9:1.[46] The most common cause of SCI was MVA (50%) followed by assault (11%) and falls (11%). Tetraplegia and paraplegia were found in 51% and 49% of cases. Cervical SCI occurred in 59%. The authors stated that problems in hospital nursing resulted in increasing number of pressure ulcer, UTI and chest infections that caused a high mortality rate.

# CARIBBEAN

## Haiti

The pattern of SCI in Haiti is unknown with the only knowledge found in reports from the 2010 earthquake. However, it is fair to expect that the epidemiologic profile of SCI in Haiti is similar to other developing countries.[47] Haiti is the poorest country in the Western Hemisphere and due to lack of health care facilities it is expected that severe SCI cases die during the first years after SCI.[47] It is estimated that the earthquake killed 250,000 to 300,000 people and resulted in 100 to 150 cases of new SCI in Haiti.[47]

# AUSTRALASIA

## Australia

In the study conducted by O'Connor, Australian SCI registry data was used to determine the incidence of SCI in Australia. [48] The age adjusted rate of persisting SCI was 14.5 per million. As expected, young adults and males had higher rates of SCI. 93% of cases were resulted from unintentional injuries and MVA was responsible for 43% of injuries. Incomplete cervical SCI was the most common type of injuries (38% of cases). These injuries mainly resulted from MVA and low falls.

In another study carried out by Walsh, prevalence of SCI in Australia was determined to be 370 cases per million in 1987.[49] O'Connor also estimated prevalence of SCI in Australia based on "historical data" on survival of SCI victims during 1986–1997. [50] According to this study, prevalence of SCI in Australia was estimated to be in the range of 8096 to 9614 cases by 1985, which increased to about 10,000 in 1997. If this trend remains unchanged, the number of SCI cases is predicted to increase to about 12,000 by 2021. However, the prevalence of SCI in Australia was estimated by Yeo et al. as 540 per million in 1998.[51]

Regarding pediatric SCI, a retrospective review was performed on spinal injuries in 340 children from 2 hospitals in Sydney which showed SCI occurred in 5.6% of cases. [52] MVA was found to be the leading cause of severe spinal injuries. Cervical spine was reported as the most common site of injury. The upper cervical spine was the most common level of serious spinal injuries in younger children. The 0 to 4 year and 9 to 12 year age groups had the highest (47%) and lowest (19%) percents of serious injuries. In the serious spinal injuries, 56% of cases were male however, in cases were younger than 13 years, the gender distribution was equal.

## New Zealand

Annually, 70 to 80 New Zealanders have a SCI resulting in varying degrees of paralysis with two-thirds of them trauma related. [53] By considering the small population of New Zealand, it seems this country has one of the highest rates for SCI among Western countries. [54] Dixon et al. used the Health Statistics Services files of New Zealand for the year 1988 to determine the epidemiology of SCI.[54] It is estimated that the annual incidence of SCI is 49.1 per million. The study demonstrated that SCI occurs more frequently in young, Caucasian men compared to other groups. MVA was the leading cause of SCI. The results of this study showed that compared to American children, in New Zealand the risk of pediatric SCI is 4 times greater. In this study, 92% of SCI's were incomplete and the number of cervical injuries increased.

# OCEANIA

## Fiji Islands

In a retrospective study carried out at a medical rehabilitation unit in the Fiji Islands from 1985 to 1994, 75 patients with traumatic SCI were included with a male to female ratio 6.5. [55] Annual incidence of SCI was 10 cases per million. Fall was the most common etiology accounting for 38.7% of injuries followed by MVA (25.3%) and sport injuries (20%). The severity of SCI was determined by the ASIA classification; 53% and 47% of cases were tetraplegic and paraplegic. There were 46.7% thoracic or lumbar SCI and 53.3% cervical SCI. Pressure ulcer, UTI and spasticity were the most common complications and were detected in 15%, 5.7% and 2.9% of cases. 47.1% of patients had multiple complications and 29.3% of cases had no complications.

# SURVIVAL AFTER SCI

Compared to developing countries, survival of cases with traumatic SCI has improved significantly in developed countries particularly for individuals with tetraplegia. One-year mortality rate following SCI is the highest in developing countries. [1]

The age at the time of injury, neurological level, extent of lesion and year of injury have been determined as predictors of survival following SCI. Among secondary complications, respiratory system failure is the leading cause of death. [56]

# PEDIATRIC SCI

Results of a systematic review by Parent et al. showed that SCI is relatively rare in pediatrics. [57] According to this systematic review, the following information can be obtained about pediatric SCI:

- Using the National Pediatric Trauma Registry over a 10-year period, Patel et al. found the overall incidence of 1.5% for cervical spine injury in pediatrics [58]
- In the study by Apple et al. 88 cases (5%) out of 1,770 pediatric injuries had SCI [59]
- Level of injury varies based on age. In pre-teen groups, C2 lesions are observed more frequently than teen group in whom C4 injuries are more common
- In younger children, MVA is the major cause of SCI while in adolescents, injuries occur mainly during sports activities [60]
- SCI seems to occur more frequently in males than females
- All-terrain vehicles are responsible for a higher injury rate in children compared to adults
- Incidence of SCIWORA was estimated to be 6% in a level I pediatric center [61]
- Neurologic recovery following SCI is better in pediatric than adults however, development of scoliosis is more frequent in pediatric group

# CONCLUSION

It should be stated that some of the studies that were used for writing this chapter were not solely designed to determine the epidemiologic pattern and incidence of SCI. Therefore, reported incidences in some countries might not be accurate. Moreover, some of these studies only reported epidemiology of SCI from a specific region of a country that might not reflect national epidemiologic patterns of SCI in those countries. Although epidemiologic patterns of SCI varies in developing and developed countries, it can be concluded that young adult males are more vulnerable to SCI. MVA and fall are the two leading causes of SCI. Among secondary complications, it appears pressure ulcer, UTI and respiratory complications are major complications in patients with SCI. Respiratory complications are considered to be one of the major causes of mortality in these patients. However, methodology diversity in reporting complications makes interpretation of reported complications difficult. Finally, it should be stated that in spite of increasing numbers of reports from developing countries, there is a persistent lack of evidence, which necessitates further research to elucidate epidemiologic patterns of SCI in these countries.

## SUGGESTED ARTICLES FOR FURTHER READING

- Cripps RA, Lee BB, Wing P, et al. A global map for traumatic spinal cord injury epidemiology: towards a living data repository for injury prevention. Spinal Cord 2011; 49(4):493-501.
- van den Berg ME, Castellote JM, Mahillo-Fernandez I, et al. Incidence of spinal cord injury worldwide: a systematic review. Neuroepidemiology 2010; 34(3):184-92.
- Sekhon LH, Fehlings MG. Epidemiology, demographics, and pathophysiology of acute spinal cord injury. Spine (Phila Pa 1976) 2001; 26(24 Suppl):S2-12.
- Ackery A, Tator C, Krassioukov A. A global perspective on spinal cord injury epidemiology. J Neurotrauma 2004; 21(10):1355-70.
- van den Berg ME, Castellote JM, de Pedro-Cuesta J, et al. Survival after spinal cord injury: a systematic review. *J Neurotrauma* 2010; 27(8):1517-28.
- Parent S, Mac-Thiong JM, Roy-Beaudry M, et al. Spinal cord injury in the pediatric population: a systematic review of the literature. J Neurotrauma 2011; 28(8):1515-24.

## REFERENCES

[1]    Cripps RA, Lee BB, Wing P, Weerts E, Mackay J, Brown D. A global map for traumatic spinal cord injury epidemiology: towards a living data repository for injury prevention. *Spinal Cord.* Apr 2011;49(4):493-501.

[2]    Biering-Sorensen E, Pedersen V, Clausen S. Epidemiology of spinal cord lesions in Denmark. *Paraplegia.* Feb 1990;28(2):105-118.

[3]    Divanoglou A, Levi R. Incidence of traumatic spinal cord injury in Thessaloniki, Greece and Stockholm, Sweden: a prospective population-based study. *Spinal Cord.* Nov 2009;47(11):796-801.

[4]    Koutsodontis I, Lavdaniti M, Sapountzi-Krepia D, et al. A study of the spinal cord injured population of the Chios island of Greece. *Int J Caring Sci.* 2011;4(2):90-96.

[5]    Pedersen V, Muller PG, Biering-Sorensen F. Traumatic spinal cord injuries in Greenland 1965-1986. *Paraplegia.* Oct 1989;27(5):345-349.

[6]    Knutsdottir S. Spinal cord injuries in Iceland 1973-1989. A follow up study. *Paraplegia.* Jan 1993;31(1):68-72.

[7]    O'Connor RJ, Murray PC. Review of spinal cord injuries in Ireland. *Spinal Cord.* Jul 2006;44(7):445-448.

[8]    Jankowski R, Zukiel R, Nowak S, Czekanowska-Szlandrowicz R, stachowska-Tomczak B. Vertebral column and spinal cord injuries: isolated and concomitant with multiple injury. *Chir Narz Ruchu Ortop Pol* 1993;58(5):353-359.

[9]    Kiwerski JE. Factors contributing to the increased threat to life following spinal cord injury. *Paraplegia.* Dec 1993;31(12):793-799.

[10]   Kiwerski JE. Traumatic lesions of the lower cervical spine in Poland. *Eur Spine J.* Jun 1993;2(1):42-45.

[11]   Martins F, Freitas F, Martins L, Dartigues JF, Barat M. Spinal cord injuries--epidemiology in Portugal's central region. *Spinal Cord.* Aug 1998;36(8):574-578.

[12] Soopramanien A. Epidemiology of spinal injuries in Romania. *Paraplegia.* Nov 1994;32(11):715-722.

[13] Fromovich-Amit Y, Biering-Sorensen F, Baskov V, et al. Properties and outcomes of spinal rehabilitation units in four countries. *Spinal Cord.* Aug 2009;47(8):597-603.

[14] Silberstein B, Rabinovich S. Epidemiology of spinal cord injuries in Novosibirsk, Russia. *Paraplegia.* Jun 1995;33(6):322-325.

[15] Kondakov EN, Simonova IA, Poliakov IV. [The epidemiology of injuries to the spine and spinal cord in Saint Petersburg]. *Zh Vopr Neirokhir Im N N Burdenko.* Apr-Jun 2002(2):50-52; discussion 52-53.

[16] Garcia-Reneses J, Herruzo-Cabrera R, Martinez-Moreno M. Epidemiological study of spinal cord injury in Spain 1984-1985. *Paraplegia.* 1991;29:180–190.

[17] Van Den Berg M, Castellote JM, Mahillo-Fernandez I, de Pedro-Cuesta J. Incidence of traumatic spinal cord injury in Aragon, Spain (1972-2008). *J Neurotrauma.* Mar 2011;28(3):469-477.

[18] Gehrig R, Michaelis LS. Statistics of acute paraplegia and tetraplegia on a national scale. Switzerland 1960-67. *Paraplegia.* Aug 1968;6(2):93-95.

[19] Augutis M, Abel R, Levi R. Pediatric spinal cord injury in a subset of European countries. *Spinal Cord.* Feb 2006;44(2):106-112.

[20] Martin BW, Dykes E, Lecky FE. Patterns and risks in spinal trauma. *Arch Dis Child.* Sep 2004;89(9):860-865.

[21] Deconinck H. The health condition of spinal cord injuries in two Afghan towns. *Spinal Cord.* May 2003;41(5):303-309.

[22] Li J, Liu G, Zheng Y, et al. The epidemiological survey of acute traumatic spinal cord injury (ATSCI) of 2002 in Beijing municipality. *Spinal Cord.* Jul 2011;49(7):777-782.

[23] Ning GZ, Yu TQ, Feng SQ, et al. Epidemiology of traumatic spinal cord injury in Tianjin, China. *Spinal Cord.* Mar 2011;49(3):386-390.

[24] Ide M, Ogata H, Tokuhiro A, Takechi H. Spinal cord injuries in Okayama Prefecture: an epidemiological study '88-'89. *J UOEH.* Sep 1 1993;15(3):209-215.

[25] Shingu H, Ohama M, Ikata T, Katoh S, Akatsu T. A nationwide epidemiological survey of spinal cord injuries in Japan from January 1990 to December 1992. *Paraplegia.* Apr 1995;33(4):183-188.

[26] Suyama T, Nihei R, Kimura T, et al. Rehabilitation of spinal cord injury in the national rehabilitation center for the disabled of Japan: profile of a spinal service. *Spinal Cord.* Nov 1997;35(11):720-724.

[27] Otom AS, Doughan AM, Kawar JS, Hattar EZ. Traumatic spinal cord injuries in Jordan--an epidemiological study. *Spinal Cord.* Apr 1997;35(4):253-255.

[28] Raibulet T, et al. Spinal Cord Injury Patients in the Physical Medicine and Rehabilitation Hospital, Kuwait – A Nine-Year Retrospective Study. *Kuwait Medical Journal.* 2001;33(3):211-215.

[29] Mena Quinones PO, Nassal M, Al Bader KI, Al Muraikhi AE, Al Kahlout SR. Traumatic Spinal Cord Injury In Qatar:An Epidemiological Study. *The Middle East Jurnal Of Emergency Medicine.* 2002;2.

[30] Mukhida K, Sharma MR, Shilpakar SK. Pediatric neurotrauma in Kathmandu, Nepal: implications for injury management and control. *Childs Nerv Syst.* Apr 2006;22(4):352-362.

[31] Al-Jadid MS, Al-Asmari AK, Al-Moutaery KR. Quality of life in males with spinal cord injury in Saudi Arabia. *Saudi Med J.* Dec 2004;25(12):1979-1985.

[32] Al-Jadid MS, Al-Asmari AK, Al-Kokani MF, Al-Moutaery KR. Quality of life in females with spinal cord injury in Saudi Arabia. *Saudi Med J.* Sep 2010;31(9):1061-1063.

[33] Don RG, Balachandran N. The pattern of traumatic spinal cord lesions in Singapore--an analysis of 70 patients admitted to the spinal unit, Department of Rehabilitation Medicine, Tan Tock Seng hospital. *Singapore Med J.* Sep 1976;17(3):174-180.

[34] Park CI, Shin JC, Kim SW, Jang SH, Chung WT, Kim HJ. Epidemiologic Study of Spinal Cord Injury. *J Korean Acad Rehabil Med.* 1999 23(2):267-275.

[35] Pajareya K. Traumatic spinal cord injuries in Thailand: an epidemiologic study in Siriraj Hospital, 1989-1994. *Spinal Cord.* Oct 1996;34(10):608-610.

[36] Kovindha A. A retrospective study of spinal cord injuries at Maharaj Nakorn Chiang Mai Hospital, during 1985-1991. *Chiang Mai Med Bull.* 1993;32(2):85-92.

[37] Kuptniratsaikul V. Epidemiology of spinal cord injuries: a study in the Spinal Unit, Siriraj Hospital, Thailand, 1997-2000. *J Med Assoc Thai.* Dec 2003;86(12):1116-1121.

[38] Chen HY, Chen SS, Chiu WT, et al. A nationwide epidemiological study of spinal cord injury in geriatric patients in Taiwan. *Neuroepidemiology.* 1997;16(5):241-247.

[39] Lan C, Lai JS, Chang KH, Jean YC, Lien IN. Traumatic spinal cord injuries in the rural region of Taiwan: an epidemiological study in Hualien county, 1986-1990. *Paraplegia.* Jun 1993;31(6):398-403.

[40] Yang NP, Deng CY, Lee YH, Lin CH, Kao CH, Chou P. The incidence and characterisation of hospitalised acute spinal trauma in Taiwan--a population-based study. *Injury.* Apr 2008;39(4):443-450.

[41] Olasode BJ, Komolafe IE, Komolafe M, Olasode OA. Traumatic spinal cord injuries in Ile-Ife, Nigeria, and its environs. *Trop Doct.* Jul 2006;36(3):181-182.

[42] Udosen A, Ikpeme A, Ngim N. A Prospective Study Of Spinal Cord Injury In The University Of Calabar Teaching Hospital, Calabar, Nigeria. *The Internet Journal of Orthopedic Surgery.* 2007;5.

[43] Velmahos GC, Degiannis E, Hart K, Souter I, Saadia R. Changing profiles in spinal cord injuries and risk factors influencing recovery after penetrating injuries. *J Trauma.* Mar 1995;38(3):334-337.

[44] Hart C, Williams E. Epidemiology of spinal cord injuries: a reflection of changes in South African society. *Paraplegia.* Nov 1994;32(11):709-714.

[45] Gosselin RA, Coppotelli C. A follow-up study of patients with spinal cord injury in Sierra Leone. *Int Orthop.* Oct 2005;29(5):330-332.

[46] Levy LF, Makarawo S, Madzivire D, Bhebhe E, Verbeek N, Parry O. Problems, struggles and some success with spinal cord injury in Zimbabwe. *Spinal Cord.* Mar 1998;36(3):213-218.

[47] Burns AS, O'Connell C, Landry MD. Spinal cord injury in postearthquake Haiti: lessons learned and future needs. *PM R.* Aug 2010;2(8):695-697.

[48] O'Connor P. Incidence and patterns of spinal cord injury in Australia. *Accid Anal Prev.* Jul 2002;34(4):405-415.

[49] Walsh J. Costs of spinal cord injury in Australia. *Paraplegia.* Dec 1988;26(6):380-388.

[50] O'Connor PJ. Prevalence of spinal cord injury in Australia. *Spinal Cord.* Jan 2005;43(1):42-46.

[51]  Yeo JD, Walsh J, Rutkowski S, Soden R, Craven M, Middleton J. Mortality following spinal cord injury. *Spinal Cord.* May 1998;36(5):329-336.

[52]  Bilston LE, Brown J. Pediatric spinal injury type and severity are age and mechanism dependent. *Spine (Phila Pa 1976).* Oct 1 2007;32(21):2339-2347.

[53]  Sullivan M, Paul CE, Herbison GP, Tamou P, Derrett S, Crawford M. A longitudinal study of the life histories of people with spinal cord injury. *Inj Prev.* Dec 2010;16(6):e3.

[54]  Dixon GS, Danesh JN, Caradoc-Davies TH. Epidemiology of spinal cord injury in New Zealand. *Neuroepidemiology.* 1993;12(2):88-95.

[55]  Maharaj JC. Epidemiology of spinal cord paralysis in Fiji: 1985-1994. *Spinal Cord.* Sep 1996;34(9):549-559.

[56]  van den Berg ME, Castellote JM, de Pedro-Cuesta J, Mahillo-Fernandez I. Survival after spinal cord injury: a systematic review. *J Neurotrauma.* Aug 2010;27(8):1517-1528.

[57]  Parent S, Mac-Thiong JM, Roy-Beaudry M, Sosa JF, Labelle H. Spinal cord injury in the pediatric population: a systematic review of the literature. *J Neurotrauma.* Aug 2011;28(8):1515-1524.

[58]  Patel JC, Tepas JJ, 3rd, Mollitt DL, Pieper P. Pediatric cervical spine injuries: defining the disease. *J Pediatr Surg.* Feb 2001;36(2):373-376.

[59]  Apple DF, Jr., Anson CA, Hunter JD, Bell RB. Spinal cord injury in youth. *Clin Pediatr (Phila).* Feb 1995;34(2):90-95.

[60]  Brown RL, Brunn MA, Garcia VF. Cervical spine injuries in children: a review of 103 patients treated consecutively at a level 1 pediatric trauma center. *J Pediatr Surg.* Aug 2001;36(8):1107-1114.

[61]  Cirak B, Ziegfeld S, Knight VM, Chang D, Avellino AM, Paidas CN. Spinal injuries in children. *J Pediatr Surg.* Apr 2004;39(4):607-612.

# INDEX

# C

# F

# G

**Q**

**R**

# S

## T

## U